BIPOLAR DISORDER IN CHILDHOOD AND EARLY ADOLESCENCE

Bipolar Disorder in Childhood and Early Adolescence

Edited by
BARBARA GELLER
MELISSA P. DELBELLO

THE GUILFORD PRESS
New York   London

© 2003 The Guilford Press
A Division of Guilford Publications, Inc.
72 Spring Street, New York, NY 10012
www.guilford.com

Printed in the United States of America

This book is printed on acid-free paper.

Last digit is print number: 9   8   7   6   5   4   3   2

Library of Congress Cataloging-in-Publication Data

Bipolar disorder in childhood and early adolescence / edited by Barbara
Geller and Melissa P. DelBello.
        p.   cm.
    Includes bibliographical references and index.
    ISBN 1-57230-837-0
    1. Manic–depressive illness in children. 2. Manic–depressive illness
in adolescence. I. Geller, Barbara. II. DelBello, Melissa P.
RJ506.D4 B575 2003
618.92′895—dc21
                                                        2002010222

About the Editors

Barbara Geller, MD, is a Professor of Psychiatry at Washington University in St. Louis, Missouri, and is an internationally recognized researcher for her groundbreaking work on prepubertal and early adolescent bipolar disorders. She is Principal Investigator on multiple National Institute of Mental Health-funded grant awards and has published over 100 articles on childhood manic–depression. Dr. Geller has served on numerous federal advisory committees and editorial boards. She is a recipient of, among other awards, the American Academy of Child and Adolescent Psychiatry Nathan Cummings Special Research Award and the National Alliance for the Mentally Ill Exemplary Psychiatrist Award.

Melissa P. DelBello, MD, is an Assistant Professor of Psychiatry and Pediatrics at the University of Cincinnati College of Medicine and Associate Director of the Bipolar and Psychotic Disorders Research Program. She is also Codirector of the Mood Disorders Clinic at Cincinnati Children's Hospital Medical Center. Dr. DelBello's primary research interests include the neurodevelopment and neuropsychopharmacology of pediatric bipolar disorder.

Contributors

David Axelson, MD, Western Psychiatric Institute and Clinic, University of Pittsburgh, Pittsburgh, Pennsylvania

Judith A. Badner, MD, PhD, Department of Psychiatry, University of Chicago, Chicago, Illinois

Linda Beringer, RN, Department of Psychiatry, Washington University School of Medicine, St. Louis, Missouri

Robinder K. Bhangoo, MD, National Institute of Mental Health, Bethesda, Maryland

Kristine Bolhofner, BS, Department of Psychiatry, Washington University School of Medicine, St. Louis, Missouri

Kiki Chang, MD, Division of Child Psychiatry and Development, Department of Psychiatry and Behavioral Sciences, Stanford University, Stanford, California

James L. Craney, MS, MPH, JD, Department of Psychiatry, Washington University School of Medicine, St. Louis, Missouri

Sandra DeJong, MD, Department of Psychiatry, McLean Hospital, Belmont, Massachusetts

Melissa P. DelBello, MD, Department of Psychiatry, University of Cincinnati, Cincinnati, Ohio

Christen M. Deveney, AB, Department of Psychology, Harvard University, Cambridge, Massachusetts

Nuri B. Farber, MD, Department of Psychiatry, Washington University School of Medicine, St. Louis, Missouri

Jean A. Frazier, MD, Department of Psychiatry, McLean Hospital, Belmont, Massachusetts

Jeanne Frazier, BSN, Department of Psychiatry, Washington University School of Medicine, St. Louis, Missouri

Mary A. Fristad, PhD, ABPP, Division of Child and Adolescent Psychiatry, Ohio State University, Columbus, Ohio

Barbara Geller, MD, Department of Psychiatry, Washington University School of Medicine, St. Louis, Missouri

Jill S. Goldberg-Arnold, PhD, Division of Child and Adolescent Psychiatry, Ohio State University, Columbus, Ohio

Martha Hellander, JD, Child and Adolescent Bipolar Foundation, Wilmette, Illinois

Daniel N. Klein, PhD, Department of Psychology, State University of New York at Stony Brook, Stony Brook, New York

Robert A. Kowatch, MD, Department of Psychiatry, University of Cincinnati, Cincinnati, Ohio

Ellen Leibenluft, MD, National Institute of Mental Health, Bethesda, Maryland

Peter M. Lewinsohn, PhD, Oregon Research Institute, Eugene, Oregon

Joan Luby, MD, Department of Psychiatry, Washington University School of Medicine, St. Louis, Missouri

Tanya K. Murphy, MD, McKnight Brain Institute, University of Florida, Gainesville, Florida

John W. Newcomer, MD, Department of Psychiatry, Washington University School of Medicine, St. Louis, Missouri

Michael J. Nickelsburg, PhD, Department of Psychiatry, Washington University School of Medicine, St. Louis, Missouri

Demitri F. Papolos, MD, Behavioral Genetics Program, Albert Einstein College of Medicine, Bronx, New York; Juvenile Bipolar Research Foundation, Pawling, New York; and private practice, New York, New York, and Westport, Connecticut

Uma Rao, MD, UCLA Neuropsychiatric Institute, Los Angeles, California

Neal D. Ryan, MD, Western Psychiatric Institute and Clinic, University of Pittsburgh, Pittsburgh, Pennsylvania

John R. Seeley, MS, Oregon Research Institute, Eugene, Oregon

Dory P. Sisson, MA, Division of Child and Adolescent Psychiatry, Ohio State University, Columbus, Ohio

Ohel Soto, MD, McKnight Brain Institute, University of Florida, Gainesville, Florida

Hans Steiner, MD, Department of Child Psychiatry, Stanford University, Stanford, California

Marlene Williams, RN, Department of Psychiatry, Washington University School of Medicine, St. Louis, Missouri

Betsy Zimerman, BSN, MA, Department of Psychiatry, Washington University School of Medicine, St. Louis, Missouri

Contents

Introduction   1
     Melissa P. DelBello, David Axelson, and Barbara Geller

1   Bipolar Disorder in Adolescents: 7
     Epidemiology and Suicidal Behavior
     Peter M. Lewinsohn, John R. Seeley, and Daniel N. Klein

2   Phenomenology and Longitudinal Course of Children   25
     with a Prepubertal and Early Adolescent Bipolar
     Disorder Phenotype
     Barbara Geller, James L. Craney, Kristine Bolhofner,
     Melissa P. DelBello, David Axelson, Joan Luby,
     Marlene Williams, Betsy Zimerman, Michael J. Nickelsburg,
     Jeanne Frazier, and Linda Beringer

3   Bipolar Disorder in Children with Pervasive   51
     Developmental Disorders
     Sandra DeJong and Jean A. Frazier

4   Bipolar Disorder and Comorbid Disorders: 76
     The Case for a Dimensional Nosology
     Demitri F. Papolos

5   Offspring Studies in Child and Early Adolescent   107
     Bipolar Disorder
     Kiki Chang and Hans Steiner

6   The Role of NMDA Receptor Hypofunction in   130
     Idiopathic Psychotic Disorders
     Nuri B. Farber and John W. Newcomer

 7 Neuroimaging in Pediatric Bipolar Disorder   158
     Melissa P. DelBello and Robert A. Kowatch

 8 Affective Neuroscience and the Pathophysiology   175
     of Bipolar Disorder
     Robinder K. Bhangoo, Christen M. Deveney,
     and Ellen Leibenluft

 9 The Immune System and Bipolar Affective Disorder   193
     Ohel Soto and Tanya K. Murphy

10 Sleep and Other Biological Rhythms   215
     Uma Rao

11 The Genetics of Bipolar Disorder   247
     Judith A. Badner

12 The Pharmacological Treatment of Child and Adolescent   255
     Bipolar Disorder
     Neal D. Ryan

13 Psychotherapy for Children with Bipolar Disorder   272
     Jill S. Goldberg-Arnold and Mary A. Fristad

14 Family Interventions for Early-Onset Bipolar Disorder   295
     Mary A. Fristad and Jill S. Goldberg-Arnold

15 Internet Support for Parents of Children   314
     with Early-Onset Bipolar Disorder
     Martha Hellander, Dory P. Sisson, and Mary A. Fristad

    Index   331

Introduction

MELISSA P. DELBELLO, DAVID AXELSON, and BARBARA GELLER

CONTROVERSIES AND NEW DIRECTIONS

Although the existence and diagnostic boundary of childhood bipolar disorder has been the focus of substantial controversy (see Chapter 2, this volume), there is evidence of a progressively growing consensus on both the existence of child mania and on the vicissitudes of age-specific research in this area (National Institute of Mental Health Research Roundtable on Prepubertal Bipolar Disorder, 2001; hereafter cited as NIMH Roundtable, 2001). The growing interest in this area has been demonstrated by the increasing number of federally funded projects on bipolar disorder in children and by the diverse areas these projects cover, including phenomenology, natural history, family studies, offspring, epidemiology, neuroimaging, treatment, and preclinical studies, as outlined in the NIMH Roundtable (2001). This book attempts to provide state-of-the-art understanding in the domains of epidemiology, diagnosis and natural history, neurobiology and genetics, and treatment.

WHY CONCEPTUALIZE CHILD AND EARLY ADOLESCENT BIPOLAR DISORDER?

As noted in the NIMH Roundtable (2001), regardless of the phenotype (conservative DSM-IV vs. broadly defined bipolar disorder not otherwise specified), there is agreement that prepubertal bipolar disorder is a chronic, mixed manic, continuously cycling disorder. Furthermore, the diagnostic and natural history similarity of prepubertal bipolar disorder to early adolescent bipolar disorder has been reported by Geller and colleagues (see

1

Chapter 2, this volume). In addition, many experts in the field view late-adolescent-onset bipolar disorder as phenomenologically similar to adult-onset bipolar disorder. In this regard, the NIMH-funded multisite study of the treatment of late-teenage-onset and adult-onset bipolar disorder, Systematic Treatment Enhancement of Bipolar Disorder (STEP-BP) includes subjects from age 15. Therefore, there is a growing consensus that prepubertal and early adolescent bipolar disorder share similar characteristics.

ORGANIZATION OF THIS BOOK

The chapters comprising this book can be divided into three sections. The first section focuses on the *diagnosis, natural history, and longitudinal course* of childhood and early adolescent bipolar disorder. In Chapter 1, Lewinsohn, Seeley, and Klein discuss their findings regarding the epidemiology, clinical characteristics, and outcome of syndromal and subsyndromal adolescent bipolar disorder. They also review their studies of the family history of psychopathology in probands with adolescent bipolar disorder. Their studies provide important insights into the risk of suicidality in early-onset bipolar disorder and the poor outcome associated with subsyndromal bipolar disorder in adolescents. Geller and colleagues, in Chapter 2, review their pioneering research examining the clinical characteristics and outcome of a prepubertal and early adolescent bipolar disorder (PEA-BP) cohort. One of the primary questions confronting the field in the early 1990s was whether children with mania were just children with "severe attention-deficit/hyperactivity disorder." Geller and colleagues compared their well-characterized PEA-BP cohort with a group of children with attention-deficit/hyperactivity disorder. The results of this study, which enlightened the field as to the differences in clinical characteristics between these populations, are described in Chapter 2. Additionally, they review the development of their Washington University in St. Louis Kiddie Schedule for Affective Disorders and Schizophrenia (WASH-U-KSADS), a modified version of the K-SADS, designed to elicit age-specific diagnostic criteria for mania. The WASH-U-KSADS is now the most widely used diagnostic assessment instrument for pediatric bipolar research. Finally, Chapter 2 addresses the prognosis and outcome of these children and raises questions for future research.

In Chapter 3, DeJong and Frazier review the relationships among early-onset bipolar disorder and the pervasive developmental disorders. Specifically, they review the phenomenological characteristics, genetics, and pharmacological treatments for children and adolescents with co-occurring pervasive developmental disorders and early-onset bipolar disorder. Finally, DeJong and Frazier describe several illustrative cases that emphasize the importance of identifying the presence of a mood disorder in a child with a pervasive developmental disorder. In Chapter 4, Papolos reviews the common comorbidities associated with early-onset bipolar disorder. Several possible explanations for the high co-occurrence between early-onset bipolar disorder and attention-deficit/hyperactivity disorder, disruptive behavior disorders, anxiety disorders, and substance use disorders are discussed. Additionally, Chapter 4 describes the methodological complications of studying comorbidities in pediatric bipolar disorder and Papolos suggests several ways in which this field can move forward. In the final chapter of this section, Chapter 5, Chang and Steiner review research involving children and adolescents of parents with bipolar disorder. This population provides an important opportunity for investigating the prodromal manifestations of early-onset bipolar disorder. Chang and Steiner provide an overview of the significance of bipolar offspring studies, discuss the methodological difficulties in studying bipolar offspring, summarize the results of bipolar offspring studies completed to date, and suggest future directions for this field of study. They also address the importance of identifying psychological and biological markers for illness development. Finally, the authors discuss preliminary results from two targeted early intervention studies.

The second section of this book focuses on the *neurobiology and genetics* of early-onset bipolar disorder. Although this field is in its infancy, this section provides important insights into innovative research that, in the near future, may clarify the biological basis of early-onset bipolar disorder. In Chapter 6, Farber and Newcomer examine the effects of N-methyl-D-Aspartate (NMDA) receptors and consider the possible role of NMDA receptor hypofunctioning in the pathophysiology of idiopathic psychotic disorders, paying particular attention to the relationship between brain maturation and development and NMDA receptor hypofunctioning. The authors propose that NMDA hypofunctioning may result in chronic severe symptoms complicated by ongoing structural brain changes and clinical deterioration. Finally, the authors discuss the implications of certain protective drugs that arrest the neurotoxicity associated with NMDA hypofunction, including olanzapine, clozapine, lamotrigine, α_2-adrenergic agonists, and perhaps antimuscarinic agents. In Chapter 7, DelBello and Kowatch examine novel neuroimaging techniques and their potential utility for investigating the neurophysiological basis of early-onset bipolar disorder. The authors also review the literature of neurostructural and neurofunctional abnormalities in children, adolescents, and adults with bipolar disorder and suggest that frontal-subcortical abnormalities may be present in children and adolescents with bipolar disorder. In Chapter 8, Bhangoo, Deveney, and Leibenluft examine the neural components of emotional processes and discuss how relevant concepts of affective neuroscience can be applied to childhood bipolar disorder. The authors also discuss methods that can be used to study theories of emotion and mood, focusing on the psychophysiological correlates of emotion that are particularly relevant to the study of early-onset bipolar disorder. In Chapter 9, Soto and Murphy use the example of PANDAS (pediatric autoimmune neuropsychiatric disorders associated with streptococcus) to describe a model for childhood neuropsychiatric illnesses with an immune system etiology. The authors also examine the role of novel therapeutic agents if the presence of an immune-mediate pathophysiology is determined for pediatric bipolar disorder and suggest directions for future research in this area. In Chapter 10, Rao discusses the relationship between circadian dysregulation and bipolar disorder and the hypothesized mechanisms that underlie these disturbances. Sleep studies provide one method for studying these disturbances. In this chapter, EEG sleep changes in unipolar and bipolar disorders are summarized, and hypothesized mechanisms for these EEG sleep changes are proposed. Finally, future areas of sleep research in pediatric bipolar disorder are suggested. In the final chapter of this section, Chapter 11, Badner reviews family, twin, and adoption studies involving bipolar probands and concludes that there is strong evidence for a genetic basis for bipolar disorder. Furthermore, the data reviewed suggest that childhood-onset affective disorders share familial factors in common with adult-onset affective disorder and do not represent an etiologically distinct group.

The third and final section of this book focuses on treatment and other aspects of support that may be provided to children and adolescents with bipolar disorder and their families. In the first chapter of this section, Chapter 12, Ryan summarizes pharmacological treatment options for this population and studies supporting their use. There is a paucity of controlled pharmacological data for children and adolescents with bipolar disorder. Future controlled trials are needed to investigate the efficacy of lithium, antiepileptic agents, and atypical antipsychotics in this population, as well as treatment options for children and adolescents with bipolar disorder and co-occurring disorders.

Chapter 13 emphasizes the importance of psychosocial treatments for children and adolescents with bipolar disorder. Specifically, in this chapter Goldberg-Arnold and Fristad describe the development of and preliminary results from a child group therapy program, developed as part of a multifamily psychoeducation program for families of preadolescent children with bipolar disorder. In Chapter 14, Fristad and Goldberg-Arnold raise the important issue of including the entire family in the treatment of patients with early-onset bipolar disorder. They outline several specific and practical family intervention strategies for helping families cope with a child with bipolar disorder. In the final chapter of this section and of the book, Hellander, Sisson, and Fristad review the literature on caregiver burden and how various forms of support can help families of children with bipolar disorder. They also provide a unique perspective on the development of a Internet-based support group for families of bipolar children, the

Child & Adolescent Bipolar Foundation, which was founded in 1999 by parents who met in early online support groups. The authors also focus on the Internet as an emerging medium for providing support services and describe the Internet's potential to create and sustain a supportive community for families raising children diagnosed with, or at risk for, bipolar disorder.

REFERENCE

National Institute of Mental Health Research Roundtable on Prepubertal Bipolar Disorder. (2001). *Journal of the American Academy of Child and Adolescent Psychiatry, 40*, 871–878.

1

Bipolar Disorder in Adolescents
Epidemiology and Suicidal Behavior

PETER M. LEWINSOHN, JOHN R. SEELEY, and DANIEL N. KLEIN

It is currently accepted that the classical form of bipolar disorder (Krae-pelin, 1921) can be manifested in children and adolescents. There is also consensus that with relatively minor modifications, the DSM-III-R and DSM-IV (American Psychiatric Association, 1987, 1994) criteria for bipolar disorder can be used with children and adolescents. Recent studies of the epidemiology of bipolar disorder in adults (Angst, 1988; Kessler, Rubinow, Holmes, Abelson, & Zhao, 1997) have indicated that the lifetime prevalence of bipolar disorder ranges from 3% to 6% across a variety of countries and cultures (Weissman et al., 1996). While data on the prevalence of bipolar disorders in community samples of older adolescents are limited, our study, the Oregon Adolescent Depression Project (OADP; Lewinsohn, Klein, & Seeley, 1995), suggests that the lifetime prevalence of bipolar disorders (primarily bipolar II and cyclothymia) is approximately 1%. An additional 5.7% of the sample reported having experienced the core manic symptom—that is, a distinct period of abnormally and persistently elevated, expansive, or irritable mood—even though they never met criteria for bipolar disorder. Lifetime prevalence of subsyndromal bipolar disorder, defined as manifesting the manic core symptom plus one other DSM-III-R manic symptom, but never having met criteria for a bipolar disorder mood disorder, was approximately 5%. While there are no community data on the prevalence of what has been called *prepubertal, juvenile,* and *pediatric bipolar disorder,* it may be relatively common in clinically referred children (Wozniak ct al., 1995).

The manifestations of childhood and adolescent mania and hypomania differ somewhat from those in adulthood. For example, the symptoms

7

of grandiosity and excessive involvement in pleasurable activities can vary as a function of age and developmental level (Bowring & Kovacs, 1992; Geller & Luby, 1997). In addition, juvenile bipolar disorder is typically characterized by high rates of rapid cycling (e.g., > 365 cycles per year) and very high rates of comorbidity with attention-deficit/hyperactivity disorder (Geller et al., 2000) and conduct disorder (Biederman et al., 1997). In addition, prepubertal bipolar disorder differs from adolescent bipolar disorder in showing nonclassical presentations such as dysphoric mania, irritability, aggressiveness, and the absence of clear-cut episodes that follow good premorbid adjustment. Juvenile bipolar disorder appears to be a much more chronic condition that has a very early onset age (Carlson, 1995). These patients are severely impaired, showing a great deal of emotional lability and impulsivity. According to Geller and colleagues (2001) the most prevalent pattern for juvenile bipolar disorder is to be ill for over 3 years during which time there are multiple episodes on a daily basis. It is important to ascertain whether the juvenile and the classical forms of manic disorder (Kraepelin, 1921) are manifestations of the same disorder or not (Biederman, 1998; Carlson, 1995, 1998).

While one of the most firmly established facts in the literature (Guze & Robins, 1970; Jamison, 1986; Robins, Murphy, Wilkinson, Gassner, & Kayes, 1959) is that adults with bipolar disorder are at very high risk for suicidal behaviors (studies report a suicide completion rate ranging from 12% to 50%), and an attempt rate from 25% to 50%, knowledge about the suicide attempt and completion rates among adolescent patients with bipolar disorder is relatively sparse (Brent et al., 1988; Kovacs, 1991; Kutcher, Robertson, & Bird, 1998; Shaffer, 1985).

In this chapter, we summarize findings from the OADP regarding (1) epidemiology and clinical characteristics of full-syndrome and subsyndromal bipolar disorder; (2) associations between suicidal behavior and bipolar disorder; (3) young adult course and outcome of adolescent bipolar disorder; (4) psychometric characteristics and predictive ability of two hypomania scales; and (5) family history of psychopathology in probands with bipolar disorder. Finally, we discuss the clinical implications of our findings and point to future directions for research in this area.

THE OREGON ADOLESCENT DEPRESSION PROJECT

The OADP is an epidemiological, family history, and follow-up study of a large cohort of community adolescents (Lewinsohn, Hops, Roberts, Seeley, & Andrews, 1993). The initial (T_1) OADP sample consisted of a randomly selected group of 1,709 high school students who were administered semistructured diagnostic interviews and completed a comprehensive battery of inventories. Approximately 1 year later (T_2), 1,507 of the adolescents were reevaluated with the same measures. At age 24 (T_3), participants with a history of major depressive disorder or nonmood disorders and a randomly selected subset of adolescents with no psychiatric diagnosis through T_2 were evaluated for a third assessment (T_3), again using semistructured diagnostic interviews (Lewinsohn, Rohde, Klein, & Seeley, 1999; Lewinsohn, Rohde, Seeley, Klein, & Gotlib, 2000). In addition, we attempted to interview all of the first-degree relatives of the probands selected to participate at T_3 about their own history of psychopathology. Direct interviews with relatives were supplemented with family history information about all relatives from the proband and family history information from a second family member for relatives who could not be interviewed (Klein, Lewinsohn, Seeley, & Rohde, 2001). Some of the results on bipolar disorder and subsyndromal bipolar disorder have been reported in greater detail in previous papers (Klein, Lewinsohn, & Seeley, 1996; Lewinsohn et al., 1995; Lewinsohn, Klein, & Seeley, 2000).

With regard to the distinction we made earlier between prepubertal and adolescent bipolar disorder, it is of interest to note that (1) review of the writeups for all of our bipolar disorder cases by our diagnostic interviewers did not reveal a single case of rapid cycling as defined by Geller and colleagues (1998); and (2) there were only three cases with an onset age less than 10. The low number of cases with prepubertal bipolar disorder may be attributable to our sample selection—that is, very few adolescents with prepubertal bipolar disorder may attend public high schools.

Another possible reason for the low number of prepubertal bipolar disorder cases, most of which have ultradian cycling (multiple cycles per day; ≥ 365 cycles/year; Geller et al., 2000), is that the version of the K-SADS (Chambers et al., 1985) that we used did not include items to detect ultradian cycling.

INCIDENCE AND PREVALENCE

The weighted first incidence of bipolar disorder through age 18 was 1.4%; from ages 19 to 23, it was 0.7%. Of the 18 cases of bipolar disorder identified in the T_1 and T_2 evaluations, two met criteria for bipolar disorder, 11 met criteria for bipolar II disorder, and five met criteria for cyclothymia. These rates are comparable to those in Carlson and Kashani's (1988) study of adolescents, and more recent community studies of bipolar disorder in adults (Kessler et al., 1997; Weissman et al., 1996).

We also examined the rates of subsyndromal bipolar disorder. The weighted lifetime prevalence of subsyndromal bipolar disorder through age 18 was 4.5%. This is roughly comparable to the rate reported in Angst's (1998) community sample of subthreshold groups. Interestingly, the rate of new cases of subsyndromal bipolar disorder in our sample decreased after age 18, as the weighted first incidence from ages 19 to 23 was only 0.9%.

The point prevalence of bipolar disorder was 0.6%, 0.5%, and 0.7% at T_1, T_2, and T_3, respectively. The point prevalence of subsyndromal bipolar disorder was 1.2%, 0.3%, and 0.0% at T_1, T_2, and T_3, respectively, again indicating that the rate of subsyndromal bipolar disorder diminishes as participants approach and enter adulthood.

There were six new cases of bipolar disorder from ages 19 to 23. Three of these cases had a history of major depressive disorder prior to age 19. However, they comprised only 1% of the adolescents with major depressive disorder in our sample, which is a lower "switch" rate than in most previous studies of major depressive disorder, which have all used clinical samples. Geller, Fox, and Clark (1994) found a rate of 32%, and Strober, Lampert, Schmidt, and Morrell (1993) found a rate of 20%. Major depressive disorder before age 19 did not significantly predict the onset of bipolar disorder during the age 19 to 23 period.

DEMOGRAPHIC CORRELATES, CLINICAL CHARACTERISTICS, AND COMORBIDITY

Adolescents with bipolar and subsyndromal bipolar disorder did not differ from adolescents with no history of mental illness on sex, age, race, or parental education. However, adolescents with bipolar disorder were significantly less likely to be living with both biological parents than adolescents with no history of mental illness.

The mean age of onset of the first affective episode for the 18 bipolar cases through T_2 was 11.8 years (range = 7–15). In the majority of cases, the first episode was depressed rather than manic. The median duration of the most recent episode was 10.8 months.

With respect to impaired role functioning, a substantial portion of adolescents with bipolar disorder exhibited impairment in social (66.7%), family (55.6%), and especially school (83.3%) functioning. Although to a lesser degree, adolescents with subsyndromal bipolar disorder also exhibited impairment in social (48.5%), family (53.6%), and school (52.6%) functioning.

While adolescents with subsyndromal bipolar disorder had fewer manic symptoms (they averaged 2.9 associated manic symptoms) than adolescents with bipolar disorder, the relative frequency of symptoms was similar in both groups, with a Spearman correlation of .74. In addition, the majority of adolescents with subsyndromal bipolar disorder had a history of major depressive disorder (48.5%) and/or dysthymia (12.4%).

Adolescents with bipolar disorder and subsyndromal bipolar disorder had high rates of comorbidity. Both groups had high lifetime rates of anxiety (32.0% and 33.3%, vs. 7.7% for the controls) and disruptive behavior disorders (18.6% and 22.2%, vs. 6.9% for the controls). In addition, adolescents with bipolar disorder and subsyndromal bipolar disorder had significantly elevated rates of substance use (22.2% and 23.7%, vs. 10.4% for the controls). It is important to note that while comorbidities with attention-deficit/hyperactivity disorder (8.2% and 11.1%, vs. 2.7%) and conduct disorder (8.2% and 3.0%, vs. 3.0%) are significantly elevated, they are substantially below those reported by Biederman and colleagues (1997) and Geller and colleagues (2000) for prepubertal cases of bipolar disorder.

Current functioning, as assessed by the DSM-III-R Axis V Global Assessment of Functioning (GAF) scale, was significantly poorer among adolescents with bipolar disorder than among those with subsyndromal bipolar disorder. In addition, both of these groups of adolescents with bipolar conditions exhibited significantly lower functioning on the GAF than adolescents with no history of mental illness and adolescents with a history of major depressive disorder. As these differences may have been due to the presence of comorbid conditions, we identified a subgroup of adolescents with subsyndromal bipolar disorder but no history of any mental disorder. This subgroup did not differ from adolescents with no history of mental illness on the GAF.

SUICIDAL BEHAVIOR

To examine the association between bipolar disorder and suicidal behavior, four groups were defined based on lifetime history of psychopathology through age 18 years: (1) bipolar disorder (n = 18), (2) subsyndromal bipolar disorder (n = 51), (3) major depressive disorder without bipolar disorder or subsyndromal bipolar disorder (n = 294), and (4) no mental disorder (n = 323). Suicidal behavior also was based on lifetime history through age 18 years via the T_1–T_3 K-SADS interview which included suicide attempt and suicidal ideation. For those who attempted suicide, group comparisons were conducted on age of first attempt, percentage with multiple attempts, suicidal intent, and medical lethality. Suicide intent was rated by the diagnostic interviewer on a 6-point scale from "no intent" to "extreme intent." Medical lethality was rated on an 11-point scale from "death was improbable" to "death was highly probable." The following planned contrasts were conducted: (1) the bipolar disorder group was compared to the no disorder, subsyndromal bipolar disorder, and major depressive disorder groups; and (2) the subsyndromal bipolar disorder group was compared to the no disorder and major depressive disorder groups.

Diagnostic group differences on the suicidal behavior measures are presented in Table 1.1.

With respect to a history of suicide attempt, the bipolar disorder group was significantly elevated (44.4%) compared to the other three groups; the subsyndromal bipolar disorder group was significantly elevated (17.6%) compared to the no disorder group (1.2%), but did not differ from the major depressive disorder group (21.8%). The bipolar disorder group was elevated also on suicide ideation compared to the no disorder and subsyndromal bipolar disorder groups, but did not differ from the major depressive disorder group; the subsyndromal bipolar disorder group was elevated only compared to the no disorder group. Concerning suicide attempt characteristics, the bipolar disorder group had a younger age of first attempt and a higher percentage of multiple attempts compared to the major depressive disorder and subsyndromal bipolar disorder groups. In addition, the bipolar disorder group had more serious suicide attempts based on the medical lethality ratings compared to the other groups. None of the above-mentioned associations were moderated by gender.

In sum, the bipolar disorder group had a greater degree of suicidal behavior compared to their major depressive disorder counterparts and compared to the subsyndromal bipolar disorder and no disorder groups. Furthermore, the subsyndromal bipolar disorder group had elevated lifetime attempts and ideation compared to the no disorder group. However, the elevation of suicide attempts and ideation in the subsyndromal bipolar disorder group could have been confounded by the above-mentioned high degree of comorbidity with other psychopathology. After removing the

TABLE 1.1. Characteristics of Suicidal Behavior by Diagnostic Group (Lifetime through Age 18 Years)

Variable	Diagnostic group				Planned contrasts	
	ND (n = 323)	MDD (n = 294)	SUB (n = 51)	BD (n = 18)	BD	SUB
Suicide attempt % (n)	1.2 (4)	21.8 (64)	17.6 (9)	44.4 (8)	ND, MDD, SUB	ND
Suicide ideation % (n)	5.9 (19)	52.4 (154)	41.2 (21)	72.2 (13)	ND, SUB	ND
Attempt characteristics						
Age of first attempt M (SD)	13.8 (2.6)	14.9 (1.8)	15.3 (1.0)	13.3 (3.3)	MDD, SUB	
Multiple attempts % (n)	50.0 (2)	51.6 (33)	22.2 (2)	87.5 (7)	MDD, SUB	
Intent scale M (SD)	2.5 (0.6)	2.8 (1.7)	3.0 (0.9)	3.0 (1.9)		
Medical lethality M (SD)	1.3 (1.0)	2.2 (2.3)	1.7 (1.7)	4.3 (3.4)	ND, MDD, SUB	

Note. ND, no disorder; MDD, major depressive disorder; SUB, subsyndromal bipolar disorder; BD, bipolar disorder. Diagnostic groups listed in the BD and SUB planned contrasts column indicate a significant difference at $p < .05$; differences between BD and SUB only appear in the BD column.

participants with comorbid subsyndromal bipolar disorder from the comparison, a significant elevation compared to the no disorder group remained for suicide attempts (12.5% vs. 1.2%), but not for suicidal ideation (12.5% vs. 5.9%).

YOUNG ADULT COURSE AND OUTCOME

Some of the adolescents who developed bipolar disorder prior to age 19 experienced a chronic/recurrent course; 35% had not remitted by age 19 and 12% had not remitted by age 24. Of those who were in remission at age 18, 27% had another episode between the ages of 19 and 24.

In order to examine the diagnostic stability of adolescent bipolar disorder in young adulthood, we compared the rates of disorders from ages 19 to 23 between adolescents with bipolar disorder, with subsyndromal bipolar disorder, with major depressive disorder, with disruptive behavior disorder, and with no mental disorder (see Lewinsohn, Klein, & Seeley, 2000, for more detail). Adolescents with bipolar disorder had a significantly higher rate of bipolar disorder in young adulthood (27.3%) than adolescents with subsyndromal bipolar disorder (2.1%), major depressive disorder (0.7%), disruptive behavior disorder (0.0%), and no history of psychopathology (0.3%). Adolescents with subsyndromal bipolar disorder experienced significantly higher rates of major depressive disorder (40.9%) and anxiety disorders (13.3%) than adolescents with no history of mental illness (18.9% and 2.3%, respectively). The groups did not differ on rates of alcohol and/or drug use disorders in young adulthood. The subgroup of adolescents with subsyndromal bipolar disorder and no lifetime history of major depressive disorder through age 18 had a significantly higher rate of first-incidence major depressive disorder during young adulthood (39.3%) than adolescents with no history of psychopathology (18.9%). Thus, it appears that even in the absence of major depressive disorder, subsyndromal bipolar disorder symptoms in adolescence are a significant risk factor for the subsequent development of a major mood disorder.

Bipolar disorder and subsyndromal bipolar disorder in adolescence also presaged significant functional impairment in young adulthood (see Table 1.2). Compared to adolescents with no history of mental illness prior to age 19, adolescents with bipolar disorder obtained significantly higher scores on a composite measure of psychosocial impairment, exhibited significantly poorer functioning on the GAF, and had significantly greater mental health treatment utilization in young adulthood. Adolescents with subsyndromal bipolar disorder also exhibited significantly greater psychosocial impairment, poorer functioning on the GAF, and greater mental health treatment utilization, and were significantly less likely to graduate from college than never mentally ill adolescents.

TABLE 1.2. Young Adulthood Functioning (Age 24) by Adolescent Diagnostic Group (Age 0–18)

Functioning measure	Diagnostic group 0–18					Planned contrasts	
	BD ($n = 17$)	SUB ($n = 48$)	MDD ($n = 275$)	DBD ($n = 49$)	ND ($n = 307$)	BD	SUB
Psychosocial impairment (M, SD)	0.27 (0.90)	0.20 (0.96)	0.25 (1.04)	0.05 (0.99)	−0.32 (0.91)	ND*	ND***
GAF (M, SD)	75.6 (9.59)	78.5 (9.0)	76.1 (10.1)	77.6 (7.9)	81.9 (7.6)	ND**	ND*
Mental health treatment utilization (%)	41.2	27.1	28.0	20.4	9.1	ND***	ND***
Suicide attempt	5.9	6.3	5.5	4.1	1.6		
Years of education (M, SD)	13.8 (2.2)	13.9 (1.8)	13.7 (1.8)	13.0 (1.8)	14.5 (1.8)		DBD*, ND*
Bachelor's degree (%)	29.4	22.9	19.6	12.2	41.7		ND*
Income (× 10K; M, SD)	2.1 (1.5)	2.3 (1.7)	2.1 (1.4)	2.4 (1.5)	2.4 (1.5)		
Unemployed (%)	5.9	4.2	7.6	2.0	6.5		
Ever married (%)	35.3	37.5	43.6	30.6	37.5		
Parent (%)	23.5	29.2	32.6	22.4	20.7		

Note. BD, bipolar disorder; SUB, subsyndromal bipolar disorder; MDD, major depressive disorder; DBD, disruptive behavior disorder; ND, no disorder. Diagnostic groups listed in the BD and SUB planned contrasts columns indicate a significant difference at $p < .05$; differences between BD and SUB only appear in the BD column (Lewinsohn, Klein, & Seeley, 2000).

*$p < .05$; **$p < .01$; ***$p < .001$.

HYPOMANIA SCALES

General Behavior Inventory

The General Behavior Inventory (GBI; Depue et al., 1981) was developed to assess bipolar and unipolar mood disorders across the full spectrum of severity, including subsyndromal conditions. Developed within the framework of the behavioral high-risk paradigm, it was hypothesized that most of the cases identified in community samples of adolescents and young adults would be at the subsyndromal level, and that these individuals would be at increased risk for subsequently developing full-syndromal mood disorders (Depue et al., 1981). In previous studies, the GBI has been shown to have high internal consistency, to have good test–retest results for stability, and to exhibit a high degree of concordance with diagnoses based on structured interviews in nonclinical and patient samples (Klein, Dickstein, Taylor, & Harding, 1989). The GBI has been extensively validated in a range of populations, including college students, psychiatric outpatients, and the offspring of bipolar I samples (Klein, Depue, & Slater, 1986).

An abbreviated GBI (Depue et al., 1981) that included eight of the original 21 GBI hypomania items (items 4, 8, 11, 15, 30, 44, 51, and 64) and four of the original seven GBI biphasic items (items 2, 19, 24, and 48) was included in the T_1 and T_2 assessments. The 12-item GBI hypomania scale scores ranged from 12 to 45 (mean = 23.6, SD = 5.5, median = 23.0), had high internal consistency (Cronbach's alpha = .80), but only moderate T_1–T_2 test–retest reliability (r = .46). The 12-item GBI scale was moderately correlated with the Eckblad and Chapman (1986) Hypomanic Personality Scale (r = .48). As expected, T_1 participants with a lifetime history of bipolar disorder or subsyndromal bipolar disorder (n = 92) were significantly elevated compared to those without a lifetime history of bipolar disorder or subsyndromal bipolar disorder (n = 1,592), mean = 27.5 versus 23.4, t (1,681) = 7.11, p < .001, and Cohen's d = .70. Participants who scored in the upper quartile of the 12-item GBI score ($\geq$ 27) were significantly more likely to have had a history of bipolar disorder or subsyndromal bipolar disorder compared to those who scored in the lower three quartiles, Likelihood Ratio χ^2 (1, N = 1,683) = 38.96, p < .001, odds ratio = 3.93, 95% confidence interval = 2.55–6.06. With respect to predicting first-onset bipolar disorder or subsyndromal bipolar disorder between T_1 and T_3, participants who scored in the upper quartile of the 12-item GBI score were significantly more likely to develop bipolar disorder or subsyndromal bipolar disorder compared to those who scored in the lower three quartiles, Likelihood Ratio χ^2 (1, N = 868) = 38.96, p < .001, odds ratio = 3.02, 95% confidence interval = 1.30–6.99.

While previous studies have supported the convergent validity of the GBI by demonstrating high levels of concordance with interview-derived diagnoses and relationships to external criteria such as informant reports, family history, and neuroendocrine dysregulation (Depue et al., 1981; Klein, Depue, & Krauss, 1986), there are few data on the inventory's predictive validity. In the only prospective study available, Klein and Depue (1984) reported that college students with elevated GBI scores continued to exhibit high levels of impairment in a 19-month follow-up. Our cross-sectional analyses of the OADP data are consistent with previous studies in finding an association between the GBI and interview-derived diagnoses. More importantly, our data extend this literature by demonstrating for the first-time that elevated GBI scores are associated with a significantly increased risk of developing a first-onset bipolar disorder or subsyndromal bipolar disorder. Thus, consistent with its original aims, the GBI may provide an economical means of screening for and identifying community-dwelling adolescents and young adults who are at elevated risk for developing bipolar disorder.

Eckblad and Chapman's Hypomanic Personality Scale

Since Kraepelin (1921), clinicians have suggested that bipolar disorder may also be manifested as a personality or temperamental type. Eckblad and Chapman (1986) developed the Hypomanic Personality Scale to assess this set of traits, and reported that college students with elevated scores on the scale exhibited increased rates of hypomanic and major depressive episodes, substance abuse, and psychotic features, and also had significantly poorer social adjustment than low-scoring students. Kwapil and colleagues (2000) followed up these students 13 years later, and found that the group with elevated scores subsequently experienced higher rates of bipolar disorder, major depressive episodes, substance use disorders, psychotic-like experiences, and borderline personality disorder features than low-scoring participants.

We extended this work by examining the distribution, correlates, and predictive validity of Eckblad and Chapman's (1986) Hypomanic Personality Scale in the OADP sample (Klein et al., 1996). The scale exhibited moderate stability ($r = .54$) in the mean 14-month period between T_1 and T_2. We divided the sample into participants with very high, moderately high, intermediate, moderately low, and very low scores on the Hypomanic Personality Scale and compared the groups on lifetime history of psychopathology at T_1. High scorers had significantly greater lifetime rates of major depressive disorder, substance use disorders, and disruptive behavior disorders. In addition, a significantly greater proportion of the highest (14%) than the lowest (0%) scoring groups reported having experienced the core symptom required for a manic or a hypomanic episode: a distinct period of abnormally and persistently elevated, expansive, or irritable mood. However, the hypomanic traits did not predict the first onset of bipolar disorder or subsyndromal bipolar disorder between T_1 and T_3.

We also examined the concurrent and predictive associations between scores on the Hypomanic Personality Scale and a number of inventory-assessed psychosocial constructs. These analyses were limited to adolescents with no lifetime history of mood disorder. At T_1, hypomanic traits were significantly associated with depressive symptomatology, internalizing and externalizing behavior problems, pessimism, excessive emotional reliance on others, less social support from family, greater conflict with parents, poorer school functioning (including lower grades, missing more days of school, being late for school more often, and failing to do homework more frequently), more major life events and daily hassles, poorer physical health, and more mental health treatment. However, hypomanic traits were also associated with greater self-reported social competence and social support from friends.

In addition, we examined the prospective associations between hypomanic traits at T_1 and the psychosocial constructs at T_2, controlling for the level of the psychosocial constructs at T_1. Hypomanic personality traits predicted significant increases in depressive symptomatology, internalizing behavior problems, emotional reliance on others, school tardiness, and major life events, and a significant decrease in social support from family, between T_1 and T_2.

Thus, our cross-sectional analyses of the OADP sample extend the Eckblad and Chapman (1986) findings in college students by indicating that elevated scores on the Hypomanic Personality Scale are associated with increased rates of major depressive disorder and substance use disorders and poorer psychosocial functioning in a large representative sample of community-dwelling adolescents. In addition, our prospective findings are consistent with Kwapil and colleagues' (2000) follow-up of Eckblad and Chapman's sample in indicating that the Hypomanic Personality Scale predicts significant increases in depressive symptoms and psychosocial impairment approximately 1 year later. However, the Hypomanic Personality Scale was not successful in predicting the development of bipolar disorder and subsyndromal bipolar disorder in individuals at either the T_2 or T_3 follow-ups.

FAMILY HISTORY OF PSYCHOPATHOLOGY

Family studies provide an important means of testing the validity of diagnostic constructs and exploring the links between disorders. Therefore, we used the family study data to explore the validity of a diagnosis of bipolar disorder in adolescents and the relationship between full-syndromal and subsyndromal bipolar disorder.

The first-degree relatives of adolescents with bipolar disorder exhibited significantly higher rates of major depressive disorder and subsyndromal bipolar disorder than the first-degree relatives of adolescents with no history of mental disorder through age 18 (see Table 1.3). In addition, the first-degree relatives of adolescents with subsyndromal bipolar disorder had significantly higher rates of bipolar disorder and major depressive disorder than the relatives of never mentally ill adolescents. Interestingly, there were also significantly higher rates of anxiety disorders in the relatives of adolescents with bipolar disorder and subsyndromal bipolar disorder than the relatives of adolescents with no history of psychopathology. However, the groups of relatives did not differ on rates of alcohol and/or drug use disorders.

These data support the validity of the diagnosis of bipolar disorder in adolescents, in that adolescent bipolar disorder is associated with an elevated rate of major depressive disorder in relatives. In addition, they indicate that subsyndromal bipolar disorder may lie on a continuum with full-syndromal bipolar disorder, as there was an elevated rate of subsyndromal bipolar disorder in the relatives of adolescents with bipolar disorder, and elevated rates of bipolar disorder and major depressive disorder in the relatives of adolescents with subsyndromal bipolar disorder.

CLINICAL IMPLICATIONS AND FUTURE DIRECTIONS

The "classical" (Kraepelin, 1921) form of bipolar disorder (as operationalized in the DSM) clearly exists in adolescence. Consistent with the early (Bleuler, 1950; Kraepelin, 1919; Kretschmer, 1936) and more recent contributors (Akiskal & Pinto, 1999; Angst, 1998), our data support the existence of a bipolar spectrum, a continuum that extends from elevated levels of hypomanic personality traits to subsyndromal, mild, and severe forms of this disorder. An implication for clinical practice is that clinicians need to be sensitive not only to the presence of the full-blown bipolar disorder syndrome, but also to the milder and less easily perceived manifestations of this disorder. It is clear that bipolar disorder even at the subsyndromal level has serious negative consequences for adolescents and also for their ability to cope with the demands for the adjustments required during young adulthood. Detecting, remediating, and, better still, preventing bipolar disorders in children and adolescents should be a high public health priority. Critical to accomplishing this goal is the availability of cost-effective screeners that can detect putative cases in a timely, nonstigmatizing, and inexpensive way.

Consistent with the literature on adult bipolar disorder, suicidal behavior was found to be highly prevalent in the OADP participants with a history of bipolar disorder (72% had suicidal ideation, 44% had attempted suicide). Moreover, the severity of the attempts were found to be even more serious among those with bipolar disorder than among those with major depressive disorder. The rates of suicidal behavior in the OADP

TABLE 1.3. Kaplan–Meier Age-Corrected (to 60 years of age) Morbid Risk Estimates of Psychiatric Disorders among First-Degree Relatives by Adolescent Diagnostic Group (Age 0–18)

Disorder	Diagnostic group 0–18					Planned contrasts[a]	
	BD (n = 52)	SUB (n = 136)	MDD (n = 774)	DBD (n = 145)	ND (n = 885)	BD	SUB
MDD % (SE)	43.3 (7.6)	40.3 (5.9)	47.4 (3.4)	48.6 (6.3)	26.9 (2.0)	ND*	ND*
BD % (SE)	3.9 (2.7)	4.8 (2.2)	1.3 (0.5)	2.1 (1.2)	1.4 (0.5)		ND*
SUB % (SE)[b]	9.6 (4.5)	2.9 (1.4)	3.8 (0.7)	4.8 (1.9)	1.7 (0.5)	ND*	
Anxiety % (SE)	24.1 (7.5)	23.1 (4.0)	15.2 (1.4)	12.6 (3.3)	10.8 (1.2)	ND*	DBD*, NND***
Alcohol abuse % (SE)	34.9 (7.2)	38.3 (4.7)	39.2 (2.1)	35.1 (4.4)	29.0 (2.1)		
Drug abuse % (SE)	27.9 (6.8)	24.2 (3.9)	20.7 (1.6)	30.1 (4.1)	13.8 (1.2)		
Antisocial PD % (SE)[b]	11.5 (5.3)	4.4 (1.7)	5.0 (0.8)	4.8 (1.7)	3.1 (0.6)	ND*	
Borderline PD % (SE)[b]	7.7 (3.5)	3.7 (1.5)	3.1 (0.6)	3.5 (1.5)	1.8 (0.4)		

Note. BD, bipolar disorder; SUB, subsyndromal bipolar disorder; MDD, major depressive disorder; DBD, disruptive behavior disorder; ND, no disorder; PD, personality disorder. Diagnostic groups listed in the BD and SUB planned contrasts columns indicate a significant difference at $p < .05$; differences between BD and SUB only appear in the BD column (Lewinsohn, Klein, & Seeley, 2000).

[a]Contrasts were based on Taylor series variance estimation and adjusted for gender of proband, gender of relative, relationship to proband, education of relative, direct interview participation, and number of informant interviews.

[b]Uncorrected rates are presented due to indeterminate age of onset.

*$p < .05$; **$p < .01$; ***$p < .001$.

participants with bipolar disorder are equal to those reported for referred cases (e.g., Leese, 1967; Pfeffer, Conte, & Plutchik, 1980). Clinicians need to be sensitive to the potential for suicidal acts among youth with subsyndromal and full-syndromal bipolar disorder.

As is well known, suicidal ideation and suicide attempts among youth almost always occur in the context of psychopathology (e.g., Lewinsohn et al., 1996). Given the elevated prevalence and seriousness of suicidal behavior among youth with bipolar disorder, it is critical that we examine, from a theoretical perspective, the potential mechanisms by which bipolar disorder potentiates suicidal behavior. As Shaffer (1985) points out, in order to determine the diagnostic specificity of suicidal behavior, it is necessary to compare the clinical characteristics of those with suicidal behavior to those without such behavior. Thus, future comparative studies should be conducted in order to identify the risk factors for a suicide attempt within the bipolar groups—that is, the factors that differentiate adolescents with bipolar disorder with a history of suicide attempt from those without such a history.

Identification of the psychosocial antecedents and consequences of prepubertal and adolescent bipolar disorder need to be pursued by future research in order to facilitate development and evaluation of preventive and therapeutic interventions. Research to delineate the psychosocial concomitants of bipolar disorder in children and adolescents is also important. What spheres of functioning are affected? In this regard we want to bring to the attention of the reader the work of Alloy and colleagues (1999), Hammen and colleagues (1990), and Miklowitz and Goldstein (1997). An understanding of the early manifestations of bipolar disorder would seem to be especially important to prevent bipolar disorder in at-risk youth at the youngest possible age. Furthermore, by means of longitudinal follow-up and family history study of the cases of prepubertal and juvenile bipolar disorder as identified, studied, and treated by Geller, Biederman, and others, it should be possible to establish whether bipolar disorder in very young children and bipolar disorder in adolescents are different manifestations of the same disorder.

We would like to end on a positive note by raising the question of whether characteristics that predispose children and adolescents to bipolar disorder bestow some advantages. We are of course referring to bipolar characteristics within the normal range of variation, not to pathological levels of intensity. As we know (Akiskal & Pinto, 1999; Andreasen, 1987; Jamison, 1995; Ludwig, 1975; Richards, Kinney, Lunde, Benet, & Merzel, 1988), highly creative individuals experience bipolar disorder more often than do other groups in the general population. The question is: What are the characteristics of the bipolar spectrum disorders that contribute to creative achievement? In her review of this literature, Jamison (1995) suggests that the following features should be considered: sharpened and unusually original thinking, high activity and energy levels, being optimistic and perhaps somewhat grandiose, verbal fluency, and enhanced motivation to work to achieve ambitious goals. To these traits, one might add the enjoyment of being with people, social competence, and the ability to persuade and to inspire others. The challenge is how to allow youngsters to take advantage of these traits while helping them to avoid escalating to destructive and pathological levels.

In conclusion, our data provide support for the existence of a bipolar spectrum. With early detection and remediation, the many adverse consequences associated with bipolar disorder, such as suicidal behavior, may be prevented. Given the pernicious course of prepubertal and adolescent bipolar disorder, such efforts should be a high public health priority.

ACKNOWLEDGMENTS

This research was supported in part by NIMH Award Nos. MH40501, MH50522, and MH52858.

REFERENCES

Akiskal, H. S., & Pinto, O. (1999). The evolving bipolar spectrum: Prototypes I, II, III, and IV. In H. Akiskal (Ed.), *Bipolarity: Beyond classic mania* (pp. 517–534). Philadelphia: Saunders.

Alloy, L. B., Reilly-Harrington, N. A., Fresco, D. M., Whitehouse, W. G., & Zechmeister, J. S. (1999). Cognitive styles and life events in subsyndromal unipolar and bipolar disorders: Stability and prospective prediction of depressive and hypomanic mood swings. *Journal of Cognitive Psychotherapy: An International Quarterly, 13,* 21–40.

American Psychiatric Association. (1987). *Diagnostic and statistical manual of mental disorders* (3rd ed., rev.). Washington, DC: Author. (Abbreviated as DSM-III-R.)

American Psychiatric Association. (1994). *Diagnostic and statistical manual of mental disorders* (4th ed.). Washington, DC: Author. (Abbreviated as DSM-IV.)

Andreasen, N. C. (1987). Creativity and mental illness: Prevalence rates in writers and their first-degree relatives. *American Journal of Psychiatry, 144,* 1288–1292.

Angst, J. (1988). Clinical course of affective disorders. In T. Helgason & R. J. Daly (Eds.), *Depressive illness: Prediction of course and outcome* (pp. 1–44). Heidelberg: Springer-Verlag.

Angst, J. (1998). The emerging epidemiology of hypomania and bipolar II disorder. *Journal of Affective Disorders, 50,* 143–151.

Biederman, J. (1998). Resolved: Mania is mistaken for ADHD in prepubertal children. *Journal of the American Academy of Child and Adolescent Psychiatry, 37,* 1091–1099.

Biederman, J., Faraone, S. V., Hatch, M., Mennin, D., Taylor, A., & George, P. (1997). Conduct disorder with and without mania in a referred sample of ADHD children. *Journal of Affective Disorders, 44,* 177–188.

Bleuler, E. P. (1950). *Dementia praecox or the group of schizophrenias.* New York: International Universities Press. (Original work published 1911)

Bowring, M. A., & Kovacs, M. (1992). Difficulties in diagnosing manic disorders among children and adolescents. *Journal of the American Academy of Child and Adolescent Psychiatry, 31,* 611–614.

Brent, D. A., Perper, J. A., Goldstein, C. E., Kolko, D. J., Allan, M. J., Allman, C. J., & Zelenak, J. P. (1988). Risk factors for adolescent suicide: A comparison of adolescent suicide victims with suicidal inpatients. *Archives of General Psychiatry, 45,* 581–587.

Carlson, G. A. (1995). Identifying prepubertal mania. *Journal of the American Academy of Child and Adolescent Psychiatry, 34,* 750–753.

Carlson, G. A. (1998). Mania and ADHD: Comorbidity or confusion. *Journal of Affective Disorders, 51,* 177–187.

Carlson, G. A., & Kashani, J. H. (1988). Manic symptoms in a non-referred adolescent population. *Journal of Affective Disorders, 15,* 219–226.

Chambers, W. J., Puig-Antich, J., Hirsch, M., Paez, P., Ambrosini, P. J., Tabrizi, M. A., & Davies, M. (1 985). The assessment of affective disorders in children and adolescents by semistructured interview: Test–retest reliability of the Schedule for Affective Disorders and Schizophrenia for School-Age Children, present episode version. *Archives of General Psychiatry, 42,* 696–702.

Depue, R. A., Slater, J. F., Wolfsetter-Kausch, H., Klein, D., Goplerud, E., & Farr, D. (1981). A behavioral paradigm for identifying persons at risk for bipolar depressive disorder: A conceptual framework and five validation studies. *Journal of Abnormal Psychology, 90,* 381–437.

Eckblad, M., & Chapman, L. J. (1986). Development and validation of a scale for hypomanic personality. *Journal of Abnormal Psychology, 95,* 214–222.

Geller, B., Craney, J., Bolhofner, K., DelBello, M. P., Williams, M., & Zimerman, B. (2001). One-year recovery and relapse rates of children with a prepubertal and early adolescent bipolar disorder phenotype. *American Journal of Psychiatry, 158,* 303–305.

Geller, B., Fox, L. W., & Clark, K. A. (1994). Rate and predictors of prepubertal bipolarity during follow-up of 6- to 12-year old depressed children. *Journal of the American Academy of Child and Adolescent Psychiatry, 33,* 461–468.

Geller, B., & Luby, J. (1997). Child and adolescent bipolar disorder: A review of the past 10 years. *Journal of the American Academy of Child and Adolescent Psychiatry, 36,* 1168–1176.

Geller, B., Williams, M., Zimerman, B., Frazier, J., Beringer, L., & Warner, K. L. (1998). Prepubertal and early adolescent bipolarity differentiate from ADHD by manic symptoms, grandiose delusions, ultra-rapid or ultradian cycling. *Journal of Affective Disorders, 51,* 81–91.

Geller, B., Zimerman, B., Williams, M., Bolhofner, K., Craney, J. L., DelBello, M. P., & Soutullo, C. A. (2000). Diagnostic characteristics of 93 cases of a prepubertal and early adolescent bipolar disorder phenotype by gender, puberty and comorbid attention deficit hyperactivity disorder. *Journal of Child and Adolescent Psychopharmacology, 10,* 157–164.

Guze, S., & Robins, E. (1970). Suicide and primary affective disorders. *British Journal of Psychiatry, 117,* 437–438.

Hammen, C., Burge, D., Burney, E., & Adrian, C. (1990). Longitudinal study of diagnoses in children of women with unipolar and bipolar affective disorder. *Archives of General Psychiatry, 47,* 1112–1117.

Jamison, K. R. (1986). Suicide and bipolar disorders. In J. J. Mann & M. Stanley (Eds.), *Psychobiology of suicidal behavior* (pp. 301–315). New York: New York Academy of Sciences.

Jamison, K. R. (1995). Manic–depressive illness and creativity. *Scientific American, 272,* 62–67.

Kessler, R. C., Rubinow, D. R., Holmes, C., Abelson, J. M., & Zhao, S. (1997). The epidemiology of DSM-III-R bipolar I disorder in a general population survey. *Psychological Medicine, 27,* 1079–1089.

Klein, D. N., & Depue, R. A. (1984). Continued impairment in persons at risk for bipolar affective disorder: Results from a 19-month follow-up study. *Journal of Abnormal Psychology, 93,* 345–347.

Klein, D. N., Depue, R. A., & Krauss, S. P. (1986). Social adjustment in the offspring of parents with bipolar affective disorder. *Journal of Psychopathology and Behavioral Assessment, 8,* 355–366.

Klein, D. N., Depue, R. A., & Slater, J. F. (1986). Inventory identification of cyclothymia: Part 9. Validation in offspring of bipolar I patients. *Archives of General Psychiatry, 43,* 441–445.

Klein, D. N., Dickstein, S., Taylor, E. B., & Harding, K. (1989). Identifying chronic affective disorders in outpatients: Validation of the General Behavior Inventory. *Journal of Consulting and Clinical Psychology, 57,* 106–111.

Klein, D. N., Lewinsohn, P. M., & Seeley, J. R. (1996). Hypomanic personality traits in a community sample of adolescents. *Journal of Affective Disorders, 38,* 135–143.

Klein, D. N., Lewinsohn, P. M., Seeley, J. R., & Rohde, P. (2001). Family study of major depressive disorder in a community sample of adolescents. *Archives of General Psychiatry, 58,* 13–20.

Kovacs, M. (1991). "Major psychiatric disorders" as risk factors in youth suicide. In L. Davidson & M. Linnoila (Eds.), *Risk factors for youth suicide* (pp. 127–143). New York: Hemisphere.

Kraepelin, E. (1919). *Dementia praecox and paraphrenia.* Edinburgh, Scotland: Livingstone. (Original work published 1913)

Kraepelin, E. (1921). *Manic–depressive insanity and paranoia.* Edinburgh, Scotland: Livingstone.

Kretschmer, E. (1936). *Physique and character* (2nd ed.). New York: Harcourt, Brace.

Kutcher, S., Robertson, H. A., & Bird, D. (1998). Premorbid functioning in adolescent onset bipolar I disorder: A preliminary report from an ongoing study. *Journal of Affective Disorders, 51,* 137–144.

Kwapil, T. R., Miller, M. B., Zinser, M. C., Chapman, L. J., Chapman, J., & Eckblad, M. (2000). A longitudinal study of high scorers on the Hypomanic Personality Scale. *Journal of Abnormal Psychology, 109,* 222–226.

Leese, M. L. (1969). Suicide behavior in twenty adolescents. *British Journal of Psychiatry, 115,* 479–480.

Lewinsohn, P. M., Hops, H., Roberts, R. E., Seeley, J. R., & Andrews, J. A. (1993). Adolescent psychopathology: Part 1. Prevalence and incidence of depression and other DSM-III-R disorders in high school students. *Journal of Abnormal Psychology, 102,* 133–144.

Lewinsohn, P. M., Klein, D. N., & Seeley, J. R. (1995). Bipolar disorders in a community sample of older adolescents: Prevalence, phenomenology, comorbidity, and course. *Journal of the American Academy of Child and Adolescent Psychiatry, 34,* 454–463.

Lewinsohn, P. M., Klein, D. N., & Seeley, J. R. (2000). Bipolar disorder during adolescence and young adulthood in a community sample. *Bipolar Disorders, 2,* 281–293.

Lewinsohn, P. M., Rohde, P., Klein, D. N., & Seeley, J. R. (1999). Natural course of adolescent major depressive disorder: Part 1. Continuity into young adulthood. *Journal of the American Academy of Child and Adolescent Psychiatry, 38,* 56–63.

Lewinsohn, P. M., Rohde, P., Seeley, J. R., Klein, D. N., & Gotlib, I. H. (2000). Natural course of adolescent major depressive disorder in a community sample: Predictors of recurrence in young adults. *American Journal of Psychiatry, 157,* 1584–1591.

Ludwig, L. D. (1975). Elation–depression and skill as determinants of desire for excitement. *Journal of Personality, 43,* 1–22.

Miklowitz, D. J., & Goldstein, M. J. (1997). *Bipolar disorder: A family-focused treatment approach.* New York: Guilford Press.

Pfeffer, C. R., Conte, H. R., & Plutchik, R. (1980). Suicidal behavior in latency-age children: An outpatient population. *Journal of the American Academy of Child and Adolescent Psychiatry, 19,* 703–710.

Richards, R., Kinney, D. K., Lunde, I., Benet, M., & Merzel, A. P. C. (1988). Creativity in manic–depressives, cyclothymes, their normal relatives, and control subjects. *Journal of Abnormal Psychology, 97,* 281–288.

Robins, E., Murphy, G. E., Wilkinson, R. H., Jr., Gassner, S., & Kayes, J. (1959). Some clinical considerations in the prevention of suicide based on a study of 134 successful suicides. *American Journal of Public Health, 49,* 888–899.

Shaffer, D. (1985). Depression, mania, and suicidal acts. In M. Rutter & L. Hersov (Eds.), *Depression, mania, and suicidal acts* (Vol. 2, pp. 698–719). Oxford, UK: Blackwell.

Strober, M., Lampert, C., Schmidt, S., & Morrell, W. (1993). The course of major depressive disorder in adolescents: Part 1. Recovery and risk of manic switching in a follow-up of psychotic and nonpsychotic subtypes. *Journal of the American Academy of Child and Adolescent Psychiatry, 32,* 34–42.

Weissman, M. M., Bland, R. C., Canino, G. J., Faravelli, C., Greenwald, S., Hwu, H. G., Joyce, P. R., Karam, E. G., Lee, C. K., Lellouch, J., Lépine, J. P., Newman, S. C., Rubio-Stipec, M., Wells, J. E., Wickramaratne, P. J., Wittchen, H. U., & Yeh, E. K. (1996). Cross-national epidemiology of major depression and bipolar disorder. *Journal of the American Medical Association, 276,* 293–299.

Wozniak, J., Biederman, J., Kiely, K., Ablon, S., Faraone, S. V., Mundy, E., & Mennin, D. (1995). Mania-like symptoms suggestive of childhood-onset bipolar disorder in clinically referred children. *Journal of the American Academy of Child and Adolescent Psychiatry, 34,* 867–876.

2

Phenomenology and Longitudinal Course of Children with a Prepubertal and Early Adolescent Bipolar Disorder Phenotype

Barbara Geller, James L. Craney, Kristine Bolhofner,
Melissa P. DelBello, David Axelson, Joan Luby,
Marlene Williams, Betsy Zimerman, Michael J. Nickelsburg,
Jeanne Frazier, and Linda Beringer

At the beginning of the 1990s, there were several key questions regarding the field of prepubertal and early adolescent bipolar disorder (PEA-BP). These included:

1. Did prepubertal mania exist?
2. If it did exist, would the pattern be similar to the typical adult episodes with relatively well-intervening periods?
3. Would the mood be only irritable?
4. Did children with mania really just have severe attention-deficit/hyperactivity disorder (ADHD) (i.e., were they children with ADHD who were having a bad day)?

This chapter presents a review of data from research in this area that address these questions. This work is from the ongoing study "Phenomenology and Course of Pediatric Bipolar Disorder," funded by the National Institute of Mental Health (NIMH), at Washington University School of Medicine in St. Louis (Geller et al., 1995; Geller, Bolhofner, et al., 2000; Geller, Craney, et al., 2001, 2002; Geller, Warner, Williams, & Zimerman, 1998; Geller, Williams, et al., 1998; Geller, Zimerman, et al., 2000a, 2000b, 2001; Geller, Zimerman, Williams, Bolhofner, et al., 2002; Geller,

Zimerman, Williams, DelBello, et al., 2002). This is a longitudinal study comparing the phenomenology of pediatric subjects with PEA-BP, ADHD, and a group of community controls (CC).

SELECTING A PHENOTYPE TO INVESTIGATE

Selecting a PEA-BP phenotype to study required taking into account two problems: (1) irritability and (2) comorbid ADHD. Several authors reported that irritability was the most common symptom of mania in their samples (e.g., Biederman, 2000; Papolos & Papolos, 1999). In spite of the fact that irritability was also one of the most common symptoms of mania in adults (Goodwin & Jamison, 1990), it was often interpreted as if it were a pathognomonic symptom of mania in children (Charney, 2000). Irritability, however, is not only *not* pathognomonic of child mania, it is also commonly present in many other child psychiatric disorders such as oppositional defiant disorder, conduct disorder, attention-deficit/hyperactivity disorder, major depressive disorder, autism, and Asperger syndrome, and it is frequently the reason for referral to psychiatric treatment (Geller, Zimerman, Williams, DelBello, et al., 2002).

This nonspecificity of irritable mood can be put into perspective by a comparison to "strep" throat (Geller, Zimerman, Williams, DelBello, et al., 2002). A sore throat is the most common symptom of strep throat, but less than 5% of sore throats are caused by streptococcal infection. By analogy, it is highly likely that only a small fraction of irritable children have mania (Geller, Zimerman, Williams, DelBello, et al., 2002). Therefore, one consideration in choosing a DSM-IV phenotype for study was to have inclusion criteria that were specific to mania so that it did not include subjects who had *only* irritable mood plus symptoms that overlapped with DSM-IV criteria for other pediatric psychiatric disorders such as ADHD.

A second consideration was how to deal with the high prevalence of comorbid ADHD in subjects with PEA-BP. In 1995, Geller and colleagues reported a pilot study in which 88.9% of subjects with mania aged ≤ 12 had comorbid ADHD, as did 29.4% of subjects ≥ 13 years. Multiple authors have reported similar findings (Geller & Luby, 1997). Therefore, studying a PEA-BP phenotype that excluded comorbid ADHD would provide a nonrepresentative group of subjects.

With these two problems in mind, the following phenotype was selected. Subjects would need to meet the DSM-IV criteria for mania or hypomania with elated mood and/or grandiosity as one criterion. Using this PEA-BP phenotype would allow diagnosing mania without using only criteria that overlapped with those for DSM-IV ADHD (e.g., hyperactivity, distractibility). Furthermore, this phenotype would ensure that the PEA-BP group had at least one of the two cardinal features of mania (i.e., elation and/or grandiosity) (Geller, Bolhofner, et al., 2000; Geller, Craney, et al., 2001, 2002; Geller, Zimerman, et al., 2000a, 2000b, 2001; Geller, Zimerman, Williams, Bolhofner, et al., 2002; Geller, Zimerman, Williams, DelBello, et al., 2002). However, it would not exclude those subjects who had comorbid ADHD.

OVERALL STUDY METHODS

This section describes the overall study methods (Geller, Craney, et al., 2001, 2002; Geller, Zimerman, et al., 2000a, 2000b, 2001; Geller, Zimerman, Williams, Bolhofner, et al., 2002).

Study Inclusion and Exclusion Criteria

The inclusion criteria for the PEA-BP group were males and females from 7 to 16 years old, in good physical health, with severity at a level of definite caseness measured by a Children's Global Assessment Scale (CGAS) score ≤ 60 (Bird, Canino, Rubio-Stipec, & Ribera, 1987; Shaffer et al., 1983). PEA-BP subjects also needed to meet DSM-IV criteria for current mania or mixed state for at least 2 weeks, or DSM-IV criteria for current hypomania for at least 2 months, with elated mood and/or grandiosity as one of the mania/hypomania criteria. Exclusion criteria for the PEA-BP group were the child was adopted; had an IQ < 70; had a diagnosis of pervasive developmental disorders, schizophrenia, epilepsy, and/or other major medical or neurological disorder; or had baseline substance dependency or pregnancy.

Inclusion criteria for the ADHD group were males and females 7 to 16 years old, in good physical health, with definite caseness (CGAS ≤ 60), who met DSM-IV criteria for ADHD (with hyperactivity, i.e., combined or hyperactive/impulsive types) with an onset before age 7 and duration ≥ 6 months. Exclusion criteria for the ADHD group were the same as those for the PEA-BP group, with the addition of major depressive disorder (MDD) and any bipolar disorder diagnosis.

The CC group was aggregately matched to the PEA-BP subjects by age, gender, socioeconomic status (SES), ethnicity, and ZIP code, were in good physical health, and had definite noncaseness (CGAS ≥ 70). Exclusion criteria for the CC group were the same as those for the PEA-BP group with the addition of any current or past bipolar disorder, major depressive disorder, or ADHD diagnoses.

The rationales for these inclusion and exclusion criteria were as follows. The duration criteria for PEA-BP were similar to conservative durations in multiple nosological schemas. Conservative durations were selected to increase the likelihood of caseness and to address the controversies in the field (National Institute of Mental Health [NIMH] Research Round-table on Prepubertal Bipolar Disorder, 2001). Current episodes of mania or hypomania were needed because this was a phenomenology study. Subjects with ultradian (continuous) rapid cycling ($\geq$ one cycle/day lasting $\geq$ 4 hours) needed to have a cycle every day for at least 2 weeks (for mania) or at least 2 months (for hypomania). The mean number of cycles/day was 3.7 (SD = 2.1), consistent with continuous rapid cycling (Geller, Zimerman, et al., 2000a). The rationale for the elation/grandiosity criterion was as given earlier. A lower age of 7 was chosen because of credibility of interview assessments and an upper age of 16 was selected so those subjects would still be teenagers at the 2-year follow-up assessment (Geller, Craney, et al., 2002). In the contrast psychiatric group, only ADHD and not attention deficit disorder was selected because the hyperactivity component was one of the major issues in differential diagnosis. Also, the subjects with ADHD (and the subjects with PEA-BP) could have conduct and/or oppositional defiant disorders because these were common comorbidities among children with ADHD, so excluding them would have produced an atypical ADHD sample. CGAS (Bird et al., 1987; Shaffer et al., 1983) scores were selected to ensure definite caseness for the bipolar disorder and ADHD groups and definite noncaseness for the CC subjects. On this scale, 100 is best and 0 is worst functioning. Scores of $\leq$ 60 were definite cases and $\geq$ 70 were definite noncases (Bird et al., 1987). At baseline only, substance use disorders and/or pregnancy were exclusion criteria to avoid confounding the diagnosis of bipolar disorder with mental status effects of substance use or gestational state. Subjects continued in the follow-up phase of the "Phenomenology" study if they developed substance use diagnoses or became pregnant after baseline. Because the mean age of the subjects with PEA-BP at baseline was 10.9 (SD = 2.6) years (Geller, Zimerman, et al., 2000a), it is unlikely that this exclusion criterion effected the generalizeability of the study findings. Adoption was an exclusion criterion due to concurrent family and genetic studies.

Subject Ascertainment

To optimize generalizeability, consecutive case ascertainment from outpatient child psychiatry and pediatric sites was used to recruit PEA-BP and ADHD subjects. These were outpatient sites because the planned inpatient sites at Barnes Hospital and at St. Louis Children's Hospital (both within the Washington University Medical Complex) closed soon after the project began. The outpatient sites were largely primary care centers for patients seeking pediatric care or the primary psychiatric center for subjects in large local HMOs. Records of every new patient at the ascertainment sites were reviewed by nonblind research nurses (i.e., different individuals than the blind research nurses who conducted the research assessments). Telephone screenings were administered to all potentially eligible cases (e.g., subjects with clear exclusionary criteria such as major medical illnesses or those not in the study age range did not receive a telephone screening). Subjects who were still eligible after the telephone screen were scheduled for in-person baseline assessments performed by blind research nurses. During the time that the 93 PEA-BP and 81 ADHD subjects were ascertained, 1,468 total new consecutive cases were seen at the pediatric and psychiatric ascertainment sites. Each of these cases was reviewed by a research nurse for any obvious study exclusionary criteria—for example, diabetes mellitus, mental retardation, or epilepsy. Of the 1,468 cases, 1,111 were from the psychiatric sites and 357 were from the pediatric sites. Eight hundred and fifty-four cases were excluded after chart review. Of the remaining 614 cases, telephone screening excluded an additional 162 cases; 144 cases refused participation at the telephone screening, and 308 remained. Thus 9.8% (144/1,468) of all consecutive new outpatients refused participation and 23.5% (144/614) of those eligible for telephone screening refused. The demography of the refusers was not significantly different from that of the nonrefusers. The 308 subjects who were not excluded were scheduled for in-person baseline assessment. During baseline evaluation, 134 cases did not fit inclusion criteria and thus were excluded, leaving the 174 cases that were entered. Thus, 6.3% (93/1,468) of consecutive new cases fit the PEA-BP phenotype.

The CC group was ascertained from a random survey that matched normal subjects to the PEA-BP subjects by age, gender, SES, ethnicity and ZIP code.

Assessment Instruments

The Washington University in St. Louis Kiddie Schedule for Affective Disorders and Schizophrenia (WASH-U-KSADS) (Geller, Williams, Zimerman, & Frazier, 1996; Geller, Williams, Zimerman, et al., 1998; Geller, Zimerman, et al., 2001) is a semistructured interview that was administered by experienced research clinicians to mothers about their children and to children about themselves. It was developed from the KSADS (Puig-Antich & Ryan, 1986) by adding (1) items to assess the lifetime and current onset and offset of each symptom and syndrome, (2) items to assess multiple DSM-IV diagnoses, and (3) items to specifically assess prepubertal and early adolescent manifestations of DSM-IV mania criteria and rapid cycling. Skip-outs were minimized to enhance collection of phenomenology data. The data collection guideline is that the narrative documentation must justify the rating with respect to onset, offset, frequency, duration, intensity, and specific examples (Geller, Zimerman, et al., 2001; Geller, Zimerman, Williams, Bolhofner, et al., 2002). Thus, the narrative next to each WASH-U-KSADS item is part of using this assessment tool (e.g., part of the narrative next to a suicidal ideation item read "cut her wrists four times with a kitchen knife and wanted to die to escape her sad feelings"). An example of the narrative documentation for a euphoric state was a child who related feeling "high, off the charts high" before "crashing right down." The elation followed by "crashing" to a state of despair was part of the narrative for cycling. Examples of prepubertal mania manifestations taken from WASH-U-KSADS interviews of children about themselves have appeared elsewhere (Geller, Zimerman, Williams, DelBello, et al., 2002). In this "examples" paper (Geller, Zimerman, Williams, DelBello, et al., 2002), the manifestations of DSM-IV symptoms in prepubertal mania were compared to normal behavior in CCs as well as to symptoms in manic adults. To score the WASH-U-KSADS items, mother and child responses were combined by using either, in accordance with the methods described by Bird, Gould, and Staghezza (1992). Excellent reliability (Geller, Zimerman, et al., 2001), stability of mania items and mania diagnoses at 6 months (Geller, Zimerman, et al., 2000a), and validity against parent and teacher reports has been shown (Geller, Williams, et al., 1998). In addition, this instrument is used in the large majority of NIMH-funded studies of children with bipolar disorder so that comparable data across studies can be facilitated (NIMH Research Roundtable, 2001). Templates to the WASH-U-KSADS to assess DSM-IV substance use disorders in childhood were also given (Geller, Cooper, Sun, et al., 1998; Geller, Cooper, Zimerman, et al., 1998).

Overlapping time periods on the WASH-U-KSADS items of mania/hypomania and major depressive disorder were used as the definition of *mixed mania*. The definition of *rapid cycling* was four episodes per year. *Ultrarapid cycling* was defined as 5 to 364 episodes and *ultradian (continuous) rapid cycling* as ≥ 365 episodes per year. In ultradian cycling, mania needed to occur for ≥ 4 hours per day (Geller et al., 1995; Geller, Craney, et al., 2001; Geller, Warner, et al., 1998; Geller, Williams, et al., 1998; Geller, Zimerman, et al., 2000b). These definitions were adapted from Kramlinger and Post (1996).

The CGAS rating (Bird et al., 1987; Shaffer et al., 1983) is a global measure of severity based on psychiatric symptomatology and impairment of adaptation in family, social, school, and work areas. It was derived by raters who performed the WASH-U-KSADS.

Psychosocial assessments were obtained with the Psychosocial Schedule for School-age Children—Revised (PSS-R) (Puig-Antich et al., 1985) administered separately to mothers about their children and to children about themselves by the research nurses who gave the WASH-U-KSADS and who were blind to group status at baseline. This semistructured tool has been shown to have good psychometrics (Lukens et al., 1983). Measurements of maternal–child and paternal–child warmth and of maternal–child and paternal–child tension/hostility are included in this instrument. Impairments given by either informant (i.e., mother or child) were used. For example, if one informant reported maternal distance and the other informant reported maternal warmth, the overall rating was maternal distance.

SES was assessed with the Hollingshead Four Factor Index of Social Status (Hollingshead, 1976).

Medication use and psychosocial therapies were coded with the treatment section of the Longitudinal Interval Follow-up Evaluation (LIFE; Keller et al., 1987), which codes by type, dose, compliance, and duration of each medication and by the type, frequency, duration, and compliance of psychosocial therapy. The LIFE was modified to weekly increments to match the time frames of the WASH-U-KSADS weekly symptom and syndrome time frames.

The Pubertal Status Questionnaire (PSQ; Duke, Litt, & Gross, 1980) was completed by subjects ≥ 10 years old at baseline.

Medical records were also obtained. Teacher ratings were obtained as previously described (Geller, Williams, et al., 1998).

To establish DSM-IV consensus diagnoses, all research materials (assessment instruments, school reports, agency records, pediatrician charts, videotapes of WASH-U-KSADS interviews of mothers and videotapes of WASH-U-KSADS interviews of children) were reviewed in consensus conferences. These conferences included Dr. Geller and the research nurses who performed the ratings (Fennig, Craig, Tanenberg-Karant, & Bromet, 1994; Klein, Ouimette, Kelly, Ferro, & Riso, 1994; Kraemer, 1992). At these meetings, narrative documentation for each WASH-U-KSADS item was reviewed to ensure that the rating was justified.

As detailed elsewhere, raters were trained to interrater reliability and recalibrated annually (Geller, Zimerman, et al., 2001). At baseline, raters were blind to group status of the subjects.

Development, Reliability, and Stability of the WASH-U-KSADS

Before beginning a diagnostic and natural history study of PEA-BP, there was a need to develop a prepubertal age mania assessment tool. The main research tool used for studies of prepubertal major depressive disorder, the KSADS (Puig-Antich & Chambers, 1978; Puig-Antich & Ryan, 1986), was developed before it was believed that prepubertal mania existed. Thus, child bipolar disorder was not as well covered as child major depressive disorder. In addition, the KSADS did not include items for onsets and offsets of each symptom and syndrome (lifetime and current), lacked items for many diagnoses including ADHD, and did not include a section to assess details of patterns of rapid cycling.

To address this need, Geller and colleagues (Geller et al., 1996; Geller, Williams, et al., 1998; Geller, Zimerman, et al., 2001) developed the WASH-U-KSADS, which has prepubertal-specific mania items, a section on rapid cycling, items for each occurrence of every symptom and syndrome, and items to assess ADHD and multiple other DSM-IV diagnoses. The semistructured format in which experienced research professionals conduct separate interviews of mothers about their children and of children about themselves has been retained.

Interrater reliability data between two blind raters on the WASH-U-KSADS mania and rapid-cycling sections were analyzed using the kappa statistic, which measures agreement beyond chance. On this scale, 0.75 or higher is considered excellent agreement. Table 2.1 presents the excellent reliability of the WASH-U-KSADS (Geller, Zimerman, et al., 2001).

The WASH-U-KSADS also has excellent 6-month stability of individual mania items (including rapid cycling) and of mania diagnoses (Geller, Zimerman, et al., 2000b).

As noted in the NIMH Research Roundtable on Prepubertal Bipolar Disorder (2001), the WASH-U-KSADS has become one of the most widely used instruments in federally funded projects on child mania. A comparison of the characteristics of this instrument to others appears in the "Roundtable" paper.

IDENTIFYING PREPUBERTAL MANIFESTATIONS OF MANIA

It is not intuitive that children can have functionally impairing, pathological happiness. Nor is it intuitive that children can be pathologically too expansive and grandiose. Below are descriptions of characteristics that differ-

TABLE 2.1. Reliability of WASH-U-KSADS Mania and Rapid Cycling Sections

DSM-IV diagnosis	% agreement	Kappa
Mania	95.0	0.90
Hypomania	95.0	0.85

WASH-U-KSADS item	Rho	Kappa
Elated mood	0.98	0.92
Grandiosity	0.96	0.82
Grandiose delusions	1.00	1.00
Flight of ideas/racing	1.00	0.95
Flight of ideas	1.00	0.93
Racing thoughts	1.00	1.00
Decreased need for sleep	1.00	1.00
Poor judgment	0.98	0.95
Hypersexuality	0.95	0.95
Daredevil acts	0.99	1.00
Silliness	1.00	1.00
Uninhibitedly seeks people	0.97	0.90

Note. From Geller, Zimerman, et al. (2001). Copyright 2001 by Lippincott Williams & Wilkins. Adapted by permission.

entiate normal versus pathological features of mania (Geller, Zimerman, Williams, DelBello, et al., 2002).

Differentiation of Normal from Pathological Elation

Normal children were extremely elated when it was the day to go to Disneyland, the grandparents were visiting, or it was Christmas morning. This mood was appropriate to context, expected by the adults, and non-impairing.

This can be compared to a child who was elated and giggling in the classroom when others were not, and who was sent to the principal and suspended from school for this behavior. In this example, the elated mood was inappropriate to context and impairing, and thus was pathological (Geller, Zimerman, Williams, DelBello, et al., 2002).

Differentiation of Normal from Pathological Grandiosity

Normal children were expansive and grandiose when playing. For example, a child played at being a firefighter after school and directed the other firefighters on what to do. Another child played being the teacher after school and directed an imaginary group of students. In these examples, the context was appropriate—that is, play after school hours—and the grandiose idea that the children were teachers and firefighters was developmentally expected. Because it was after school and only in an imaginary play situation, the behavior is nonimpairing.

Compare the above to the following two situations. In one instance, a child got up during the class and began instructing the teacher on how to educate the class and telling the students what they should learn. In another, the child went to the principal and demanded that the principal fire his teacher. In these examples, the grandiosity was not in play after school but was acted upon inappropriately in real-life situations. It was impairing in that it disrupted the class and led to school punishments (Geller, Zimerman, Williams, DelBello, et al., 2002).

What Are Prepubertal Equivalents of Manifestations of Adult-Onset Mania?

Children developmentally cannot present with many of the manifestations of mania observed in late-teenage-/adult-onset mania (e.g., children will not "max out credit cards" or engage in serial marriages). Therefore, child-age behaviors that were equivalent to those observed in older age groups needed to be described. Tables 2.2–2.6 present examples of manifestations of mania criteria in normal children, PEA-BP children, and adults with bipolar disorder (Geller, Zimerman, Williams, DelBello, et al., 2002).

TABLE 2.2. Examples of Elated Mood in Subjects with Prepubertal and Early
Adolescent Bipolar Disorder, Normal Children, and Adults with Bipolar Disorder

Normal child	Child mania	Adult mania
Child was superhappy on days family went to Disneyland, on Christmas morning, and during grandparents' visits. Child's joy was appropriate to context. Child's behavior was not impairing.	A 7-year-old boy was repeatedly taken to the principal for clowning and giggling in class (when no one else was), and was suspended from school. He had to leave church with his family for similar behaviors. A 9-year-old girl continually danced around at home stating, "I'm high, over the mountain high" after suspension from school.	A 40-year-old male giggled infectiously while being placed in restraints in the emergency room. A 50-year-old male in the emergency room was infectiously amusing as he described multiple hospitalizations, losing jobs, and losing family ties.

Note. From Geller, Zimerman, Williams, DelBello, et al. (2002). Copyright 2002 by Mary Ann Liebert, Inc. Adapted by permission.

COMPARISON OF DSM-IV CRITERIA IN PEA-BP, ADHD, AND NORMAL CONTROL SUBJECTS

Characteristics of Study Subjects

The PEA-BP and CC groups were well matched and not significantly different on age, gender, puberty status, ethnicity, SES, and ZIP code, consistent with the ascertainment schema. The ADHD group was significantly younger and had a higher percent of males than the PEA-BP or CC groups. It was decided not to force age, puberty, and gender matches between the PEA-BP and ADHD groups because that would have produced a highly skewed, nonrepresentative ADHD group. These differences were controlled for in the statistical analyses.

Details of PEA-BP subject characteristics, comorbid ADHD and oppositional defiant disorder/conduct disorder and comparison of prepubertal to pubertal subjects were reported in Geller, Zimerman, and colleagues (2000a). In brief, 87.1% of the PEA-BP subjects had comorbid ADHD and 76.3% had comorbid oppositional defiant disorder/conduct disorder. The only symptom or course feature that was significantly different between pre- and postpubertal subjects was more frequent ADHD in prepubertal subjects.

Age of Onset and Duration of Current PEA-BP Episode

PEA-BP subjects were 10.9 (SD = 2.6) years old at baseline and were 7.3 (SD = 3.5) years old at onset of the baseline episode. Therefore, the duration of the baseline episode was 3.6 (SD = 2.5) years, consistent with a

TABLE 2.3. Examples of Grandiose Behaviors in Subjects with Prepubertal and Early Adolescent Bipolar Disorder, Normal Children, and Adults with Bipolar Disorder

Normal child	Child mania	Adult mania
A 7-year-old boy played at being a fireperson, directing other fire people and rescuing victims. Child was not calling the firestation to tell them what to do. Play was during after-school hours; it was age-appropriate and not impairing.	A 7-year-old boy stole a go-cart because he just wanted to have it. He knew stealing was wrong, but he did not believe it was wrong for him to steal. When the police arrived, the child thought the officers had come to play with him. An 8-year-old girl opened a paper flower store in her classroom and was annoyed and refused to do class work when asked by the teacher. An 8-year-old girl, failing at school, spent her evenings practicing for when she would be the first lady president. She was also planning how to train her husband to be the first gentleman. When asked how she could fail school and still be president, she said she just knew.	An adult male kept his family in increasing debt due to multiple unrealistic business ventures. A 21-year-old male believed he could commit a homicide and not be arrested because the laws would not pertain to him. An 18-year-old woman rang the city mayor's home doorbell because she knew they were engaged. When asked if she had ever met the mayor, she stated that did not matter.

Note. From Geller, Zimerman, Williams, DelBello, et al. (2002). Copyright 2002 by Mary Ann Liebert, Inc. Adapted by permission.

TABLE 2.4. Examples of Decreased Need for Sleep in Subjects with Prepubertal and Early Adolescent Bipolar Disorder, Normal Children, and Adults with Bipolar Disorder

Normal child	Child mania	Adult mania
Normal children sleep approximately 8–10 hours a night and are tired the next day if they sleep fewer hours than usual.	An 8-year-old boy chronically stayed up until 2:00 A.M. rearranging the furniture or playing games. Then he awoke at 6:00 A.M. for school and was energetic during the day without evident tiredness or fatigue. A 7-year-old girl knocked on a friend's door daily at 6:00 A.M. ready to play.	A 25-year-old woman worked both day and evening full-time jobs seemingly without fatigue. A husband noted that his wife "parties" for days in a row and then "sleeps" for days in a row.

Note. From Geller, Zimerman, Williams, DelBello, et al. (2002). Copyright 2002 by Mary Ann Liebert, Inc. Adapted by permission.

TABLE 2.5. Examples of Hypersexual Behaviors in Subjects with Prepubertal and Early Adolescent Bipolar Disorder, Normal Children, and Adults with Bipolar Disorder

Normal child	Child mania	Adult mania
A 7-year-old child played doctor with a same-age friend. A 12-year-old boy looked at his father's pornographic magazines.	An 8-year-old boy imitated a rock star by gyrating his hips and rubbing his crotch during a research interview. A 9-year-old boy drew pictures of naked ladies in public, stating they were drawings of his future wife. A 14-year-old girl passed notes to boys in class asking them to f___ her. Another girl faxed a similar note to the local police station. A 7-year-old girl touched the teacher's breasts and propositioned boys in class. A 10-year-old boy used explicit sexual activity language in restaurants and other public places. Another child called 1-900 sex lines, which his parents discovered when the phone bill arrived at the end of the month.	Numerous adults who had four or more marriages not due to death of spouses or who had multiple extramarital affairs.

Note. From Geller, Zimerman, Williams, DelBello, et al. (2002). Copyright 2002 by Mary Ann Liebert, Inc. Adapted by permission.

chronic, unremitting course (Geller, Craney, et al., 2001; Geller, Zimerman, et al., 2000a).

Comparisons of DSM-IV Mania Symptoms

Figure 2.1 shows the comparisons for four of the five symptoms (elated mood, grandiosity, decreased need for sleep, flight of ideas/racing thoughts) that provided the best discrimination between the PEA-BP and the ADHD groups. These four symptoms and the hypersexuality symptom described below and in Table 2.5 and Figure 2.2 are mania-specific, that is, they are DSM-IV symptoms for mania but are not DSM-IV symptoms for ADHD (Geller, Zimerman, Williams, Bolhofner, et al., 2002).

Figure 2.2 demonstrates the comparisons for the WASH-U-KSADS symptoms that are used to rate the DSM-IV poor judgment criterion. Although the overall prevalences of the poor judgment criterion were signifi-

TABLE 2.6. Examples of Racing Thoughts in Subjects with Prepubertal and Early Adolescent Bipolar Disorder, Normal Children, and Adults with Bipolar Disorder

Normal child	Child mania	Adult mania
Normal subjects did not give affirmative responses to inquiries about "racing thoughts."	Unlike manic adults, children gave concrete answers to describe their "racing thoughts." Examples are a girl pointed to the middle of her forehead and stated "I need a stoplight up there." Other children noted the following: "It's like an Energizer Bunny in my head." "Too much stuff is flying around up there." "I don't know what to think first." "My thoughts broke the speed limit." "My thoughts broke the sound barrier of my mind."	Adults conceptually understand "racing thoughts" and can describe them using the word "racing."

Note. From Geller, Zimerman, Williams, DelBello, et al. (2002). Copyright 2002 by Mary Ann Liebert, Inc. Adapted by permission.

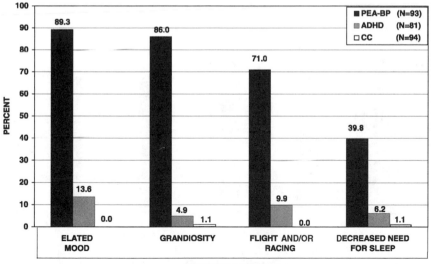

FIGURE 2.1. DSM-IV mania-specific symptoms in 93 PEA-BP, 81 ADHD, and 94 CC subjects. From Geller, Zimerman, Williams, Bolhofner, et al. (2002). Copyright 2002 by Mary Ann Liebert, Inc. Adapted by permission. All comparisons between the PEA-BP and ADHD groups were significant at $p < .0001$. Details of these and other comparisons appear in Geller, Zimerman, Williams, Bolhofner, et al. (2002).

cantly different between subjects with PEA-BP and subjects with ADHD, poor judgment was a less clinically useful discriminator because it also occurred in 44.4% of the ADHD group. By contrast, the hypersexuality symptom provided excellent discrimination between subjects with PEA-BP and subjects with ADHD (Geller, Zimerman, Williams, Bolhofner, et al., 2002). As reported by Geller, Zimerman, Williams, DelBello and colleagues (2000), only 1% of the subjects with PEA-BP had a history of sexual abuse. This disparity between history of abuse and occurrence of hypersexual symptoms supports the need to include mania in the differential diagnosis of hypersexual behaviors.

Figure 2.3 presents comparisons for DSM-IV symptoms that are included in DSM-IV for both the PEA-BP and ADHD categories. Therefore, these symptoms are not mania-specific because they occur in both the DSM-IV mania and ADHD categories. In addition, Figure 2.3 shows the data for irritability. Even though there were statistically significant differences, these nonspecific mania symptoms were poor discriminators because they were frequent in both the PEA-BP and the ADHD groups (Geller, Zimerman, Williams, Bolhofner, et al., 2002).

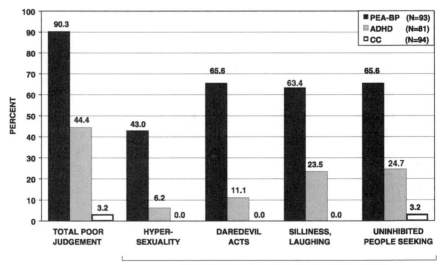

FIGURE 2.2. DSM-IV mania poor judgment symptoms in 93 PEA-BP, 81 ADHD, and 94 CC subjects. From Geller, Zimerman, Williams, Bolhofner, et al. (2002). Copyright 2002 by Mary Ann Liebert, Inc. Adapted by permission. All comparisons between the PEA-BP and ADHD groups were significant at $p < .0001$. Details of these and other comparisons appear in Geller, Zimerman, Williams, Bolhofner, et al. (2002).

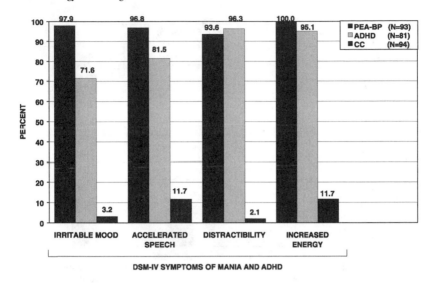

FIGURE 2.3. DSM-IV mania nonspecific symptoms in 93 PEA-BP, 81 ADHD, and 94 CC subjects. From Geller, Zimerman, Williams, Bolhofner, et al. (2002). Copyright 2002 by Mary Ann Liebert, Inc. Adapted by permission. The PEA-BP and ADHD groups were not significantly different on any item in this figure except irritability (p = .0002). All comparisons between PEA-BP and CC and between ADHD and CC groups were significant at p < .0001. Details of these and other comparisons appear in Geller, Zimerman, Williams, Bolhofner, et al. (2002).

Concurrent Elation and Irritability

Coexisting elated mood and irritability occurred in 87.1% (n = 81) of the subjects with PEA-BP (Geller, Zimerman, Williams, Bolhofner, et al., 2002), similar to the percent of concurrent elation and irritable mood reported for adults with bipolar disorder (Goodwin & Jamison, 1990).

Suicidality, Psychosis, Mixed Mania, and Rapid Cycling

Figure 2.4 presents rapid-cycling moods including elation, depression, and irritability in the group with PEA-BP. It can be seen that no subject had only four episodes per year. Rather, continuous rapid cycling was the most prevalent pattern. Unlike adults with bipolar disorder, rapid cycling was not more frequent in females in the PEA-BP group (Geller, Zimerman, Williams, Bolhofner, et al., 2002).

Figure 2.5 presents the prevalence of psychotic and suicidal symptoms and of mixed mania and rapid-cycling course features in the group with PEA-BP. Psychosis-only included malignant, pathological hallucinations and delusions. For example, hearing a voice call your name was not counted, but hearing a voice telling you to kill yourself was counted. It was

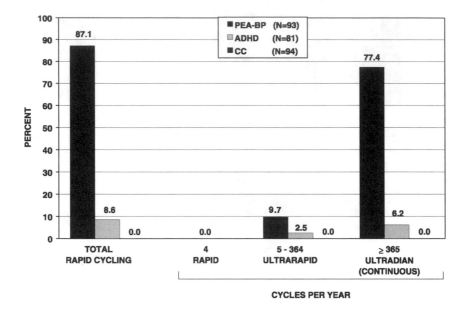

FIGURE 2.4. PEA-BP subjects with rapid cycling, ultra rapid cycling, and continuous rapid (ultradian) cycling. From Geller, Zimerman, Williams, Bolhofner, et al. (2002). Copyright 2002 by Mary Ann Liebert, Inc. Adapted by permission. The PEA-BP group had significantly greater total and ultradian (continuous) rapid cycling than the ADHD group ($p < .0001$). Details of these and other comparisons appear in Geller, Zimerman, Williams, Bolhofner, et al. (2002).

previously shown that these items did not differ by age or gender within the group with PEA-BP (Geller, Zimerman, et al., 2000a).

Longitudinal Diagnostic Validation

In contrast to multiple studies of the naturalistic course of late-teenage- and adult-onset bipolar disorders, little was known about the longitudinal outcome of child-onset mania (Geller, Craney, et al., 2001, 2002). Clearly, ethical mandates precluded withholding long-term treatment to study natural history. Nevertheless, natural history studies of late-teenage- and adult-onset mania have been highly informative about diagnostic outcomes (Geller, Craney, et al., 2001, 2002). Naturalistic studies of adult-onset mania have also increased our knowledge of the outcome of lithium treatment on suicidality, social functioning, and number of hospitalizations (Geller, Craney, et al., 2001, 2002).

In our natural history study subjects with PEA-BP were assessed at 6-month intervals in the research unit but received all of their clinical care

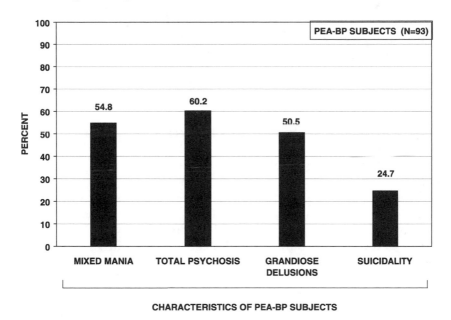

FIGURE 2.5. DSM-IV mania features in 93 PEA-BP subjects. From Geller, Zimerman, Williams, Bolhofner, et al. (2002). Copyright 2002 by Mary Ann Liebert, Inc. Adapted by permission.

from their own community practitioners. Treatments provided by their community practitioners were collected and used in data analyses.

Recovery and Relapse in the PEA-BP Group

For examining the 2-year outcome, recovery was defined as at least 8 consecutive weeks without meeting DSM-IV criteria for mania or hypomania. Remission was defined as 2–7 weeks without meeting DSM-IV criteria for mania or hypomania. These definitions were adapted from Frank et al. (1991) to provide comparability across outpatient pediatric and adult studies. Relapse after recovery was defined as 2 consecutive weeks of meeting DSM-IV criteria for mania or hypomania with clinically significant impairment evidenced by a CGAS ≤ 60.

At the 2-year time point, 98.1% of the 268 probands were retained in the study. This included 95.7% of the subjects with PEA-BP (Geller, Craney, et al., 2002).

Table 2.7 shows the percent of subjects who recovered and relapsed at the 6-, 12-, 18-, and 24-month time points.

Fifty-eight subjects recovered during the 2 years. Thirty-two of these

58 subjects relapsed after recovery. Time to recovery was 36.0 (SD = 25.0) weeks. Relapse after recovery occurred at 28.6 (SD = 13.2) weeks (Geller, Craney, et al., 2002).

Predictors of Recovery and Relapse

There were no significant differences in baseline characteristics between the 58 (65.2%) recovered subjects by the 2-year time point and the 31 (34.8%) unrecovered subjects after correction for multiple comparisons (Geller, Craney, et al., 2002).

Figure 2.6 presents the rates of recovery by subjects living in an intact biological family versus those in other living situations as assessed with the Psychosocial Schedule for School-age Children—Revised (PSS-R) as described in the Overall Study Methods section. Living with their intact biological family significantly predicted recovery. Based on the Cox modeling hazard ratio, subjects living with their intact biological families were 2.2 (95% confidence interval [CI] = 1.2–3.8) times more likely to recover than those in other living situations (Geller, Craney, et al., 2002).

Figure 2.7 demonstrates the rates of relapse after recovery by maternal–child warmth assessed with the PSS-R. Low maternal warmth significantly predicted relapse; based on the Cox modeling hazard ratio, subjects with low maternal–child warmth were 4.1 (95% CI = 1.7–10.1) times more likely to relapse after recovery (Geller, Craney, et al., 2002).

No other baseline characteristics (e.g., major depressive disorder, CGAS, mixed mania, continuous cycling, psychosis, oppositional defiant disorder/conduct disorder) predicted recovery or relapse (Geller, Craney, et al., 2002).

Relatively poor outcomes of these subjects may be due to their phenotypic resemblance to severely ill adults with bipolar disorder who have mixed mania, continuous rapid cycling, psychosis, and treatment resistance. The lower effectiveness of mood stabilizers in children cannot be ruled out.

TABLE 2.7. Recovery and Relapse After Recovery in Subjects with a Prepubertal and Early Adolescent Bipolar Disorder Phenotype

Time points (months)	Total n	Recovery		Relapse after recovery	
		%	n	%	n
6	91	14.3	13	15.4	2
12	89	37.1	33	27.3	9
18	89	56.2	50	40.0	20
24	89	65.2	58	55.2	32

Note. From Geller, Craney, et al. (2002). Copyright 2002 by the American Psychiatric Association. Adapted by permission.

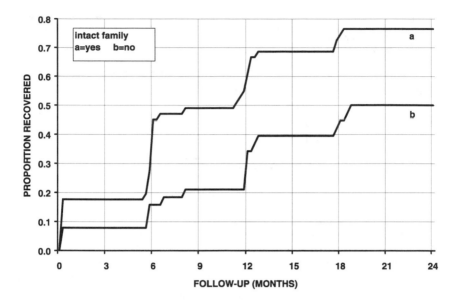

FIGURE 2.6. Two-year rate of recovery by living situation in subjects with a pre-pubertal and early adolescent bipolar disorder phenotype. From Geller, Craney, et al. (2002). Copyright 2002 by the American Psychiatric Association. Adapted by permission. Fifty-eight of the 89 subjects recovered by 24 months. There was a significant difference between the 39 recovered subjects who lived with their intact biological families and the 19 who resided in other living situations (Cox model χ^2 = 7.40, df = 1, p = .007). The K-M estimates for recovery in intact families was 76.5% (95% CI = 64.8–88.1) and for recovery in other living situations was 50.0% (95% CI = 34.1–65.9).

Although the maternal warmth predictor is consistent with reports in adult mania, the intact family predictor may be unique to child mania (Geller, Craney, et al., 2002).

Outcome of Hypomania

Eight of the 10 subjects with hypomania at baseline developed mania during the 24-month follow-up. Also, eight subjects with baseline hypomania recovered; four of these eight relapsed after recovery. The number of hypomanic subjects was too small for separate analyses (Geller, Craney, et al., 2002).

Other Diagnoses During Recovery

Proportions of recovered subjects who had ADHD, oppositional defiant disorder/conduct disorder, and/or major depressive disorder at any time during recovery were 32.8%, 24.1%, and 29.3%, respectively. No subject

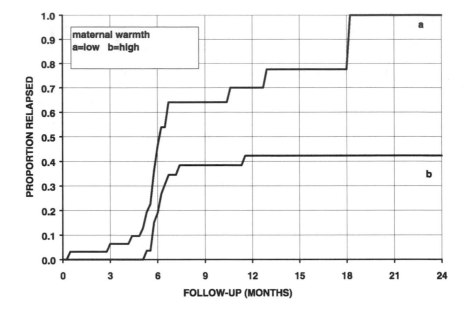

FIGURE 2.7. Two-year rate of relapse after recovery by high versus low maternal–child warmth in subjects with a prepubertal and early adolescent bipolar disorder phenotype. From Geller, Craney, et al. (2002). Copyright 2002 by the American Psychiatric Association. Adapted by permission. Thirty-two of the 58 recovered subjects relapsed after recovery. There was a significant difference between the 21 relapsers with low maternal–child warmth and the 11 with high maternal–child warmth (Cox model χ^2 = 9.84, df = 1, p = .002). The K-M estimates for relapse by low maternal–child warmth was 100.0% (95% CI = not applicable when K-M 100.0%) and by high maternal–child warmth was 42.2% (95% CI = 23.2–61.2).

developed a substance dependency disorder during the 2-year follow-up (Geller, Craney, et al., 2002).

Treatment by Community Practitioners

Subjects were assessed in the research unit, but received all of their treatment from their own community practitioners (see Figure 2.8). Findings are described in detail in Geller, Craney, and colleagues (2001, 2002). In brief, by the 2-year time point, less than half (47%) of the subjects were prescribed any antimanic medication (lithium, an anticonvulsant, or a neuroleptic) by their community practitioners. This relatively low rate may be because community practitioners do not yet recognize prepubertal and early adolescent mania. Of subjects who received antimanic medications for at least 2 consecutive weeks, no medication class was predictive of recovery or relapse, with the following exception: subjects who received a

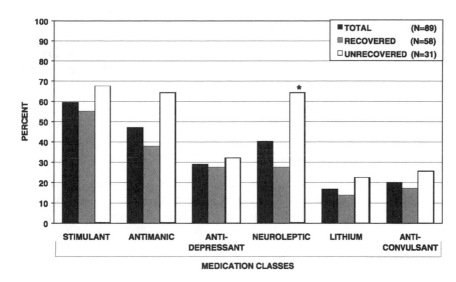

FIGURE 2.8. Baseline to 2-year psychotropic medications in 89 subjects with PEA-BP treated by their own community practitioners. Subjects who received a neuroleptic drug between baseline and recovery were significantly *less* likely to recover (χ^2 = 13.27, p = .0003). Further discussion of community practitioner-provided treatment appears in Geller, Zimerman, et al. (2000b) and Geller, Craney, et al. (2002).

neuroleptic were less likely to recover. The lower recovery rate may be because neuroleptics were administered significantly more frequently to subjects who had higher rates of psychosis, comorbid oppositional defiant disorder/conduct disorder, and major depressive disorder at baseline. There was no difference in outcome between psychotic subjects who received a neuroleptic compared to those who did not. There was no difference in the rate of recovery of subjects who received lithium compared to those who received anticonvulsants. Community physicians prescribed antidepressants to 29% of the subjects and stimulants to 60% of the subjects during the 2-year follow-up. Neither antidepressants nor stimulants had a significant effect (positive or negative) on recovery or on relapse.

Community practitioners gave 54% of subjects individual and/or group therapy at some point over the follow-up period (Geller, Craney, et al., 2002). These subjects were significantly less likely to recover. However, subjects receiving individual and/or group therapy were also significantly more likely to be ascertained at a psychiatric site, so that they may have had more treatment-resistant disorders. In addition, 21% of the subjects received family therapy; family therapy was not predictive of recovery or relapse (Geller, Craney, et al., 2002).

Psychosocial Functioning in Subjects with PEA-BP Compared to Subjects with ADHD and Normal Subjects

Details of these psychosocial data appear in Geller, Zimerman, Williams, DelBello, and colleagues (2002). In brief, compared to both ADHD and CC subjects, PEA-BP cases had significantly greater impairment on items that assessed maternal–child warmth, maternal–child and paternal–child tension, and peer relationships.

Comparison to Course of Adult Mania

Table 2.8 presents a comparison of PEA-BP to late-teenage-/adult-onset bipolar disorder. The percents for adults are from Goodwin and Jamison (1990) and those for children are from Geller and colleagues (Geller Craney, et al., 2001, 2002; Geller, Zimerman, et al., 2000a, 2000b; Geller, Zimerman, Williams, Bolhofner, et al., 2002).

Comparison to Reports from Other Investigators

Comparisons between the "Phenomenology" study data on a PEA-BP phenotype and that of other groups can be problematic due to methodological differences. For example, Faraone, Biederman, Mennin, Wozniak, and Spencer (1997) did not interview the children about themselves, used lay raters, did not use prepubertal age-specific mania items, did not require a cardinal mania criterion (i.e., elation and/or grandiosity) for diagnosing mania, and used an instrument designed for epidemiology studies and ascertained for a study of ADHD.

SUMMARY AND DISCUSSION

The PEA-BP phenotype was validated by reliable assessment, 6-month stability, and 1- and 2-year longitudinal diagnostic outcome. Poor prognosis

TABLE 2.8. Comparison of Late Teenage/Adult Bipolar Disorder (BP) to Prepubertal and Early Adolescent BP (PEA-BP)

Episode	Typical adult	Severe adult[a]	Typical PEA-BP[b]
Type	Mania or MDD	Mixed 40%	Mixed 54.8%
Duration	2–8 months discrete	Continuous, rapid cycling (20%)	Continuous, rapid cycling (77.4%) for 3.6 (2.5) years
Treatment	Responsive	Resistant	?

[a] Statistics for severe adults were from Goodwin and Jamison (1990).

[b] Statistics for typical PEA-BP subjects were from Geller, Zimerman, et al. (2000b), Geller, Craney, et al. (2001, 2002), and Geller, Zimerman, Williams, Bolhofner, et al. (2002).

over a 24-month period was evidenced by low rates of recovery and high rates of relapse. Counterintuitively, typical 7-year-old children with PEA-BP were more severely ill than typical 27-year-olds with late-teenage-/adult-onset mania. Thus, PEA-BP resembled the severest form of late-teenage-/adult-onset mania by presenting with a chronic, mixed manic, psychotic, continuously cycling picture.

Data also showed that the prevalence of comorbid ADHD is very high even in subjects selected for DSM-IV mania with the cardinal symptoms of elation and/or grandiosity. This high rate of ADHD in PEA-BP is dissimilar to late-teenage-/adult-onset bipolar disorder.

As noted in the data, pathological elated mood and grandiosity can be identified in children with mania by using age-appropriate assessments. Furthermore, similar to adults with bipolar disorder, subjects with PEA-BP had a high rate of coexisting elated mood and irritability.

FUTURE RESEARCH QUESTIONS

One of the key issues for future study is whether the subjects with PEA-BP will continue to resemble severely ill adults with bipolar disorder or begin to present with the more typical late-teenage/adult pattern of discrete episodes of mania or depression, often with sudden onsets, and with intervening relatively well periods of functioning. In this regard, future predictors of recovery and relapse, including medication administration, will be important to assess. Furthermore, later follow-ups can address whether the prevalence of comorbid ADHD will decrease as these subjects reach late adolescence and adulthood.

ACKNOWLEDGMENTS

This work was supported by National Institute of Mental Health Grant No. R01 MH-53063 (to Barbara Geller).

REFERENCES

Biederman, J. (2000). Advances in the psychopharmacology of pediatric bipolar disorder and ADHD. *Journal of Child and Adolescent Psychopharmacology, 10*, 153–154.

Bird, H. R., Canino, G., Rubio-Stipec, M., & Ribera, J. C. (1987). Further measures of the psychometric properties of the Children's Global Assessment Scale. *Archives of General Psychiatry, 44*, 821–824.

Bird, H. R., Gould, M. S., & Staghezza, B. (1992). Aggregating data from multiple informants in child psychiatry epidemiological research. *Journal of the American Academy of Child and Adolescent Psychiatry, 31*, 78–85.

Charney, D. S. (2000). Bipolar disorder: Can studies of natural history help us define clinically and neurobiologically relevant subtypes? *Biological Psychiatry, 48,* 427.

Duke, P. M., Litt, I. F., & Gross, R. T. (1980). Adolescents' self-assessment of sexual maturation. *Pediatrics, 66,* 918–920.

Faraone, S. V., Biederman, J., Mennin, D., Wozniak, J., & Spencer, T. (1997). Attention-deficit hyperactivity disorder with bipolar disorder: A familial subtype? *Journal of the American Academy of Child and Adolescent Psychiatry, 36,* 1378–1387.

Fennig, S., Craig, T. J., Tanenberg-Karant, M., & Bromet, E. J. (1994). Comparison of facility and research diagnoses in first-admission psychotic patients. *American Journal of Psychiatry, 151,* 1423–1429.

Frank, E., Prien, R. F., Jarrett, R. B., Keller, M. B., Kupfer, D. J., Lavori, P. W., Rush, A. J., & Weissman, M. M. (1991). Conceptualization and rationale for consensus definitions of terms in major depressive disorder. *Archives of General Psychiatry, 48,* 851–855.

Geller, B., Bolhofner, K., Craney, J. L., Williams, M., DelBello, M. P., & Gundersen, K. (2000). Psychosocial functioning in a prepubertal and early adolescent bipolar disorder phenotype. *Journal of the American Academy of Child and Adolescent Psychiatry, 39,* 1543–1548.

Geller, B., Cooper, T. B., Sun, K., Zimerman, B., Frazier, J., Williams, M., & Heath, J. (1998). Double-blind placebo controlled study of lithium for adolescent bipolar disorders with secondary substance dependency. *Journal of the American Academy of Child and Adolescent Psychiatry, 37,* 171–178.

Geller, B., Cooper, T. B., Zimerman, B., Frazier, J., Williams, M., Heath, J., & Warner, K. (1998). Lithium for prepubertal depressed children with family history predictors of future bipolarity: A double-blind, placebo-controlled study. *Journal of Affective Disorders, 51,* 165–175.

Geller, B., Craney, J. L., Bolhofner, K., DelBello, M. P., Williams, M., & Zimerman, B. (2001). One-year recovery and relapse rates of children with a prepubertal and early adolescent bipolar disorder phenotype. *American Journal of Psychiatry, 158,* 303–305.

Geller, B., Craney, J. L., Bolhofner, K., Nickelsburg, M. J., Williams, M., & Zimerman, B. (2002). Two year prospective follow-up of children with a prepubertal and early adolescent bipolar disorder phenotype. *American Journal of Psychiatry, 159,* 927–933.

Geller, B., & Luby, J. (1997). Child and adolescent bipolar disorder: A review of the past 10 years. *Journal of the American Academy of Child and Adolescent Psychiatry, 36,* 1168–1176.

Geller, B., Sun, K., Zimerman, B., Luby, J., Frazier, J., & Williams, M. (1995). Complex and rapid-cycling in bipolar children and adolescents: A preliminary study. *Journal of Affective Disorders, 34,* 259–268.

Geller, B., Warner, K., Williams, M., & Zimerman, B. (1998). Prepubertal and young adolescent bipolarity versus ADHD: Assessment and validity using the WASH-U-KSADS, CBCL and TRF. *Journal of Affective Disorders, 51,* 93–100.

Geller, B., Williams, M., Zimerman, B., & Frazier, J. (1996). *Washington University in St. Louis Kiddie Schedule for Affective Disorders and Schizophrenia (WASH-U-KSADS).* St. Louis, MO: Department of Psychiatry, Washington University.

Geller, B., Williams, M., Zimerman, B., Frazier, J., Beringer, L., & Warner, K. L. (1998). Prepubertal and early adolescent bipolarity differentiate from ADHD by manic symptoms, grandiose delusions, ultrarapid or ultradian cycling. *Journal of Affective Disorders, 51*, 81–91.

Geller, B., Zimerman, B., Williams, M., Bolhofner, K., Craney, J. L., DelBello, M. P., & Soutullo, C. A. (2000a). Diagnostic characteristics of 93 cases of a prepubertal and early adolescent bipolar disorder phenotype by gender, puberty and comorbid ADHD. *Journal of Child and Adolescent Psychopharmacology, 10*, 157–164.

Geller, B., Zimerman, B., Williams, M., Bolhofner, K., Craney, J. L., DelBello, M. P., & Soutullo, C. A. (2000b). Six-month stability and outcome of a prepubertal and early adolescent bipolar disorder phenotype. *Journal of Child and Adolescent Psychopharmacology, 10*, 165–173.

Geller, B., Zimerman, B., Williams, M., Bolhofner, K., Craney, J. L., DelBello, M. P., & Soutullo, C. A. (2001). Reliability of the Washington University in St. Louis Kiddie Schedule for Affective Disorders and Schizophrenia (WASH-U-KSADS) mania and rapid cycling sections. *Journal of the American Academy of Child and Adolescent Psychiatry, 40*, 450–455.

Geller, B., Zimerman, B., Williams, M., Bolhofner, B., Craney, J. L., Frazier, J., & Beringer, L. (2002). DSM-IV mania symptoms in a prepubertal and early adolescent bipolar disorder phenotype compared to attention-deficit hyperactive and normal controls. *Journal of Child and Adolescent Psychopharmacology, 12*, 11–25.

Geller, B., Zimerman, B., Williams, M., DelBello, M. P., Frazier, J., & Beringer, L. (2002). Phenomenology of prepubertal and early adolescent bipolar disorder: Examples of elated mood, grandiose behaviors, decreased need for sleep, racing thoughts and hypersexuality. *Journal of Child and Adolescent Psychopharmacology, 12*, 3–9.

Goodwin, F. K., & Jamison, K. R. (Eds.). (1990). *Manic-depressive illness.* New York: Oxford University Press.

Hollingshead, A. B. (1976). *Four Factor Index of Social Status.* New Haven, CT: Yale University Press.

Keller, M. B., Lavori, P. W., Friedman, B., Nielsen, E., Endicott, J., McDonald-Scott, P., & Andreasen, N. C. (1987). The Longitudinal Interval Follow-up Evaluation: A comprehensive method for assessing outcome in prospective longitudinal studies. *Archives of General Psychiatry, 44*, 540–548.

Klein, D. N., Ouimette, P. C., Kelly, H. S., Ferro, T., & Riso, L. P. (1994). Test–retest reliability of team consensus best-estimate diagnoses of axis I and II disorders in a family study. *American Journal of Psychiatry, 151*, 1043–1047.

Kraemer, H. C. (1992). How many raters?: Toward the most reliable diagnostic consensus. *Statistics in Medicine, 11*, 317–331.

Kramlinger, K. G., & Post, R. (1996). Ultra-rapid and ultradian cycling in affective illness. *British Journal of Psychiatry, 168*, 314–323.

Lukens, E., Puig-Antich, J., Behn, J., Goetz, R., Tabrizi, M., & Davies, M. (1983). Reliability of the Psychosocial Schedule for School-Age Children. *Journal of the American Academy of Child and Adolescent Psychiatry, 22*, 29–39.

National Institute of Mental Health Research Roundtable on Prepubertal Bipolar Disorder. (2001). *Journal of the American Academy of Child and Adolescent Psychiatry, 40*, 871–878.

Papolos, D. F., & Papolos, J. (1999). *The bipolar child: The definitive and reassuring guide to childhood's most misunderstood disorder.* New York: Broadway Books.

Puig-Antich, J., & Chambers, W. (1978). *The Schedule for Affective Disorders and Schizophrenia for School-age Children (Kiddie-SADS)–1978.* New York: New York State Psychiatric Institute.

Puig-Antich, J., Lukens, E., Davies, M., Goetz, D., Brennan-Quattrock, J., & Todak, G. (1985). Psychosocial functioning in prepubertal major depressive disorders: Part I. Interpersonal relationships during the depressive episode. *Archives of General Psychiatry, 42,* 500–507.

Puig-Antich, J., & Ryan, N. (1986). *The Schedule for Affective Disorders and Schizophrenia for School-age Children (Kiddie-SADS)–1986.* Pittsburgh, PA: Western Psychiatric Institute and Clinic.

Shaffer, D., Gould, M. S., Brasic, J., Ambrosini, P., Fisher, P., Bird, H., & Aluwahlia, S. (1983). A Children's Global Assessment Scale (C-GAS). *Archives of General Psychiatry, 40,* 1228–1231.

3

Bipolar Disorder in Children with Pervasive Developmental Disorders

SANDRA DEJONG and JEAN A. FRAZIER

Children and adolescents with pervasive developmental disorders (PDDs), including Asperger's disorder, also known as syndrome, frequently present to pediatricians, family physicians, pediatric neurologists, and child psychiatrists with a variety of emotional and behavioral disturbances (Chiu & Frazier, 2002; Frazier et al., 1999). Aggression and self-injury are the two most common reasons for presentation. These behaviors are often due to an underlying comorbid psychiatric condition, particularly one of the mood disorders, rather than due to the developmental disorder. Unfortunately, comorbid psychiatric diagnoses are often overlooked or under-identified in this population.

There has been ongoing debate about whether or not individuals with PDDs can also have comorbid mood disorders (Reid, 1972). However, over the past several years, due to clearer assessment criteria and diagnostic tools designed specifically for this population, it is more commonly accepted that comorbid mood disorders (major depressive disorder, bipolar disorder) occur in the developmentally disabled (Sovner & Parry, 1993; Ruedrich, 1993). Nonetheless, individuals with PDDs can suffer from treatable comorbid mood disorders for years despite frequent medical assessments and developmental evaluations.

Early identification of mood disorders in children with PDDs is crucial in order to reduce the problematic behaviors and symptoms that can further impair their overall functioning. In particular, since PDDs are associated with long-term disability and no specific pharmacological treatment, it is imperative that *treatable* comorbid disorders such as bipolar disorder be recognized and treated appropriately. Proper pharmacological intervention can lead to more optimal functioning and improved quality of life (Frazier, Doyle, Chiu, & Coyle, 2002).

This chapter discusses the overlap between mood disorders, particularly bipolar disorder, and PDDs, highlighting the extant literature regarding phenomenology, genetic liability, and pharmacology. Finally, several representative cases have been included to illustrate the importance of diagnosing bipolar disorder in children and adolescents with PDDs who clearly have signs and symptoms of the disorder, and providing them with the appropriate interventions.

DEFINITIONS AND EPIDEMIOLOGY

PDDs are a group of five disorders including autistic disorder, Rett's disorder, childhood disintegrative disorder, Asperger's disorder, and pervasive developmental disorder not otherwise specified (see Table 3.1) (American Psychiatric Association, 1994). These disorders share severe impairments in several areas of development: reciprocal social interaction skills, communication skills, and/or behaviors and interests (often circumscribed or stereotyped).

Asperger's disorder, which is especially relevant to the discussion of comorbid bipolar disorder, is on the autistic disorders spectrum, but includes relatively normal speech and intelligence, later age of onset (older than age 2 years), lower incidence of stereotypic movements, and better overall prognosis. For example, individuals with Asperger's disorder often do attend college and start their own families. Asperger's disorder is often considered a form of high-functioning autism, although this is controversial: some authors choose to emphasize an autistic continuum, whereas others suggest that Asperger's disorder should be regarded as a separate entity to avoid diagnostic confusion (Schopler, 1985; Szatmari, Bartolucci, Finlayson, & Krames, 1986; Wing, 1991). The current edition of the DSM includes Asperger's disorder for the first time as a diagnostic entity.

Pediatric bipolar disorder is a diagnosis that is under active discussion in the literature (Biederman, Klein, Pine, & Klein, 1998; National Institute of Mental Health [NIMH] Research Roundtable, 2001; Stein, Roizen, & Leventhal, 1999). Many investigators have described children with many of the hallmarks of bipolar disorder in their prepubertal years (Carlson, Loney, Salisbury, Kramer, & Arthur, 2000; Geller et al., 2000; Strober et al., 1998; Wozniak et al., 1995). A National Institute of Mental Health roundtable of experts on bipolar disorder met in April 2000 to better delineate the phenomenology of juvenile-onset bipolar disorder. Investigators studying bipolar I and bipolar II phenotypes that fit DSM-IV criteria in prepubertal children noted that the most frequent course is a long-duration episode with rapid cycling (ultradian or continuous cycling as the predomi-

TABLE 3.1. Characteristics of Pervasive Developmental Disorders

Diagnosis	Age of onset	Social	Communication	Behavior
PDDNOS	Varies	Impaired reciprocal social interaction	Impaired verbal and nonverbal communication	Atypical patterns of interest, unusual intensity
Autism	18 months	Gross and sustained impairment	Delay in or failure to develop spoken language	Restricted/stereotyped patterns of interest, rituals, motor mannerisms, preoccupation with parts of objects
Rett's syndrome	5–48 months; females only	Loss of interest in social environment	Nonverbal	Loss of purposeful hand movements, stereotypic hand movements, psychomotor retardation
Disintegrative disorder	2–10 years	Loss of social skills	Loss of communication skills	Loss of previously acquired play, motor, or adaptive behavior skills
Asperger's disorder	Preschool to early grade school	Impairment in nonverbal behaviors, peer relationships, and social/emotional reciprocity	Development on time (odd intonation, perseveration)	Motorically clumsy; restricted play and interests; preoccupation with routines, rituals

nant type) and mixed mania (i.e., co-occurring mania and depression) (NIMH Research Roundtable, 2001). Furthermore, children who met DSM-IV criteria were similar to those adults who have a history of continuous psychopathology with few well periods (< 20% of adults with bipolar disorder) (Geller et al., 2000).

PREVALENCE OF PERVASIVE DEVELOPMENTAL DISORDERS AND PEDIATRIC BIPOLAR DISORDER

The reported prevalence of autism has varied over the past decade. Autism was initially estimated to occur at a rate of 2–5 per 10,000 (Wing, 1993). When the diagnostic category was expanded to include all categories of PDDs, rates increased to 12–15 per 10,000 (Kemper & Baumann, 1998; Wing, 1993). More recently, the estimated prevalence has been placed at 1 out of 500 (Filipek et al., 2000; Tanguay, 2000). In one English survey conducted from July 1998 to June 1999 on 15,500 children (age range = 2.5–6.5 years), the prevalence rate for autism was found to be 16.8 per

10,000 and 45.8 per 10,000 for other PDDs (Chakrabarti & Fombonne, 2001).

The reported prevalence of Asperger's disorder has also varied, in part because of confusion and controversy regarding the diagnostic concept of Asperger's disorder (see Table 3.2). For example, Wing and Gould (1979) studied all physically and mentally disabled children under the age of 15 years in a section of London, and found two cases of Asperger's disorder (0.6 in 10,000). They identified four other cases (1.1 in 10,000) that early on appeared autistic in their presentation, but over time developed into cases of Asperger's disorder. In a 1991 population study of Asperger's disorder in Sweden (1,519 children; age range 7–16 years), Ehlers and Gillberg (1993) reported a prevalence rate of 0.36% (36.0 per 10,000) using conservative criteria and 0.71% (71 per 10,000) with broader criteria. In the study of preschool children reported by Chakrabarti and Fombonne (2001), Asperger's disorder was estimated to occur in 8.4 per 10,000. In yet another report, the prevalence was 1 out of 1,000 (Tanguay, 2000).

While the prevalence rate of Asperger's disorder or other PDDs is not clear, the estimated prevalence of pediatric bipolar disorder, given the ongoing phenomenological discussions, is even less clear. Depending on the diagnostic criterion utilized and the age range of the youth considered, it may be higher than the 1% previously described by Lewinsohn, Klein, and Seeley (1995). The Lewinsohn and colleagues study focused only on older adolescents and therefore does not adequately capture the prevalence of bipolar disorder in prepubertal children.

TABLE 3.2. Prevalence Rates

Diagnosis	Prevalence
PDD (Wing 1993; Kemper & Bauman, 1998; Filipek et al., 2000; Tanguay, 2000; Chakrabarti & Fombonne, 2001)	12–15/10,000 1 out of 500 45.8/10,000
Autism (Wing, 1993; Chakrabarti & Fombonne, 2001)	2–5/10,000 16.8/10,000
Asperger's (Wing & Gould, 1979; Ehlers & Gillberg, 1993; Tanguay, 2000; Chakrabarti & Fombonne, 2001)	0.6/10,000 8.4/10,000 36–71/10,000 1/1,000
Adolescent BPD (Lewinsohn et al., 1995)	100/10,000
PDD + BPD (Wozniak et al., 1997)	1.9% in a pediatric psychopharmacology clinic
Autism + BPD	?
Asperger's + BPD	?

Prevalence rates of comorbid PDDs, specifically Asperger's disorder and bipolar disorder, are even more difficult to ascertain. Wing (1991) reported that nearly half of the children with Asperger's disorder she followed into adolescence developed mood disorders. In a more recent study, Wozniak and colleagues (1997) looked at the entire group of children with PDDs who were referred to a specialized pediatric psychopharmacology program due to accompanying behavioral and emotional problems. They reported that out of a total of 727 children, 52 met criteria for PDDs, 114 met criteria for mania, and 14 out of 52 children with a PDD (1.9%) met criteria for both a PDD and mania (Wozniak et al., 1997). Clearly, these data suggest that there is an overrepresentation of children with PDDs in the overall bipolar disorder group as well as an overrepresentation of children with bipolar disorder in the PDDs group. However, there are a number of methodologic weaknesses in this study that limit the generalizability of these data. For example, the study does not specify the type of PDD (including Asperger's disorder) in each case. In addition, the study utilized indirect structured interviews that were administered by raters who were not trained mental health professionals. Finally, the children in this study were referred to a specialized pediatric psychopharmacology clinic for problematic behaviors, and therefore may not be representative of the general population nor even of a general psychiatry clinic. To date, there is little known about the prevalence of mood disorders in an unselected population of children with PDDs.

GENETICS

The genetics of autism are still being elucidated. The concordance rate in monozygotic twins for autism is 60% and for a broader autism phenotype is 90% (Bailey et al., 1995; Folstein & Rutter, 1977). In one study, the recurrence risk for autism (i.e., the frequency of autism in subsequently born siblings) was estimated at 6–8%, or up to 200 times the risk in the general population (Ritvo et al., 1989). However, a more complicated analysis of the same data utilizing a mixed model method (i.e., using a major-gene model, a polygenic model, a sibling-effect model, and a mixed model consisting of major-gene and shared-sibling effects) estimates that the relative recurrence risk of autism is only 4.5%, or no higher than 65 times the risk in the normal population.

PDDs and Asperger's disorder may be highly heritable. For example, a recent familial aggregation study demonstrated that in families of children with PDDs (34 with two affected children, 44 with one affected child, and 14 with an adopted child with a PDD), all components of the lesser variant of the PDD (or PDD-like traits) were more common in biological relatives than in nonbiological relatives. These results suggest a familial aggregation for traits. In this same study, children who had an increased risk of family members affected were those with a higher level of functioning and who came from families with two children affected with a PDD (Szatmari et al., 2000). However, the genetics of Asperger's disorder, in particular among the PDDs, have not been well studied. Future research needs to focus on the specific genetics of this disorder and those of each of the PDDs.

Relationship between Asperger's Disorder and Pediatric Bipolar Disorder

A possible genetic link between bipolar disorder and the PDDs has been explored. (See Table 3.3 for a summary of studies.) In general, children with PDDs are two to six times more likely to develop a comorbid psychiatric condition than their developmentally normal peers (Frazier et al., 1999; Matson, 1985; Matson & Bamberg, 1998; Rutter, Tizard, Yule, & Graham, 1976). In particular, some genetic studies suggest a link between autism spectrum disorders (ASDs) and bipolar disorder. For example, a recent study of five patients with a fragile site at 16Dq22-23 (associated with some developmental disabilities) reported that three had mental retardation, one had autistic disorder, and two had bipolar disorder (Kerbershian, Severud, Burd, & Larson, 2000). The authors hypothesized a possible etiological similarity in patients with bipolar disorder, Tourette's syndrome, and autistic disorder. Moreover, Gillberg and Wahlstrom (1985) found fragile sites in 25 of 66 cases (38%) of "autism and other childhood psy-

TABLE 3.3. Literature that Investigates the Relationship between Asperger's Disorder and Pediatric BPD

DeLong (1978)	Similar special abilities found in children with BPD as in ASD children with FH of BPD
DeLong & Dwyer (1988)	Incidence of BPD in relatives of autistic individuals 4.2% (4–5 times greater than the general population)
Gillberg (1989)	4/23 (17%) children with AS have FH of affective disorder
Piven (1991)	Lifetime prevalence of depression higher in parents of autistic individuals (27%), but not BPD
DeLong & Nohria (1994)	Different presentation in cases of autistic spectrum disorder with FH of BPD vs. without family history of BPD
Wozniak et al. (1997)	14/52 (21%) PDD clinic-referred patients also met criteria for mania

chosis." The site was at 16D in 13% of the 25 with fragile sites. However, at the time of the report, the authors had been unable to replicate these findings. Such studies are clearly very preliminary, and much work remains to be done. The results of the Human Genome Project may be very helpful in this regard

Several studies point to a relationship between bipolar disorder and the PDDs, particularly in those youth with a PDD and a positive family history of affective illness. However, not all of these studies are explicit about the number of children included that have Asperger's disorder. In some cases, the studies predate DSM-IV, which included the diagnostic criteria for Asperger's disorder for the first time.

DeLong and Nohria (1994) studied a group of 40 clinic-referred children with ASDs in repeated interviews over time. They included children with autism (as defined by the *Diagnostic and Statistical Manual of Mental Disorders*, 3rd ed., rev. [DSM-III-R]; American Psychiatric Association, 1987) Asperger's disorder (as defined by Wing [1981]), and pervasive developmental disorder, not otherwise specified (DSM-III-R). Thirty-three of 40 children had been diagnosed independently before referral, the majority using the Childhood Autism Rating Scale (CARS; Schopler, Reichler, & Renner, 1986). The remainder of the children were diagnosed by other developmental evaluation units. The authors looked for evidence of underlying neurological disease that could account for the developmental delays (using neurological exam, electroencephalogram [EEG], biochemical studies, computed tomography [CT], magnetic resonance imaging [MRI], positive emission tomography [PET], and karyotyping where indicated), and they assessed for a positive family history of psychopathology, particularly mood disorders. Fifty-two relatives were interviewed directly by clinicians who were blinded to the children's diagnoses (minimum of one from each family). Psychiatric history was obtained about 420 first- and second-degree relatives. Neuropsychiatric diagnoses were recorded according to the Family History Research Diagnostic Criteria, which is similar to the DSM-III-R (Andreasen, Endicott, Spitzer, & Winoker, 1977). Descriptive criteria, history of psychiatric hospitalizations, diagnosis by a psychiatrist, use of psychotropic medication, and other clinical information about each relative were recorded. This information was reviewed and a diagnosis was given to the relative only if the history was consistent with having a psychiatric disorder (Thompson, Orvaschel, Prusoff, & Kidd, 1982).

Twenty of the 40 children examined had neurological signs that were identifiable on exam (including encephalopathy with epilepsy, tuberous sclerosis, and fragile X), while the other 20 probands had no neurological signs. Those without neurological signs were overall higher functioning, and this group included three children with pervasive developmental disorder not otherwise specified, four with Asperger's disorder, and 13 with autism. Only two out of 20 (10%) children with ASDs with neurological signs had a positive family history of major affective disorders. In sharp contrast, 14 out of 20 (70%) of the group of children with ASDs without neurological signs had a positive family history of major affective disorders. The difference between the two groups was highly significant (χ^2 = 12.5, p < .001). Ten of the 14 (71.4%) "nonneurological" cases with a positive family history of affective illness had a parent with bipolar disorder. In these families, the overall proportion of relatives having major affective disorder was 26.8% (33 of 123).

DeLong (1994) also looked at the clinical features of 40 cases of idiopathic (i.e., "nonneurological") ASD with a positive family history of bipolar disorder (17 from the study discussed above). He contrasted the clinical features of these children with children diagnosed with bipolar disorder (DSM-III-R) and with children diagnosed with autism (DSM-III-R) with associated neurological etiologies (Younes, DeLong, Nieman, & Rosner, 1986). In consecutive interviews over time, an "exhaustive description" of behavioral features was recorded and behavioral features were analyzed. The children without a family history of bipolar disorder did not have marked cyclic variations in behavior and showed less florid agitation, fearfulness, and aggression than those with a positive family history of bipolar disorder. This study, as well as the other work by DeLong, includes data that are suggestive of a relationship between PDDs and bipolar disorder, but the studies are limited by the wide inclusion criteria for ASDs and the lack of clear criteria and use of validated instruments in the assessment of the bipolar disorder symptomatology. DeLong (1994) discussed three other studies of youth with ASDs plus a positive family history of affective disorder (Coryell, Endicott, Andreasen, & Keller, 1985; Fieve, Go, Dunne, & Elston, 1984; Gershon et al., 1982). The Gershon and colleagues (1992) study reported a similar total morbid risk of affective disorder (24%) DeLong concluded that there might be two groups of children with ASDs, positing that one group, the higher functioning one, might be an expression of early-onset bipolar disorder. In addition, the authors state that early-onset bipolar disorder may in fact impair affective and cognitive development and result in an affective deficit that manifests in the social remoteness, the severe obsessionality, and/or the manic–depression seen in some children with ASDs (DeLong & Nohria, 1994).

In an earlier report, DeLong and Aldershof (1988) documented that children with bipolar disorder had especially high rates of special abilities such as hyperlexia, calendar calculation, and obsessive interests. The authors found similar features in some children with autism or other PDDs who also had a family history of bipolar disorder. The behavior of those with ASDs without signs of neurological illness plus a positive family history of affective disorder differed from the children with ASDs with underlying neurological illness (DeLong & Nohria, 1994). The children in the latter group were lower functioning (by IQ), did not have cyclical behavioral patterns or affectively lability, and did not have special abilities or complex obsessional interests

The finding of a positive family history of bipolar disorder in children with PDDs, as suggested by DeLong, is consistent with other studies and case reports. For example, Gillberg (1985) described a case of Asperger's disorder with recurrent psychosis in an individual with a family history of bipolar disorder. Komoto, Usui, and Harate (1984) described three autistic children with comorbid affective disorders plus a positive family history of depression or bipolar disorder. DeLong and Dwyer (1988) looked at relatives of individuals with autism and found that the incidence of bipolar disorder was 4.2%, four to five times greater than in the general population. Despite the compelling evidence in the above studies and case series of an increased rate of bipolar disorder in children affected by ASDs and of an increased rate of bipolar disorder in the first-degree relatives of these children, other studies have not found such associations. For example, Gillberg (1989) found that only four out of 23 (17%) children with Asperger's disorder (age range = 5–18 years) and three out of 23 (13%) children with autism (same ages) had a positive family history of major affective disorder; this rate is similar to the rate of affective disorders in the general population. In addition, Piven and colleagues (1991) found a higher lifetime prevalence of major depression but not of bipolar disorder in the parents of autistic probands (27%) in comparison with population norms.

A relationship between Asperger's disorder-type symptoms and mood disorders was also suggested by Rourke's (1989) study of individuals with nonverbal learning disability (NVLD). NVLD is a disorder characterized by neuropsychological deficits in visual–spatial organization, nonverbal problem solving, psychomotor coordination, and other facets of social and communication skills (Rourke, 1989). Many children with Asperger's disorder share neuropsychological profiles similar to the profile seen in children with NVLD. Some investigators contend that there is an overlap between the diagnostic groups of those with Asperger's disorder and those with NVLD and/or that these two groups of individuals may be on a diagnostic continuum (Klin, Volkmar, Sparrow, Cicchetti, & Rourke, 1995). It is noteworthy that Ritvo and colleagues (1989) found an increased risk of mood disorder in children with NVLD compared to the general population.

In a retrospective case–control study of the neurodevelopmental antecedents of early-onset bipolar disorder (Sigurdsson, Fombonne, Sayal, & Checkley, 1999), an association was found between early-onset bipolar disorder and delayed language, social, and motor development (none of these youth met criteria for full autism). In addition, subjects with early-onset bipolar disorder had lower mean IQs than those with mild-to-moderate forms of juvenile affective illness. Finally, the authors also found that adolescents with early-onset bipolar disorder with developmental anteced-ents were at higher risk for developing psychotic symptoms.

NEUROBIOLOGY

In 1978, Damasio and Maurer postulated a mesolimbic model for autism. This mesolimbic model is supported by a study done by Bachevalier (1994), who was able to demonstrate deficits in social reciprocity and an increased rate of circumscribed behaviors in nonhuman primates who had their amygdalo–hippocampal complex lesioned during infancy.

The amygdala is a limbic structure that is a critical component in the loop in the brain that regulates affect. The amygdala has also been impli-cated, in neuropathological and neuroimaging studies, as one structure that may be affected in individuals who carry the diagnoses of Asperger's disorder and autism. For example, one neuropathological study done by Kemper and Bauman (1998) pointed to abnormalities in the distribution of pyramidal cells in the medial temporal lobe in pathological samples of indi-viduals with ASDs. In a structural anatomical brain MRI study, Abell and colleagues (1999) found left amygdalar enlargement in young adults with Asperger's disorder (12 males, three females; mean age = 28 years ± 9 months) when compared to 15 matched healthy controls. In addition, those with Asperger's disorder had a decrease in gray matter volume in the right paracingulate sulcus, the left occipitotemporal cortex, and the left in-ferior frontal sulcus, as well as increased volumes in the following struc-tures: the left amygdala/periamygdaloid cortex, the right inferior temporal gyrus, and the left middle temporal gyrus. The authors noted that these ar-eas of abnormal gray matter volume form part of the circuit that is cen-tered on the amygdala (Abell et al., 1999). These increases in volume may in fact correspond to studies of macrocephaly in children with autism. Such studies have reported that macrocephaly is common in this popula-tion and is usually not present at birth, but rather appears to become ab-normal in early and middle childhood in some children with autism (Bailey et al., 1995; Bolton et al, 1994; Lainhart et al., 1997).

Functional MRI studies (fMRI) have also been done in individuals with high-functioning PDDs or Asperger's disorder. For example, Baron-Cohen and colleagues (1999) used fMRI to study the "social intelligence" network, which consists of the orbito-frontal cortex, superior temporal gyrus, and amygdala. Six adults with autism or Asperger's disorder (mean age = 26.3 years) and 12 comparison subjects (six male, six female) were scanned while performing a task that required them to judge from the ex-pression of another's eyes what a person might be thinking or feeling.

While performing the task, the superior temporal gyrus and amygdala and some parts of the orbito-frontal cortex showed activation in the comparison subjects, while the fronto-temporal regions and not the amygdala were activated in the subjects with Asperger's disorder. In yet another fMRI study (Critchley et al., 2000), investigators did a case–control study of high-functioning individuals with autism (*n* = 9) versus healthy controls (*n* = 9) looking at activation while performing two tasks of reading specific facial expressions (one explicit and one implicit). During the explicit task, subjects with ASDs showed increased activation in the right amygdalo-hippocampal junction, right fusiform gyrus, anterior cingulate/medial prefrontal cortex, left dorsolateral prefrontal cortex, left superior temporal gyrus, and posterior cingulate/precuneus. During the explicit task, comparison subjects activated the left middle temporal gyrus (a cortical "face area"), but the subjects with ASDs did not. Implicit (unconscious) processing of facial expression in subjects with autism or Asperger's disorder was associated with significant activation in the left superior and middle temporal gyrus, cerebellar vermis, and left anterior insula. Notably, the left cerebellum and left amygdalo-hippocampal regions were activated in controls, but not in the subjects with ASDs. The authors postulated that individuals with autism had neurodevelopmental problems in the areas that did not activate during these tasks.

In general, the neuroimaging studies involving individuals with autism have tended to find left-sided abnormalities, while studies involving subjects with Asperger's disorder point to right-sided deficits (Hendren, De Backer, & Pandina, 2000). The involvement of the amygdala and the limbic system plus the apparently right-sided findings in subjects with Asperger's disorder may suggest areas of overlap with bipolar disorder, which has been described as a disorder with right hemispheric dysfunction (Weinberg, Harper, & Brumback, 1995).

ASSESSMENT AND DIAGNOSIS

Sovner (1986) clearly described how persons with mental retardation and developmental disabilities have different clinical presentations of psychiatric symptoms than cognitively normal individuals. Sovner focused much of his efforts on the population with PDDs, including individuals with Asperger's disorder. Sovner noted that there are four specific domains of functioning in individuals with PDDs that may be compromised at baseline but may be further affected by the existence of a comorbid affective illness, making the task of diagnostic formulation difficult and often resulting in the phenomenon called *diagnostic overshadowing*. Diagnostic overshadowing occurs when a comorbid psychiatric diagnosis is missed in an individual who is developmentally disabled and when the problematic behaviors that have arisen or worsened as a result of the coexistent psychiatric disorder are ascribed to the underlying developmental disorder (Chiu & Frazier, 2002). The four domains, as outlined by Sovner, that can be further compromised by a comorbid psychiatric disorder, particularly mood disorders, are (1) intellectual distortion, (2) psychosocial masking, (3) cognitive disintegration, and (4) baseline exaggeration.

Intellectual distortion consists of poor communication skills and concrete thinking, both of which limit a developmentally disabled person's ability to label or accurately describe complicated internal experiences. *Psychosocial masking* implies a further impoverishment of already compromised social skills by the affective illness. The increased impairment in this domain can be easily missed or misattributed. The result of psychosocial masking can be a bland presentation—for example, "delusions may look like nonspecific fears of young children," or manic expansiveness may lack the type of grandiosity that would be expected in an intellectually normal individual. Sovner (1986) noted that "when the normal person becomes manic, he thinks he's God. When the MR [mentally retarded] person becomes manic, he thinks he's not retarded." A similar situation can develop in children with PDDs. Furthermore, *cognitive disintegration* that occurs during an affective episode leads to stress-induced disruption of information processing, which can cause the patient to appear more psychotic than mood-disordered. Finally, *baseline exaggeration* refers to the exacerbation of preexisting cognitive deficits and maladaptive behaviors, making it difficult to recognize that the increased symptoms are actually a function of psychiatric illness rather than of the developmental disorder.

Clinicians therefore face many challenges in accurately making diagnoses, identifying target symptoms, and establishing outcome measurements in the population that is developmentally delayed. As Sovner (1986) underscored, in individuals with PDDs and comorbid mania, persistent poor judgment and distractibility can be key features of the psychiatric illness and may not be due to the developmental disability. In order to help delineate target symptoms in the population with PDDs, Sovner collected information on observable behaviors seen in these individuals who also suffered from mood disorders. These behaviors did not rely on the affected individual's self-report but rather on staff or caretaker observations of the affected individual's behaviors. For example, Sovner included the following as diagnostic criteria for depression in the population that is developmentally delayed: the onset of increased self-injurious behaviors, apathy, and loss of activities of daily living skills (e.g., onset of urinary incontinence). For mania, the following criteria were included: onset of or increase in the rate or frequency of verbalizations, overactivity, distractibility, and noncompliance.

TREATMENT

For an overview of medication treatment of pediatric bipolar disorder, please see Chapter 12 in this text. Here we review the literature that pertains only to children who have both bipolar disorder and a PDD.

The importance of accurate assessment and diagnosis cannot be over-emphasized in a discussion of optimal treatment, particularly in children and adolescents with a PDD or Asperger's disorder and comorbid mood disorders. These children need to be evaluated for underlying medical problems initially. Once a psychiatric disorder is diagnosed, the intervention strategies should be multimodal in nature (including all of the necessary interventions for the underlying developmental disability, close communication with caretakers, supportive psychotherapy, cognitive-behavioral therapy, family work, parental support, and psychopharmacology). Selection of medications for treating unwanted behaviors requires careful observation of the child with ASDs over a period of time, owing to the patient's limited ability to express problems verbally. Proper formulation needs to occur prior to initiating treatment.

Controlled medication studies for the treatment of mood disorders in the population with PDDs are lacking. Moreover, no controlled, randomized work has been done on pharmaceutical treatment in patients with ASDs and comorbid bipolar disorder. Below is a summary of some of the existing psychopharmacological literature in youth with PDDs and affective dysregulation, mood disorders, and/or bipolar disorder, which consists primarily of case reports and open trials that include only small numbers of patients.

Antidepressants

Clomipramine

One double-blind comparison of clomipramine (CMI) (mean dose = 152 mg/day), imipramine, and placebo in children with PDDs with anger and mood dysregulation demonstrated superiority of the active agents over placebo in decreasing stereotypies, compulsive behaviors, and anger (Gordon, State, Nelson, Hamburger, & Rapoport, 1993); however, a subsequent open-label study of CMI (in a younger group of children with PDDs) demonstrated little response and in fact reported that six out of the seven children worsened symptomatically while on CMI (Sanchez et al., 1996).

Fluoxetine

An open study of fluoxetine (dose range = 20–80 mg/day) in 17 patients with mild-to-profound mental retardation, reported improvement in six out of the eight youth who also had moodiness and impulse control problems (Cook, Rowlett, Jaselskis, & Leventhal, 1992).

Mood Stabilizers

Lithium

There are case reports indicating that lithium can be quite helpful in the treatment of bipolar symptoms in children with PDDs (Komoto et al., 1984; Steingard & Biederman, 1987). In addition, DeLong (1994) reported that four out of seven children with Asperger's disorder and comorbid bipolar disorder *plus* a positive family history of bipolar disorder had a good response to lithium.

In all of the above reports, lithium was well tolerated.

Valproate

In a study of five adults with both PDDs and comorbid mood disorders, Sovner (1989) found that four out of the five had a marked positive response to divalproex sodium and the fifth had a moderate response. Two of these individuals were diagnosed with autism, the first with rapid-cycling bipolar mood disorder and the second with "classic" bipolar disorder. Some of these patients were on thioridazine before switching over to divalproex; their deterioration during the medication crossover suggested that thioridazine had been helpful in controlling some bipolar symptoms. However, the divalproex ultimately controlled the symptoms better, according to staff reports, behavioral data, clinical interviews, and the Clinical Global Impressions Scale.

Divalproex (serum level = 64–124 µg/ml) was studied in an open fashion in 18 patients (age range = 8–18 years) with moderate-to-profound mental retardation who were irritable and self-injurious; 12 out of 18 (67%) improved (Kastner et al., 1993).

Finally, divalproex (mean dose = 892 mg; mean level = 75 µg/ml) was studied using a 10-month open retrospective design of 14 patients with PDDs with associated mood lability, impulsivity, and aggression. Ten of the 14 (71%) patients were rated as responders, with noted decrease in mood lability, impulsivity, aggression, and repetitive behaviors, and noted improvement in social relatedness and language (Hollander, Dolgoff-Kaspar, Cartwright, Rawitt, & Novotny, 2000).

Antipsychotics

Typical antipsychotics have long been used clinically to treat children with developmental disabilities. Several double-blind studies have demonstrated that these agents are effective in decreasing problematic behaviors in the population with PDDs.

Haloperidol

For example, haloperidol reduced anger, hyperactivity, and stereotypies in the dose range of 0.25–4 mg/day (Campbell et al., 1984).

Historically, children with developmental disabilities have been reported to have high rates of dyskinesias (29.7%) (Campbell, Adams, Perry, Spencer, & Overall, 1988) when treated with neuroleptics. However, when 16 neuroleptic-naive autistic children were assessed at baseline for stereotypies, mannerisms, or dyskinetic movements, 25% were found to have abnormal movements (Campbell et al., 1988). In addition, the blinded raters in this study were unable to distinguish these baseline abnormal movements from dyskinesias that other children with autism had developed during treatment with neuroleptics. Despite the possible high rates of dyskinesias in this population in general, medication-induced dyskinesias remain a concern, especially when considering the use of typical antipsychotics in this population.

Therefore, the atypical agents, with their lower incidence of dyskinesias, offer much promise for the pharmacotherapy of these children (Frazier et al., 1999; McDougle et al., 1997).

Risperidone

McDougle and colleagues (1997) reported that an open trial of risperidone (mean optimal dose = 1.8 ± 1.0 mg/day) led to significant improvement in repetitive behavior, aggression, impulsivity, and some elements of social relatedness in 18 children with ASDs (mean age = 10.2 ± 3.7 years; 78% IQs < 70).

Several open-label trials of risperidone in youth with PDDs who were affectively dysregulated have demonstrated that this agent may be effective in decreasing aggression and mood instability (Buitelaar, 2000). For example, Buitelaar (2000) administered risperidone (dose range = 0.5–4 mg) to 26 hospitalized aggressive subjects (age range = 10–18 years). All patients had some reduction in aggression; 14 (54%) had marked reduction and 10 had moderate reduction.

Although not yet published, a large-scale controlled double-blind study of risperidone in the population with PDDs fortunately has recently been completed (Arnold et al., 2000).

Independently, the effectiveness of risperidone in treating bipolar disorder in youth *without* PDDs was evaluated in a retrospective chart review. Risperidone was found to be helpful in decreasing mania, psychosis, and aggression in youth with bipolar disorder (Frazier et al., 1999).

Olanzapine

A recent open pilot comparison of olanzapine (mean dose = 6.5 ± 2.2 mg/day) and haloperidol (mean dose = 1.6 ± 0.9 mg/day) in 11 children with PDDs (age range = 4.5–11.8 years) showed both agents were effective in reducing problematic behaviors such as social withdrawal, hyperactivity, anger, mood lability, and stereotypic behaviors. The olanzapine-treated group gained significantly more weight (Malone, Sheikh, Choudhury, Luthra, & Delaney, 2000).

An open trial of olanzapine (mean dose = 9.8 mg/day) that has been recently reported suggests that this agent may be effective in the treatment of bipolar disorder in youth (Frazier et al., 2001). Although promising, both the efficacy and safety of the atypical agents for use with children with disorders in the PDD spectrum need to be investigated through longitudinal double-blind treatment studies. Although these agents are less likely to cause tardive dyskinesia, they have their own set of concerning side effects, notably hyperprolactinemia and pronounced weight gain, with its attendant morbidities. The weight gain seen on atypical agents occurs far more frequently than the tardive dyskinesia seen in children treated with the older antipsychotics. Therefore, studies assessing the long-term effects of these agents need to be done in this population. Finally, there are a couple of recently approved atypical agents that purportedly have less associated hyperprolactinemia and weight gain (quetiapine and ziprasidone). These agents also need to be assessed in a systematic fashion in children with PDDs.

CASE VIGNETTES

Case 1

J. V. is a boy who first presented to the outpatient clinic at age 13.5 years. He carried a diagnosis of Asperger's disorder, although both parents suspected issues beyond this diagnosis.

J. V.'s history revealed impairments in the following areas of social interaction (including nonverbal communication), interests, and behavior—despite grossly normal development—that are consistent with Asperger's disorder: Starting when J. V. was about 2 years old, his parents felt he was different from other children. Although his speech development was on time, he tended to speak in a loud voice, with odd prosody. While bright and verbally precocious, he exhibited pronominal reversals and repeated nonsensical words. He would engage in lengthy pedantic monologues regarding his circumscribed topics of interest. He had little capacity for reciprocal interaction or empathy. He had difficulties making friends because he was so controlling and bossy. He often preferred the company of adults and did not relate well with his peers. His eye contact was only fair. He also tended to be preoccupied with objects to the exclusion of people. For example, as a preschooler, he was preoccupied with his stuffed animals; as an adolescent, he was preoccupied with trains and he focused on mechanical items such as electrical sockets and washing machines.

At 6 years of age, J. V. had psychological testing. His Verbal IQ was 111 and his Performance IQ was 97 (normal range). He had difficulties grasping a pencil and was noted to have troubles placing pegs in the Klove Pegboard with one hand alone (consistent with fine-motor difficulties sometimes noted in children with Asperger's disorder, although not a diagnostic criterion). He had difficulties "reading" the emotional content of the Children's Apperception Test pictures (which contains drawings of familiar social situations, like a father sitting in a chair with a boy next to him). J. V. had consistent difficulty labeling the feelings shown in the pictures accurately and perceiving the social interactions taking place. The examiner concluded that he had a "social learning disability."

Features in the presentation and the history also pointed toward a diagnosis of juvenile-onset bipolar disorder: He suffered from ongoing mood disturbance, with frequently recurring episodes of mixed sadness and irritability, consistent with the findings reported in studies of juvenile-onset bipolar disorder. J. V. displayed sleep disturbance; loud, pressured speech; racing thoughts; distractibility; and heightened activity (his parents reported frenzied, intense behavior such as staying up all night washing clothes)—all criteria for a manic episode. In addition, J. V. showed evidence of psychosis, including a delusional belief regarding a girlfriend and the conviction that God could read his mind. His parents also reported increased aggression, which resulted in almost daily restraints at school.

J. V. was hospitalized at age 8 years. Since that initial hospitalization, he had been given multiple diagnoses, including conduct disorder, intermittent explosive disorder, and multiple anxiety disorders. One psychiatrist questioned whether he had a mood disorder and initiated lithium, which was stopped after a brief trial due to diarrhea. EEG, MRI, and a fragile X test were all negative. Past treatment included various selective serotonin reuptake inhibitors (SSRIs), imipramine, methylphenidate, and lithium, all of which led to side effects (predominantly sleep disturbance, agitation, and aggression). At the time of presentation, J. V.'s medications included clonidine (0.25 mg/day) and thioridazine (125 mgs/day), which had been started during a recent hospitalization for suicidal ideation.

J. V. was healthy and had no past history of head trauma, seizures, or motor or vocal tics. Of note, the family psychiatric history was positive for major depression in the father. There was also a history of hyperactivity in an uncle and probable alcoholism in both maternal grandparents. There was no family history of anxiety disorder, obsessive–compulsive disorder, developmental disorders, psychosis, bipolar disorder, or any neurologic disorders. Birth and developmental history were unremarkable except as described above.

J. V. was given the diagnosis of Asperger's disorder and bipolar disorder, mixed, with psychotic features, and features of obsessive–compulsive disorder. After an additional hospitalization and a number of different medication trials, he was stabilized on the combination of clonazepam, lithium up to 2,100 mg (levels of 1.0), and risperidone up to 3 mg a day. He has required no further hospitalizations over the past 3 years; in addition, J. V. will graduate from high school in 1 year, currently has a part-time job, and just got his driver's license.

Case 2

R. B. first presented as a 9-year-old boy with a diagnosis of high-functioning autism; he had a history of impaired communication (delayed language, with only three-word sentences at age 3), restricted interests (he was preoccupied with weather, geography, music, and numbers), failure to develop appropriate peer relationships, a lack of social and emotional reciprocity, and difficulties with nonverbal communication. His mother also described him as hyperactive, moody and irritable, quick to tantrum and get out of control, with a tendency to become giddy or silly. She noted a pattern of several months of difficulty with coping accompanied by increased tearfulness and aggression, followed by several months of improved ·behavior, affect, and coping skills. He presented as an inattentive young man with a slightly euphoric affect and a somewhat tangential thought process. Speech was notable for echolalia.

R. B. had a history of treatment with fluoxetine, which resulted in a hypomanic response. He also had a trial of clonazepam, with unknown effect. Perinatal history was notable for mother's hospitalization for kidney stones at 8 months gestation and a precipitous delivery. Medical history was significant for dental problems (four root canals of primary teeth), mild asthma, constipation, strabismus, and primary nocturnal enuresis. Past MRI and EEGs were normal. Family psychiatric history included depression in mother, bipolar disorder in grandmother, suicidality and paranoia in a paternal uncle, and anxiety on the mother's side.

R. B.'s presentation was consistent not only with mild autism (not Asperger's disorder because of the language delay), but also with bipolar disorder due to his chronic cyclical mixed mood disturbance, distractibility, psychomotor agitation, and loose thought process. R. B. was initiated on a trial of buproprion SR up to 150 mg twice a day and valproate up to 125 mg twice a day. Due to persistent irritability, a trial of risperidone was added, with resulting decrease in aggression, mood lability, and oppositionality and improved eye contact, sociability, and conversationality. When irritability reoccurred, olanzapine was initiated with good effect. He has been maintained on olanzapine alone since.

Case 3

L. Q. presented as a 9-year-old boy who carried a diagnosis of Asperger's disorder, attention-deficit/hyperactivity disorder, and obsessive–compulsive disorder. He was a young boy who had poor eye contact, early speech development with occasional pronominal reversals and some echolalia, a pedantic-pattern to his speech, lack of empathy for the feelings of others, preoccupation with mechanical things, poor peer relationships, poor fine-motor skills, difficulties with change in routine, and a history of needing to line his toys up over and over again as well as other compulsive behaviors. Mother described the appearance of daily temper outbursts over the past few months marked by irritability and episodes of hitting his head on a bedpost. In addition, he had tremendous difficulty falling asleep. On the Young Mania Rating Scale (Young, Biggs, Ziegler, & Meyer, 1978), his mother endorsed elevated and expansive mood, increased activity with little or no fatigue, and a marked increase in goal-directed activities. There had never been evidence of psychosis. On exam, he had very pressured speech and racing thoughts.

He had been treated in the past with methylphenidate up to 25 mg a day, which led to sleep disturbance and the emergence of tics. He also had had a fluvoxamine trial, which resulted in increasingly explosive behavioral outbursts.

Medical history was noncontributory. Birth and developmental history were unremarkable. Family history was significant for mood swings and alcoholism in the father and panic disorder in the mother.

He was given a diagnosis of Asperger's disorder, attention-deficit/ hyperactivity disorder, and obsessive–compulsive disorder. He also was diagnosed with bipolar disorder, mixed, due to the history of chronic cyclical mood disturbance with more than week-long episodes of both depression and irritability associated with sleep disturbance, increased activity, psychomotor agitation, impaired concentration, distractibility, pressured speech, and racing thoughts. He was started on a combination of mood stabilizer and antipsychotic, initially gabapentin and olanzapine, and most recently risperidone and lithium. Although he continues to struggle with irritability, the temper outbursts, pressured speech, and racing thoughts are considerably improved.

CONCLUSION

Comorbidity of bipolar mood disorder and affective illness in general in the PDDs has been described in the literature; however, systematic research regarding the comorbidity and its treatment is relatively sparse. More research is needed to better establish prevalence of this comorbidity and to characterize the clinical presentation. Accumulating genetic data suggests a link between bipolar disorder and high-functioning ASDs; however, more research is needed to delineate this relationship.

In addition, it is crucial for more controlled medication trials to take place in the populations of individuals with PDDs and ASDs, in general, and in those with comorbid affective disorders, in particular, to better identify effective and safe treatment modalities. The cornerstone of effective treatment, however, ultimately lies in careful diagnosis and assessment, with an emphasis on the consideration of comorbid affective disorders, particularly bipolar disorder, in this population.

REFERENCES

Abell, F., Krams, M., Ashburner, J., Passingham, R., Friston, K., Frackowiak, R., Rappe, F., Frith, C., & Frith, U. (1999). The neuroanatomy of autism: A voxel-based whole brain analysis of structural scans. *NeuroReport, 10*(83), 1647–1651.

American Psychiatric Association. (1987). *Diagnostic and statistical manual of mental disorders* (3rd ed., rev.). Washington, DC: Author.

American Psychiatric Association. (1994). *Diagnostic and statistical manual of mental disorders* (4th ed.). Washington, DC: Author.

Andreasen, N. C., Endicott, J., Spitzer, R. L., & Winokur, G. (1977). The family history method using diagnostic criteria: Reliability and validity. *Archives of General Psychiatry, 34*, 1229–1235.

Arnold, L. E., Aman, M. G., Martin, A., Collier-Crespin, A., Vitello, E., Tierney, E., Asarnow, R., Bell-Bradshaw, F., Freeman, E. J., Gates-Ulanet, P., Klin, A., McCracken, J. T., McDougle, C. J., McGough, J. J., Posey, D. J., Scahill, L., Swiezy, N. E., Ritz, L., & Volkmar, F. (2000). Assessment in multisite randomized clinical trials of patients with autistic disorder: The Autism RUPP Network. Research Units on Pediatric Psychopharmacology. *Journal of Autism and Developmental Disorders, 30*(2), 99–111.

Bachevalier, J. (1994). Medial temporal lobe structures and autism: A review of clinical and experimental findings. *Neuropsychologia, 32*, 627–648.

Bailey, A., Le Couteur, A., Gottesman, I., Bolton, P., Simonoff, E., Yuzda, E., & Rutter, M. (1995). Autism as a strongly genetic disorder: Evidence from a British twin study. *Psychological Medicine, 25*(1), 63–78.

Baron-Cohen, S., Ring, H. A., Wheelwright, S., Bullmore, E. G., Brammer, M. J., Simmons, A., & Williams, S. C.R. (1999). Social intelligence in the normal and autistic brain: An fMRI study. *European Journal of Neuroscience, 11*, 1891–1898.

Biederman, J., Klein, R. G., Pine, D. S., & Klein, D. F. (1998). Resolved: Mania is mistaken for ADHD in prepubertal children. *Journal of the American Academy of Child and Adolescent Psychiatry, 37*, 1091–1099.

Bolton, P., Macdonald, H., Pickles, A., Rios, P., Goode, S., Crowson, M., Bailey, A., & Rutter, M. (1994). A case–control family history study of autism. *Journal of Child Psychology and Psychiatry, 35*, 877–900.

Buitelaar, J. K. (2000). Open-label treatment with risperidone of 26 pychiatrically-hospitalized children and adolescents with mixed diagnoses and aggressive behavior. *Journal of Child and Adolescent Psychopharmacology, 10*(1), 19–26.

Campbell, M., Adams, P., Perry, R., Spencer, E. K., & Overall, J. E. (1988). Tardive and withdrawal dyskinesia in autistic children: A prospective study. *Psychopharmacology Bulletin, 24,* 251–255.

Campbell, M., Small, A. M., Green, W. H., Jennings, S. J., Perry, R., Bennett, W. G., & Anderson, L. (1984). Behavioral efficacy of haloperidol and lithium carbonate. *Archives of General Psychiatry, 41,* 650–656.

Carlson, G., Loney, J., Salisbury, H., Kramer, J. R., & Arthur, C. (2000). Stimulant treatment in young boys with symptoms suggesting childhood mania: A report from a longitudinal study. *Journal of Child and Adolescent Psychopharmacology, 10,* 175–184.

Chakrabarti, E., & Fombonne, E. (2001). Pervasive developmental disorders in preschool children. *Journal of the American Medical Association, 285*(24), 3093–3099.

Chiu, S., & Frazier, J. A. (2002). Autism, Asperger's and schizophrenia. In L. Finberg (Ed.), *Saunders manual of pediatric practice* (pp. 191–195). Philadelphia: Saunders.

Cook, E. H., Rowlett, R., Jaselskis, C., & Leventhal, B. L. (1992). Fluoxetine treatment of children and adults with autistic disorder and mental retardation. *Journal of the American Academy of Child and Adolescent Psychiatry, 31,* 739–745.

Coryell, W., Endicott, J., Andreasen, N., & Keller, M. (1985). Bipolar I, bipolar II, and nonbipolar major depression among the relatives of affectively ill probands. *American Journal of Psychiatry, 142,* 817–821.

Critchley, H. D., Daly, E. M., Bullmore, E. T., Williams, S. C. R., Van Amelsvoort, T., Robertson, D. M., Rowe, A., Phillips, M., McAlonan, G., Howlin, P., & Murphy, D. G. M. (2000). The functional neuroanatomy of social behavior: Changes in cerebral blood flow when people with autistic disorder process facial expressions. *Brain, 123,* 2203– 2212.

Damasio, A. R., & Maurer, R. G. (1978). A neurological model for childhood autism. *Archives of Neurology, 35,* 777–786.

DeLong, G. R. (1978). Lithium carbonate treatment of select behavior disorders in children suggesting manic–depressive illness. *Journal of Pediatrics, 93,* 689–694.

DeLong, G. R., & Dwyer, J. T. (1988). Correlation of family history with specific autistic subgroups: Asperger's syndrome and bipolar affective disease. *Journal of Autism and Developmental Disorders, 18,* 593–600.

DeLong, R. (1994). Children with autistic spectrum disorder and a family history of affective disorder. *Developmental Medicine and Child Neurology, 36,* 674–688.

DeLong, R., & Aldershof, A. L. (1988). An association of special abilities with juvenile manic-depressive illness. In L. K. Obler & D. Fein (Eds.), *The exceptional brain: Neuropsychology of talent and special abilities* (pp. 387–398). New York: Guilford Press.

DeLong, R., & Nohria, C. (1994). Psychiatric family history and neurological disease in autistic spectrum disorders. *Developmental Medicine and Child Neurology, 36,* 441–448.

Ehlers, S., & Gillberg, C. (1993). The epidemiology of Asperger syndrome: A total population study. *Journal of Child Psychology and Psychiatry, 34,* 1327–1350.

Fieve, R. R., Go, R., Dunne, D. L., & Elston, R. (1984). Search for biological/genetic markers in a long-term epidemiological and morbid risk study of affective disorders. *Journal of Psychiatric Research, 18,* 425–445.

Filipek, P. A., Accardo, P. J., Ashwal, S., Baranek, G. T., Cook, E. H., Jr., Dawson, G.,

Gordon, B., Gravel, J. S., Johnson, C. P., Kallen, R. J., Levy, S. E., Minshew, N. J., Ozonoff, S., Prizant, B. M., Rapin, I., Rogers, S. J., Stone, W. L., Teplin, S. W., Tuchman, R. F., & Volkmar, F. R. (2000). Practice parameter: Screening and diagnosis of autism. Report of the Quality Standards Subcommittee of the American Academy of Neurology and Child Neurology Society. *Neurology, 55,* 468–479.

Folstein, S. E., & Rutter, M. (1977). Infantile autism: A genetic study of 21 twin pairs. *Journal of Child Psychology and Psychiatry and Allied Disciplines, 18,* 297–321.

Frazier, J. A., Doyle, R., Chiu, S., & Coyle, J. (2002). Treating a child with Asperger's disorder and comorbid bipolar disorder? *American Journal of Psychiatry, 159,* 13–21.

Frazier, J. A., Biederman, J., Tohen, M., Feldman, P. D., Jacobs, T. G., Toma, V., Rater, M. A., Tarazi, R. A., Kim, G. S., Garfield, S. B., Sohma, M., Gonzales-Heydrich, J., Risser, R. C., & Nowlin, Z. M. (2001). A prospective open-label treatment trial of olanzapine monotherapy in children and adolescents with bipolar disorder. *Journal of Child and Adolescent Psychopharmacology, 11,* 239–250.

Frazier, J. A., Meyer, M. D., Biederman, J., Wozniak, J., Wilens, T., Spencer, T., Kim, G., & Shapiro, S. (1999). Risperidone treatment for juvenile bipolar disorder: A retrospective chart review. *Journal of the American Academy of Child and Adolescent Psychiatry, 8,* 960–965.

Geller, B., Zimerman, B., Williams, M., Bolhofner, K., Craney, J. L., DelBello, M. P., & Soutullo, C. A. (2000). Diagnostic characteristics of 93 cases of prepubertal and early adolescent bipolar disorder phenotype by gender, puberty and comorbid attention deficit hyperactivity disorder. *Journal of Child and Adolescent Psychopharmacology, 10,* 157–164.

Gershon, E. S., Hamovit, J., Guroff, J. J., Dibble, E., Leckman J. F., Sceery, W., Targum, S. D., Nurnberger, J. I., Jr., Goldin, L. R., & Bunney, W. E., Jr. (1982). A family study of schizoaffective, bipolar, bipolar II, unipolar, and normal control probands. *Archives of General Psychiatry, 39,* 1157–1167.

Gillberg, C. (1989). Asperger syndrome in 23 Swedish children. *Developmental Medicine and Child Neurology, 31,* 520–531.

Gillberg, C., & Wahlstrom, J. (1985). Chromosome abnormalities in infantile autism and other childhood psychoses: A population study of 66 cases. *Developmental Medicine and Child Neurology, 27,* 293–304.

Gordon, C. T., State, R. C., Nelson, J. E., Hamburger, S. D., & Rapoport, J. L. (1993). A double-bind comparison of clomipramine, desipramine, and placebo in the treatment of autistic disorder. *Archives of General Psychiatry, 50,* 441–447.

Hendren, R. L., De Backer, I., & Pandina, G. J. (2000). Review of neuroimaging studies of child and adolescent psychiatric disorders from the past 10 years. *Journal of the Academy of Child and Adolescent Psychiatry, 39*(7), 815–828.

Kemper, T. L., & Bauman, M. (1998). Neuropathology of infantile autism. *Journal of Neuropathology and Experimental Neurology, 57*(7), 645–652.

Kerbershian, J., Severud, R., Burd, L., & Larson, L. (2000). Peek-a-boo fragile site at 16D associated with Tourette syndrome, bipolar disorder, autistic disorder, and mental retardation. *American Journal of Medical Genetics (Neuropsychiatric Genetics), 96,* 69–73.

Klin, A., Volkmar, F. R., Sparrow, S. S., Cicchetti, D. V., & Rourke, B. P. (1995). Validity and neuropsychological characterization of Asperger syndrome: Convergence with nonverbal learning disabilities syndrome. *Journal of Child Psychology and Psychiatry and Allied Disciplines, 35*(1), 118–123.

Komoto, J., Usui, S., & Hirata, J. (1984). Infantile autism and affective disorder. *Journal of Autism and Developmental Disorders, 14*(1), 81–85.

Lainhart, J. L., Piven, J., Wzorek, M., Landa, R.,, Santangelo, S., Coon, H., & Folstein, S. (1997). Macrocephaly in children and adults with autism. *Journal of the American Academy of Child and Adolescent Psychiatry, 36*(2), 282–290.

Lewinsohn, P. M., Klein, D. N., & Seeley, J. R. (1995). Bipolar disorders in a community sample of older adolescents: Prevalence, phenomenology, comorbidity, and course. *Journal of the American Academy of Child and Adolescent Psychiatry, 34*, 454–463.

Malone, R. P., Sheikh, R. M., Choudhury, M. S., Luthra, V., & Delaney, M. A. (2000). Olanzapine vs. haloperidol in PDD: An open pilot study. *Journal of Child and Adolescent Psychopharmacology, 4*, 253.

Matson, J. R. (1985). Emotional problems in the mentally retarded: The need for assessment and treatment. *Psychopharmacology Bulletin, 21*(2), 258–261.

Matson, J. L., & Bamberg, J. W. (1998). Reliability of the assessment of dual diagnosis (ADD). *Research in Developmental Disabilities, 19*, 89–95.

McDougle, C. J., Holmes, J. P., Bronson, M. R., Anderson, G. M., Volkmar, F. R., Price, L. H., & Cohen, D. J. (1997). Risperidone treatment of children and adolescents with pervasive developmental disorders: A prospective, open-label study. *Journal of the American Academy of Child and Adolescent Psychiatry, 36*, 685–693.

National Institute of Mental Health Research Roundtable on Prepubertal Bipolar Disorder. (2001). Special communication. *Journal of the American Academy of Child and Adolescent Psychiatry, 40*, 871–878.

Piven, J., Gayle, J., Chase, G. A., Fink, B., Landa, R., Wzorek, M., & Folstein, S. E. (1991). Psychiatric disorders in parents of autistic individuals. *Journal of the American Academy of Child and Adolescent Psychiatry, 30*, 471–478.

Reid, A. H. (1972). Psychoses in adult mental defectives: Part 1. Manic depressive psychosis. *British Journal of Psychiatry, 120*, 205–212.

Ritvo, E. R., Freeman, B. J., Pingree, C., Mason-Brothers, A., Jorde, L., Jenson, W. R., Petersen, P. B., Mo, A., & Ritvo, A. (1989). The UCLA–University of Utah epidemiologic survey of autism: Prevalence. *American Journal of Psychiatry, 146*, 194–199.

Ritvo, E. R., Jorde, L. B., Mason-Brothers, A., Freeman, B. J., Pingree, C., Jones, M. B., McMahon, W. M., Petersen P. B., Jenson W. R., Mo, A., & Ritvo, A. (1989). The UCLA–University of Utah Epidemiologic Survey of Autism: Recurrence risk estimates and genetic counseling. *American Journal of Psychiatry, 146*, 1032–1036.

Rourke, B. P. (1989). *Nonverbal learning disabilities: The syndrome and the model.* New York: Guilford Press.

Ruedrich, S. (1993). Bipolar mood disorders in persons with mental retardation: Assessment and diagnosis. In R. J. Fletcher & A. Dosen (Eds.), *Mental health aspects of mental retardation: Progress in assessment and treatment* (pp. 111–129). New York: Lexington Books.

Rutter, M., Tizard, J., Yule, W., & Graham, 0. (1976). Research report, Isle of Wight studies, 1964–1974. *Psychological Medicine, 6,* 313–332.

Sanchez, L. E., Campbell, M., Small, A. M., Cueva, J. E., Armenteros, J. L., & Adams, P. B. (1996). A pilot study of clomipramine in young autistic children. *Journal of the American Academy of Child and Adolescent Psychiatry, 25,* 537–544.

Schopler, E. (1985). Convergence of learning disabilities, higher-level autism, and Asperger's disorder. *Journal of Autism and Developmental Disorders, 15,* 359.

Schopler, E., Reichler, R. J., & Renner, B. R. (1986). *The Childhood Autism Rating Scale (CARS): For diagnostic screening and classification of autism.* New York: Irvington.

Sigurdsson, E., Fombonne, E., Sayal, K., & Checkley, S. (1999). Neurodevelopmental antecedents of early-onset bipolar affective disorder. *British Journal of Psychiatry, 174,* 121–127.

Singh, R. N., & Aman, M. G. (1990). Ecobehavioral assessment of pharmacotherapy. In S. R. Schroeder (Ed.), *Ecobehavioral analysis in developmental disabilities* (pp. 182–200). New York: Springer-Verlag.

Singh, R. N., Ellis, C. R., & Wechsler, H. (1997) Psychopharmacoepidemiology of mental retardation: 1966–1995. *Journal of Child and Adolescent Psychopharmacology, 7(4),* 255–266.

Sovner, R. (1986). Limiting factors in the use of DSM-III criteria with mentally ill/ mentally retarded persons. *Psychopharmacology Bulletin, 22(4),* 1055–1059.

Sovner, R. (1989). The use of valproate in the treatment of mentally retarded persons with typical and atypical bipolar disorders. *Journal of Clinical Psychiatry, 50(3),* 40–43.

Sovner, R., & Parry, R. J. (1993). Affective disorders in developmentally disabled persons. In J. L. Matson & R. P. Barrett (Eds.), *Psychopathology in the mentally retarded* (2nd ed., pp. 87–147). Needham Heights, MA: Allyn & Bacon.

Stein, M. R., Roizen, N. M., & Leventhal, B. L. (1999). Bipolar disorder and ADHD [Letter to the editor]. *Journal of the American Academy of Child and Adolescent Psychiatry, 38,* 1208–1209.

Steingard, R., & Biederman, J. (1987). Lithium-responsive manic-like symptoms in two individuals with autism and mental retardation. *Journal of the American Academy of Child and Adolescent Psychiatry, 26,* 932–935.

Strober, M. (1992). Relevance of early age-of-onset in genetic studies of bipolar affective disorder. *Journal of the American Academy of Child and Adolescent Psychiatry, 31,* 606–610.

Strober, M., Morrell, W., Burroughs, J., Lampert, C., Danforth, H., & Freeman, R. (1998). A family study of bipolar I disorder in adolescence: Early onset of symptoms linked to increased familial loading and lithium resistance. *Journal of Affective Disorders, 15,* 255–268.

Szatmari, P., Bartolucci, G., Finlayson, A., & Krames, L. (1986). A vote for Asperger's disorder. *Journal of Autism and Developmental Disorders, 15,* 515–517.

Szatmari, P., MacLean, J. E., Jones, M. B., Bryson, S. E., Zwaigenbaum, L., Bartolucci, G., Mahoney, W. J., & Tuff, L. (2000). The familial aggregation of the lesser variant in biological and nonbiological relatives of PDD probands: A family history study. *Journal of Child Psychology and Psychiatry, 41,* 579–586.

Tanguay, P. E. (2000). Pervasive development disorders: A 10-year view. *Journal of the American Academy of Child and Adolescent Psychiatry, 39(9),* 1079–1095.

Thompson, W. D., Orvaschel, H., Prusoff, B., & Kidd, K. (1982). An evaluation of the family history method for ascertaining psychiatric disorders. *Archives of General Psychiatry, 39*, 53–58.

Weinberg, W. A., Harper, C. R., & Brumback, R. A. (1995). Neuroanatomic substrate of developmental specific learning disabilities and select behavioral syndromes. *Journal of Child Neurology, 10*(Suppl.), S78–S80.

Wing, L. (1991). The relationship between Asperger's disorder and Kanner's autism. In U. Frith (Ed.), *Autism and Asperger syndrome* (pp. 93–121). Cambridge, UK: Cambridge University Press.

Wing, L. (1993). The definition and prevalence of autism: A review. *European Child and Adolescent Psychiatry, 2*, 61–74.

Wing, L., & Gould, J. (1979). Severe impairments of social interaction and associated abnormalities in children: Epidemiology and classification. *Journal of Autism and Developmental Disorders, 9*, 11–29.

Wozniak, J., Biederman, J., Faraone, S., Frazier, J., Kim, J., Millstein, R., Gershon, J., Thornell, A., Cha, K., & Snyder, J. B. (1997). Mania in children with pervasive developmental disorder revisited. *Journal of the American Academy of Child and Adolescent Psychiatry, 36*, 1552–1559.

Wozniak, J., Biederman, J., Kiely, K., Ablon, J. S., Faraone, S. V., Mundy, E., & Mennin, D. (1995). Mania-like symptoms suggestive of childhood-onset bipolar disorder in clinically referred children. *Journal of the American Academy of Child and Adolescent Psychiatry, 34*, 867–876.

Younes, R. P., DeLong, G. R., Nieman, G., & Rosner, B. (1986). Manic-depressive illness in children: Treatment with lithium carbonate. *Journal of Child Neurology, 1*, 364–368.

Young, R. C., Biggs, J. T., Ziegler, V. E., & Meyer, D. A. (1978). A rating scale for mania: Reliability, validity and sensitivity. *British Journal of Psychiatry, 133*, 429–435.

4

Bipolar Disorder and Comorbid Disorders
The Case for a Dimensional Nosology

DEMITRI F. PAPOLOS

Over the last decade, mood disorders in children and adolescents have received much wider recognition as a number of research studies and clinical reports have clearly documented that these conditions are diagnosable entities in youth (Biederman et al., 2000; Carlson, 1984; Egeland, Hostetter, Pauls, & Sussex, 2000; Faedda et al., 1995; Geller et al., 1998; Kovacs & Pollock, 1995; Papolos & Papolos, 1999; Strober, 1998; Weller, Weller, & Fristad, 1995; Wozniack et al., 1995). However, in contrast to a growing body of literature on attention-deficit/hyperactivity disorder, oppositional defiant disorder, conduct disorder, obsessive–compulsive disorder, and other anxiety disorders, bipolar disorder has been relatively neglected, and its diagnosis in youth remains the subject of some controversy, particularly regarding prepubertal children.

A host of problems have contributed to the current state of affairs—not the least of which is the misconception that bipolar disorders in the pediatric age group are rare and unlikely to be seen before puberty. From at least the 1930s onward, standard clinical textbooks have omitted reference to the condition (Faedda et al., 1995). This prevailing view persists to the present day, despite clinical observations of mania and melancholia in the young since ancient times, as well as compelling reports from general population and family studies that have found a secular trend toward progressively earlier onset mood disorders in successive generations since 1940 (Adams, 1856; Kraepelin, 1921; Joyce, Oakley-Brown Wells, Bushnell, & Hornblow, 1990; Lavori et al., 1987). Indeed, estimates of the prevalence of bipolar disorder in youth are limited by the paucity of general population studies that have even included the possibility of this diagnosis within juvenile samples, as well as a strong historical bias against diagnosing the condition in this age group. Findings from current clinical and epidemiological research strongly suggest that juvenile mania may not be rare at all, but that it is difficult to diagnose, and rather than identify bipolar disorder in childhood, clinicians instead diagnose one or more of its multiple comorbidities (Biederman, Mick, et al., 2000; Lewinsohn, Klein, & Seeley, 1995; Papolos & Papolos, 1999).

Adult-onset and juvenile-onset forms of bipolar disorder have certain similar features and comorbidities as well as important and potentially misleading dissimilarities. In the juvenile form of the disorder, the complexities wrought by the frequent overlap of evidently nonspecific symptoms with other disorders commonly diagnosed in childhood, and the lack of wide recognition of major differences in the frequency and duration of mood/energy cycles between adult- and childhood-onset forms, have had a confounding affect on clinical diagnostic practice for many years (Biederman, Faraone, Chu, & Wozniak, 1999; Carlson, 1998; Faedda et al., 1995; Geller, Williams, et al., 1998; Kruger, Cooke, Hasey, Jorna, & Persad, 1995; Papolos & Papolos, 1999; Weller et al., 1995; Wozniack, Biederman, Kiely, et al., 1995; Wozniack, Biederman, Mundy, et al., 1995). Difficulties in diagnosing early, especially prepubertal-onset, bipolar disorder are not specific to the past half century. As early as 1931, Kasanin reported that nearly 25% of childhood-onset cases were misdiagnosed.

A 1995 meta-analysis of 2,168 cases by Faedda and colleagues was the first large-scale review of the world literature that took issue with prevailing diagnostic practices. Faedda and colleagues concluded that while clinical features of pediatric and adult bipolar disorder have similarities, pediatric cases cannot be defined solely by features characteristic of the adult disorder as delineated in contemporary international diagnostic systems such as the American Psychiatric Association's (1994) *Diagnostic and Statistical Manual of Mental Disorders*, fourth edition (DSM-IV), or the World Health Organization's International Classification of Diseases, 10th edition (ICD-10). This review, as well as subsequent diagnostic and family/genetic studies, have paved the way for a reevaluation of apparent myths that have largely obscured our understanding of the condition and its substantial prevalence in the general population.

Since the mid-1990s, several systematic clinical investigations and family/genetic studies have begun to shed light on the presentation and naturalistic course of the condition in childhood, suggesting a developmentally different presentation of bipolar disorder in young children as compared to its adult and even adolescent forms (Biederman, Faraone, Mick, et al., 1996; Farone, Biederman, Jetton, et al., 1997; Geller et al., 1998; Papolos & Papolos, 1999; Wozniack & Biederman, 1997). In addition to differences in phenomenology, course, and cycling pattern from adult bipolar disorder, symptomatic overlap and comorbidity with other conditions, including attention-deficit/hyperactivity disorder, oppositional defiant disorder, conduct disorder, obsessive–compulsive disorder, separation anxiety disorder, and other anxiety disorders, poses a major problem in clinical diagnosis (Biederman et al., 1999; Kovacs & Pollock, 1995; Papolos & Papolos, 1999).

BIPOLAR DISORDER AND COMORBID CONDITIONS

Historically, child and adult psychiatry have evolved as discrete disciplines. Indeed, the psychiatric profession has maintained this division by providing fellowship training programs and credentialing for child and adolescent psychiatry, as well as specialty journals defined by the developmental stage of patients of interest. This separation of child and adult psychopathology, while useful in the facilitation of developmentally appropriate treatment approaches for patients, has unwittingly led to ambiguity and discontinuities in diagnosis across the life cycle. A number of clinical diagnoses have been obscured by this practice. Attention-deficit/hyperactivity disorder, for example, was for many years rarely diagnosed in adulthood, as it was viewed as a condition that always started before the age of 7, and attenuated by late adolescence, and so was not within the province of adult psychiatry. More recently, longitudinal studies that followed children through childhood and adolescence into adulthood have contradicted this assumption, and led to changes in the DSM diagnostic nomenclature to recognize attention-deficit/hyperactivity disorder as a disorder that can present throughout the life cycle.

Comorbidity studies have found elevated rates of attention-deficit/hyperactivity disorder in adults diagnosed with bipolar disorder (Sachs, Baldassano, Truman, & Guille, 2000; Wender, 1998). Similarly, recent studies have found high rates of childhood-onset bipolar disorder in children originally diagnosed with attention-deficit/hyperactivity disorder (Papolos & Papolos, 1999; West, McElroy, Strakowski, Keck, & McConville, 1995; Wozniack, Biederman, Kiely, et al., 1995). This diagnostic discontinuity, based on myth rather than on clinical or epidemiological data, has had major effects on clinical diagnostic practice, and likely on treatment outcomes in child psychiatry for at least the past 3 decades.

Over the last 10 years, comorbidity research in childhood-onset disorders has focused primarily on attention-deficit/hyperactivity disorder and its multiple associated comorbid conditions. More recently, reports of *elevated* rates of comorbidity with attention-deficit/hyperactivity disorder have been found in individuals receiving primary diagnoses of bipolar disorder, obsessive–compulsive disorder, oppositional defiant disorder/conduct disorder, Tourette's syndrome, pervasive developmental disorder, and obsessive–compulsive disorder and other anxiety disorders (DeLong, 1999; Geller, Biederman, Griffin, Jones, & Lefkowitz, 1996; Kerbeshian, Burd, & Klug, 1995; Kovacs & Pollock, 1995). Over the past 2 decades, numerous investigations have examined the epidemiology, genetic basis, phenomenology, course, and treatment outcome of bipolar disorder in the adult population (Akiskal et al., 1995; Baldessarini, Tohen, & Tondo, 2000; Coryell et al., 1995; Egeland, 1988; Regier et al., 1990; Winokur, Tsuang, & Crowe, 1982). Until relatively recently, studies of rates of comorbid conditions in adults with bipolar disorder have been limited largely to reports of high rates of substance abuse, particularly alcoholism and polysubstance abuse (Regier et al., 1990). The discovery of elevated rates of panic disorder and obsessive–compulsive disorder in adult bipolar disorder has awaited more recent epidemiological catchment area studies and studies of large clinical samples (Chen & Dilsaver, 1995a, 1995b; Schurhoff et al., 2000).

So, for both adult and childhood-onset bipolar disorder, the complex issues surrounding comorbidity and the thorny diagnostic boundary issues that they raise have come relatively recently to the field of psychiatry. Diagnostic manuals such as the American Psychiatric Association's *Diagnostic and Statistical Manual* (DSM) and the World Health Organization's International Classification of Diseases (ICD) describe psychiatric disorders as separate illnesses. From the outset, the DSM endorsed the view that there was a diagnostic hierarchy—if two conditions co-occured, the disorder lower on the hierarchy could not be diagnosed. For example, in the DSM-III, panic disorder could not be diagnosed if panic attacks occurred within the same time frame as periods of major depression. Over time, with the advent of greater clinical experience and further epidemiological research, DSM-IV has been modified to encompass the view that the co-occurance of two or more disorders—*psychiatric comorbidity*—in the same patient is more the rule than the exception. Because the National Institute of Mental Health (NIMH) Epidemiologic Catchment Area and subsequent epidemiological studies of children and adults found extensive comorbidity, clinical views and the DSM have shifted away from diagnostic hierarchies, and have begun to accept a more empirical approach to diagnosis that allows for the possibility of multiple co-occuring conditions, without assuming the primacy of one condition over another. Epidemiological studies provide only one piece of the puzzle: they demonstrate that comorbidity is a valid phenomenon, but they do not clarify the psychiatric phenotype or the boundaries between distinct categories of symptoms. Uncertainties about the best definition of disease phenotype, variable expression of the illness, difficulties in the assessment of lifetime diagnosis, and the perplexities of variable age of onset are among the critical issues that play a confounding role not only in the clinical realm, but also in the performance of genetic studies. Perhaps the most significant confounding factor is genetic heterogeneity and the accompanying problem of establishing more homogeneous subtypes for the disorder. Taken together, these factors may in large measure, along with variable reported age of onset of illness, account for the lack of replication of studies that have reported positive associations between the illness and a linked genetic marker (Baron et al., 1993; Egeland, 1988; Kelsoe et al., 1988; Pauls et al., 1991).

In the genetic study of the Old Order Amish conducted by Janice Egeland and colleagues (Egeland, 1988), a highly positive LOD score on chromosome 11 was lost when a 40-year-old Amish man had an unexpectedly late onset, significantly altering the results of the study (Pauls et al., 1991). Subsequent studies have found that age at onset of bipolar disorders may be a key indicator for identifying more homogeneous clinical subtypes. Schurhoff and colleagues (2000), from a consecutively recruited sample of 210 patients diagnosed with bipolar disorder, compared early-onset (n = 58) and late-onset (n = 39) forms using cutoff points at age at onset before 18 years and after 40 years for the two subgroups. These investigators found that the early-onset group had the most severe form of bipolar disorder, with more psychotic features, more mixed episodes, and greater comorbidity with panic disorder. First-degree relatives of early-onset patients also had a higher risk of affective disorders, particularly bipolar disorder, suggesting that early- and late-onset bipolar disorder differ in clinical expression and degree of familial risk, and therefore may constitute distinct variants of the condition.

Within the general category of juvenile-onset bipolar disorder there appear to exist various subtypes that represent either sets of comorbid conditions with unique but partially shared genetic or other diatheses, or a spectrum of conditions that share discrete symptoms, possibly expressed in a developmental sequence, with different sets of symptoms waxing and waning chronologically, perhaps in response to environmental factors and central nervous system maturation.

COMORBIDITY OF BIPOLAR DISORDER WITH ATTENTION-DEFICIT/HYPERACTIVITY DISORDER

Attention-deficit/hyperactivity disorder is comorbid with a variety of psychiatric disorders. These include oppositional defiant disorder and conduct disorder, as well as affective, anxiety, and learning disorders (Pliszka et al., 2000). Considerable debate has surrounded the meaning of this overlap. Does it occur by chance, or is it an artifact of referral bias? Are the comorbid conditions secondary to the attention-deficit/hyperactivity disorder, or does their co-occurance represent a chronological sequence on a developmental continuum? Alternatively, attention-deficit/hyperactivity disorder may exist as distinct subtypes, each with selective comorbidities. Three of the seven DSM-IV criteria for bipolar disorder are shared with attention-deficit/hyperactivity disorder: distractibility, physical restlessness, and over-talkativeness. Therefore, distinguishing children with attention-deficit/hyperactivity disorder from childhood-onset bipolar disorder by clinical assessment alone is difficult. Many (perhaps most) children later diagnosed with bipolar disorder originally present with symptoms and behaviors that support a simultaneous diagnosis of attention-deficit/hyperactivity disorder (Biederman, Faraone, Mick, et al., 1996). Wozniack, Biederman, Mundy, and colleagues (1995) found that 94% of a sample of 43 children aged 12 or younger evaluated with current or previous mania also met DSM-III-R criteria for attention-deficit/hyperactivity disorder, while only 19% with a diagnosis of attention-deficit/hyperactivity disorder also met criteria for current or previous mania. Furthermore, when the diagnoses of attention-deficit/hyperactivity disorder and bipolar disorder in children with both conditions were reassessed after removing overlapping symptoms, the majority of children continued to meet diagnostic criteria for both conditions.

Because of concerns about the validity of the diagnosis of mania in children, Biederman and colleagues (1995) followed their initial work with systematic evaluations of external validators that addressed issues of assessor bias, symptom overlap, and familial aggregation. The Child Behavioral Checklist (CBCL) was used to examine children who received the clinical diagnosis of mania. Using this well-validated instrument, it was possible to discriminate between attention-deficit/hyperactivity disorder and childhood-onset bipolar disorder patients, as these investigators found excellent convergence between CBCL scales; clinical scales of Delinquent Behavior, Aggressive Behavior, Somatic Complaints, Anxious/Depressed, and Thought Problems; and the structured diagnostic interview-derived diagnosis of mania. Confirmation that the CBCL discriminates juvenile mania from attention-deficit/hyperactivity disorder was recently independently reported by Hazell, Lewin, and Carr (2000).

Further progress toward the clarification of the difficult clinical distinction between these two conditions was made by Geller, Williams, and colleagues (1998) who, using data collected from 60 individuals with bipolar disorder, 60 individuals with attention-deficit/hyperactivity disorder, and 90 community controls, found that elated mood, grandiosity, hypersexuality, decreased need for sleep, racing thoughts, and all other mania items except excess energies and distractibility were significantly and substantially more frequent among bipolar disorder than attention-deficit/hyperactivity disorder cases (e.g., elation: 86.7% bipolar disorder vs. 5.0% attention-deficit/hyperactivity disorder; grandiosity: 85.0% bipolar disorder vs. 6.7% attention-deficit/hyperactivity disorder). In the bipolar disorder group, 55.0% had grandiose delusions, 26.7% had suicidality with plan/intent, and 83.3% were rapid, ultrarapid, or ultradian cyclers.

The nature of attention-deficit/hyperactivity disorder as a prodromal feature, phenocopy, comorbid condition, or misdiagnosis may become clearer with long-term follow-up of attention-deficit/hyperactivity disorder cases to determine if comorbid diagnoses predict course and prognosis, and by the application of family/genetic studies, which are uniquely suited for the evaluation of complex patterns of comorbidity. Wozniack and her colleagues (Wozniack, Biederman, Mundy, et al., 1995) were the first to apply this approach to examine the strikingly high rates of comorbidity between attention-deficit/hyperactivity disorder and childhood-onset bipolar disorder. They performed diagnostic assessments of the families of their sample of children diagnosed with both mania and attention-deficit/hyperactivity disorder, and found that (1) first-degree relatives of probands diagnosed with childhood-onset bipolar disorder and attention-deficit/hyperactivity disorder and relatives of probands with attention-deficit/hyperactivity disorder alone were at significantly greater risk for attention-deficit/hyperactivity disorder than relatives of normal controls subjects; and, more specifically, that (2) an elevated risk for bipolar disorder was observed only among relatives when the child proband had both bipolar disorder and attention-deficit/hyperactivity disorder but not in those with attention-deficit/hyperactivity disorder alone. This observation of cosegregation, whereby the two disorders segregate together in families, suggests that childhood-onset bipolar disorder and attention-deficit/hyperactivity disorder may be transmitted together, not independently, at least in a subgroup of families, and that childhood-onset bipolar disorder *plus* attention-deficit/hyperactivity disorder may represent a distinct diagnostic subtype. If these findings are confirmed by independent family/genetic studies, they would suggest that this comorbid syndrome may have a specific genotype as well as course, treatment response, and outcome, and therefore may represent a unique condition.

The findings of elevated rates of comorbidity in both childhood- and adult-onset bipolar disorder parallel similar findings in several other major diagnostic categories in child and adolescent psychiatry (DeLong, 1999; Faraone, Biederman, Jetton, & Tsuang, 1997; Geller et al., 1996; Kerbesian et al., 1995; Kovacs & Pollock, 1995; Pliska, Sherman, Barrow, & Irick, 2000). From a clinical perspective, these emerging data underscore the need to eschew any notions of hierarchical diagnosis, and, furthermore, to begin to call into question categorical views of diagnosis as they are now promulgated in the DSM. The political debate and current controversy surrounding the existence of childhood-onset bipolar disorder appears, at least in part, to be centered around the issue of what to call these entities that meet multiple diagnostic categories and, more pointedly, which condition takes precedence in terms of instituting treatment.

COMORBIDITY OR SYMPTOM OVERLAP OF OPPOSITIONAL DEFIANT DISORDER AND CONDUCT DISORDER WITH CHILDHOOD-ONSET BIPOLAR DISORDER AND ATTENTION-DEFICIT/HYPERACTIVITY DISORDER

Oppositional defiant disorder is a common clinical diagnosis that has attracted little research interest. Indeed, doubts about its validity as a distinct category remain (Rey, 1993). The diagnostic construct underwent substantial changes between DSM-III-R and DSM-IV. Current evidence supports a distinction between the symptoms of oppositional defiant disorder and many symptoms of conduct disorder, but there has been a continuing controversy about whether aggressive symptoms should be considered to be part of oppositional defiant disorder or of conduct disorder. A proportion of children with oppositional defiant disorder later develop conduct disorder, and a proportion of those with conduct disorder later meet criteria for antisocial personality disorder; moreover, oppositional defiant disorder and conduct disorder frequently co-occur with other psychiatric conditions.

In a meta-analysis of the literature, Rey (1993) reported that one-third of all community-based children with any psychiatric condition had a diagnosis of oppositional defiant disorder, that symptoms of oppositional defiant disorder appear to be stable over time, and that oppositional defiant disorder has a developmental profile and sex distribution different from those of conduct disorder. Rey also reported that the reliability of the diagnosis of oppositional defiant disorder is low, and that while there was some support for oppositional defiant disorder as a category that reflects an oppositional–aggressive psychological dimension, which is different from a delinquent dimension, he found little evidence in the literature for making oppositional defiant disorder a part of the construct of conduct disorder.

In a follow-up study that examined psychiatric predictors of the onset of conduct disorder in a clinic-referred sample of 177 preadolescent boys who were studied for a period of 6 years, Loeber, Green, Keenan, and Lahey (1995) found that of all conduct disorder symptoms, physical fighting, low socioeconomic status (SES) of the parent, oppositional defiant disorder, and parental substance abuse best predicted the onset of conduct disorder. Degree of lack of control over aggressive impulses, low SES, and drug abuse in parents (all measurable predictors) indicate that genetic and environmental influence combine to influence this transformation from what is termed oppositional defiant disorder to the more severe conduct disorder.

What environmental and genetic factors might influence the switch from attention-deficit/hyperactivity disorder to bipolar disorder or the transformation of a subgroup of individuals initially diagnosed with attention-deficit/hyperactivity disorder to develop conduct disorder and substance abuse disorder, while others with attention-deficit/hyperactivity disorder progress through adolescence without the same temperamental expression in behavior that runs up against authority? It is well known that approximately one-third of children with attention-deficit/hyperactivity disorder show aggressive and antisocial behavior. Almost all children younger than age 12 who meet criteria for oppositional defiant disorder or conduct disorder meet criteria for attention-deficit/hyperactivity disorder (Reeves, Werry, Elkind, & Zametkin, 1987; Szatmari, Boyle, & Offord, 1989). It has also been established that the siblings of attention-deficit/hyperactivity disorder probands have an expected prevalence of conduct disorder, and that their parents show higher than expected levels of antisocial personality disorder. In a seminal study, Biederman, Faraone, Hatch, and colleagues (1997) assessed 140 children with attention-deficit/hyperactivity disorder and 120 normal controls at baseline and 4 years later to evaluate the overlap between attention-deficit/hyperactivity disorder and oppositional defiant disorder and to address whether oppositional defiant disorder is a subsyndromal form of conduct disorder, and, if so, whether it is a precursor or prodromal syndrome of conduct disorder. They found that of children who had attention-deficit/hyperactivity disorder at baseline, 65% had comorbid oppositional defiant disorder and 22% had comorbid conduct disorder. Among those with oppositional defiant disorder, 32% had comorbid conduct disorder. Children with both oppositional defiant disorder and conduct disorder had more severe symptoms of oppositional defiant disorder, and more comorbid psychiatric disorders, particularly bipolar disorder. These investigators concluded that two subtypes of oppositional defiant disorder were associated with attention-deficit/hyperactivity disorder: one is prodromal to conduct disorder and another is subsyndromal to conduct disorder but not likely to progress into conduct disorder in later years. These oppositional defiant disorder subtypes have different correlates, course, and outcome.

A growing literature suggests that attention-deficit/hyperactivity disorder with antisocial comorbidity may be nosologically distinct from other forms of attention-deficit/hyperactivity disorder (Faraone et al., 1998). A similar pattern has been observed for attention-deficit/hyperactivity disorder and bipolar disorder. In a study that retrospectively examined the evolution of symptoms in a group of 120 children and adolescents (age range = 3–18) diagnosed with bipolar disorder, using an 85-item questionnaire containing all DSM-IV symptoms of bipolar disorder, attention-deficit/hyperactivity disorder, oppositional defiant disorder, and conduct disorder, 96% met DSM-IV criteria for attention-deficit/hyperactivity disorder, 97% met criteria for oppositional defiant disorder, and 65% met criteria for both oppositional defiant disorder and conduct disorder (Papolos & Papolos, 1999). This finding supports the idea that attention-deficit/hyperactivity disorder *plus* conduct disorder *plus* bipolar disorder may be a separate diagnostic entity with a definable phenotype.

Faraone and colleagues (1998) used data from their study of 140 families with attention-deficit/hyperactivity disorder and 120 control families to determine if conduct and bipolar disorders in boys with attention-deficit/hyperactivity disorder should be considered alternative manifestations of the same familial disorder. Families were stratified into bipolar, antisocial, and other types, and investigators examined the risk to relatives separately for probands with and without the comorbid conditions, and divided the group of attention-deficit/hyperactivity disorder-conduct disorder probands into those with and without bipolar disorder. Their results provide fairly consistent support for the hypothesis that antisocial-attention-deficit/hyperactivity disorder and bipolar-attention-deficit/hyperactivity disorder subtypes are different manifestations of the same familial condition.

In a sample of 224 child twins (140 monozygotic, 84 dizygotic), Coolidge, Thede, and Young (2000) examined the heritability and comorbidity of attention-deficit/hyperactivity disorder with conduct disorder, oppositional defiant disorder, and executive function deficits. The results of their multivariate twin analysis suggest that attention-deficit/hyperactivity disorder shares most of its genetic liability with conduct disorder, oppositional defiant disorder, and executive function deficits. This strategy goes beyond the examination of a genetic association between comorbid conditions to include specific and measurable neuropsychological deficits that have been found to be commonly associated with attention-deficit/hyperactivity disorder and other disruptive disorders of childhood. The fact that three categorical diagnoses, as delineated in DSM-IV, and a specific set of measurable deficits in cognitive performance, were all found to share a common genetic liability in twin pairs underscores the possibility that diagnostic boundaries, as currently defined by the DSM, may need to be expanded to encompass comorbid conditions, specified criteria from different diagnostic groupings, and objectively measured cognitive deficits.

COMORBIDITY OF SUBSTANCE USE DISORDER WITH BIPOLAR DISORDER

Population-based studies have documented that among all patients with major psychiatric disorders, those with bipolar disorder have the highest prevalence of comorbid substance abuse and dependence. In an epidemiological survey (Kessler et al., 1994), the lifetime prevalence for any mood disorder was 19.3%, and for any substance use disorder was 26.6%. In the NIMH Epidemiologic Catchment Area Study (ECA), mood disorders (major depression, dysthymia, bipolar disorder) had an overall prevalence of 8.3%. Bipolar disorder was associated with the highest risk (odds ratio = 6.6) of any Axis I disorder for coexistence with drug or alcohol abuse. Among the bipolar I disorder group, 60.7% had a comorbid substance use disorder: 46% had an alcohol diagnosis and 40.7% had a drug-abuse or drug-dependence diagnosis (Regier et al., 1990).

While it is inherently difficult to diagnose bipolar disorder, particularly in its milder forms, it is considerably more difficult in the context of substance use disorder because of the ability of drug abuse to mimic almost any major psychiatric disorder. Research studies have found that patients with comorbid bipolar disorder and substance use disorder have more lifetime psychiatric hospitalizations than those with bipolar disorder who do not abuse substances. In addition, Sonne and Brady (1999) found that substance abusers have a much earlier age of onset of bipolar disorder, indicating that the mood disorder preceded the substance abuse and therefore may have contributed to the initial appeal of addictive drugs. Certainly, clinical evidence suggests that untreated bipolar disorder dramatically lessens the likelihood of abstinence from drugs of abuse. Some clinical investigators have suggested that the undertreatment of these conditions may be a significant cause of relapse from efforts at detoxification. However, there are no controlled studies that have examined this question.

The analysis of patterns of co-occurrence and cotransmission of affective disorders and alcoholism in families may provide clues for understanding the excess comorbidity of these conditions in clinical settings and in the general population (Winokur et al., 1994). In a family study of the relatives of patients with bipolar disorder, unipolar depression, alcoholism, and combinations thereof, Maier and Merikangas (1996; Maier, Lichterman, Minges, Delmo, & Heun, 1995) observed an excess comorbidity between affective disorders and alcoholism in all groups of relatives studied. However, the sharing of familial etiological components was not a major contributor to the excess comorbidity between affective disorders and alcoholism. Unipolar depression and alcoholism segregated independently in families, but modest correlation between familial components of alcoholism and bipolar disorder was observed.

Todd, Geller, Neuman, Fox, and Hickok (1996) conducted a study of 6- to 12-year-olds with major depressive disorder ($n = 76$) and matched normal controls ($n = 31$). Over 30% of patients originally diagnosed with major depressive disorder switched to bipolar disorder after 2 to 5 years of follow-up (Geller, Fox, & Clark, 1994). In this sample, the prevalence of alcoholism among the relatives of the major depressive disorder and bipolar probands was found to be two to three times that reported for control relatives and twice that reported for the relatives of adult major depressive disorder and bipolar probands. Mood disorders and maternal alcoholism were independently transmitted, while paternal alcoholism increased the risk for mood disorder in offspring. Papolos and Papolos (1999), in a study of 120 families of children with bipolar disorder ages 5–18, found that over 80% of children with onset of bipolarity before age 9 had family histories of bilineal transmission of mood disorder and alcoholism. Taken together, these findings raise the possibility that high rates of assortative mating between individuals with mood disorder, particularly those individuals with bipolar disorder, and alcoholism, may be primary risk factors for pediatric-onset bipolar disorder.

In one of the few studies to assess the risk for substance use disorder in child- versus adolescent-onset bipolar disorder with attention to comorbid psychopathology, Wilens and colleagues (1999) found that, after stratification of the sample by age, patients with adolescent-onset bipolar disorder had an 8.8 times higher risk for substance use disorder than those with childhood-onset bipolar disorder. While bipolar disorder has emerged as a risk factor for substance use disorder in youth, as well as in adults, the association between bipolar disorder and substance use disorder in youth is complicated by comorbidity with conduct disorder. Using familial risk analysis to attempt to unravel associations among the three disorders, Biederman, Faraone, Wozniak, and Monuteaux (2000) compared relatives of four proband groups: (1) conduct disorder *plus* bipolar disorder, (2) bipolar disorder *without* conduct disorder, (3) conduct disorder *without* bipolar disorder, and (4) control subjects without bipolar disorder or conduct disorder. They found that the effects of bipolar disorder and conduct disorder in probands combined additively to predict the risk for substance use disorders in relatives, and that the combination of conduct disorder *plus* bipolar disorder in youth predicts especially high rates of substance use disorders in relatives.

Pliszka and colleagues (2000) sought to determine the prevalence of major mental disorders and substance abuse in adolescents admitted to a juvenile detention center. They administered the Diagnostic Interview Schedule for Children to 50 youths (age range = 11–17 years). They found a high rate of affective disorder (42%) in this group: 10 (20%) met criteria for mania, another 10 met criteria for major depressive disorder, and one met criteria for bipolar disorder, mixed type. Thirty (60%) met criteria for conduct disorder. Moreover, very high rates of alcohol, marijuana, and other substance dependence were found. There was also a strong association between affective disorders and conduct disorder. Adolescents with mania had much higher rates of reported abuse of substances other than alcohol or marijuana, confirming earlier findings by Willens and colleagues (1999). Further studies are needed to examine the relationship of affective disorder to substance abuse as well as to antisocial behavior in the adolescent population.

COMORBIDITY OF BIPOLAR DISORDER WITH OBSESSIVE–COMPULSIVE DISORDER, PANIC DISORDER, AND SOCIAL PHOBIA

Apparently, regardless of age, a majority of individuals with mood disorders have co-occuring disorders, and this phenomenon has also been found to occur with obsessive–compulsive disorder, panic, and other anxiety disorders. In their systematic review of the literature, Geller and colleagues (1996) found that over 69% of children diagnosed with obsessive–compulsive disorder by DSM-IV criteria had an associated mood disorder. In data from adult general population studies, obsessive–compulsive disorder often coexists with mood disorders, with high rates of co-occurance (Chen & Dilsaver, 1995a). The ECA database supports the conclusion that the lifetime rate of comorbidity for obsessive–compulsive disorder is particularly high among bipolar subjects, and that, in adults with bipolar disorder, obsessive–compulsive disorder is also associated with panic disorder. The lifetime rates of obsessive–compulsive disorder among adult subjects with bipolar and unipolar disorders have been reported by Chen and Dilsaver (1995a) to be 21.0% and 12.2%, respectively. The probability of both disorders occurring within the same individual by chance would be 0.000312% if the two disorders are independent. Since the observed rate of concurrence was 22% and the ages of onset of both disorders were remarkably close, this high rate suggests that their co-occurence is the product of a single underlying diathesis.

Interestingly, using the same database, Chen and Dilsaver (1995b) found that the rates of panic disorder among adult subjects with bipolar disorder who did and did not meet the criteria for obsessive–compulsive disorder were 37.1% and 16.7%, respectively. These data highlight the fact that obsessive–compulsive disorder and panic disorder co-occur with bipolar disorder in a sizable subgroup of adult patients and raise the possibility that these separate comorbidities bipolar disorder *plus* panic disorder *plus* obsessive–compulsive disorder and bipolar disorder *plus* obsessive–compulsive disorder may represent distinct phenotypes paralleling the subtypes reported in studies of children: bipolar disorder *plus* attention-deficit/hyperactivity disorder *plus* conduct disorder and bipolar disorder *plus* attention-deficit/hyperactivity disorder. Both groupings, perhaps, are differentiated by unique environmental and genetic risk factors that occur on a developmental continuum.

Perugi and colleagues (1997) examined this complex pattern of comorbidity with bipolar disorder (bipolar disorder *plus* obsessive–compulsive disorder) in a consecutive series of 315 adult outpatients with obsessive–compulsive disorder, and found that 15.7% had such comorbidity (mostly with bipolar II disorder). In an effort to further delineate this specific phenotype along clinical lines, they found that several features distinguished the bipolar *plus* obsessive–compulsive disorder group from the nonbipolar *plus* obsessive–compulsive disorder group. In their sample, bipolar disorder *plus* obsessive–compulsive disorder patients had a more gradual onset of obsessive–compulsive disorder symptoms, which pursued a more episodic course with a high number of concurrent major depressive episodes, and a significantly higher rate of sexual and religious obsessions, and a lower rate of checking rituals. These investigators concluded that when comorbidity occurs with bipolar and unipolar affective disorders, it has a differential impact on the clinical characteristics, comorbidity, and course of obsessive–compulsive disorder. From a clinical point of view, these investigators suggest that major depression in obsessive–compulsive disorder is incidental, as obsessive–compulsive disorder in such cases dominates the course and dictates treatment choice. By contrast, when bipolar and obsessive–compulsive disorders coexist, bipolarity should take precedence in diagnosis, course, and treatment considerations.

Savino and colleagues (1993) systematically explored the spectrum of intraepisodic and longitudinal comorbidity of 140 adult patients diagnosed with panic disorder, 67.1% of whom concomitantly met DSM-III-R criteria for agoraphobia. Patients enrolled in the study were consecutively admitted to the outpatient department of a university psychiatric clinic over a 2-year period. Comorbidity of patients with panic disorder *plus* agoraphobia with strictly defined anxiety disorders (i.e., not explained as mere symptomatic extensions of panic disorder) was relatively uncommon, and included simple phobia (10.7%), social phobia (6.4%), generalized anxiety disorder (3.6%), and obsessive–compulsive disorder (4.2%). Comorbidity with major depression—strictly limited to the melancholic subtype—occurred in 22.9% of the sample. Comorbidity with bipolar disorder included 2.1% with mania, 5% with hypomania, and 6.4% with cyclothymia, for a total of 13.5%. Although the comorbid subgrouping panic disorder *plus* agoraphobia *plus* bipolar disorder, as currently defined, only numbered 13.5%, an additional 34.3% of patients with panic disorder met criteria for hyperthymic temperament. This finding raises the provocative question, Are temperamental features such as hyperthymia, behavioral inhibition, rejection sensitivity, and poor control over aggressive impulses critical factors in the assessment of comorbidity in psychiatric phenotypes? This question should be assessed in studies of comorbidity in clinical, epidemiological samples, as well as in the diagnostic ascertainment of family pedigrees for genetic studies.

Perugi and colleagues (1999), following this line of inquiry, investigated lifetime comorbidity in adults between panic disorder with or without agoraphobia, social phobia, or obsessive–compulsive disorder, on the one hand, and mood disorder, on the other. They found significantly higher numbers of anxiety disorders in those with lifetime comorbidity with bipolar (especially bipolar II) disorder. When the sample was sorted by specific anxiety disorder diagnosis, compared with panic disorder, social phobia, and obsessive–compulsive disorder showed significantly higher numbers of comorbid anxiety and mood disorders. In addition, social phobia and obsessive–compulsive disorder were significantly more likely to co-occur with each other than with panic disorder.

If bipolar disorder is genetically heterogeneous, it may be possible to discern clinically heterogeneous familial subtypes based on differential risk of psychiatric comorbidity. For example, emerging trends in family and genetic studies underscore high rates of comorbid panic disorder. MacKinnon, MacMahon, Simpson, McInnis, and DePaulo (1997) evaluated 528 members of 57 families ascertained for a genetic linkage study of bipolar disorder. Families were assorted according to the panic disorder diagnosis of bipolar probands, and the rates of panic and other disorders in relatives were compared. Of the 41 subjects with panic disorder, 88% had bipolar disorder. Panic disorder was diagnosed in 18% of family members with bipolar disorder. Ten of 57 bipolar probands had panic disorder. Their bipolar first-degree relatives had a significantly higher prevalence of panic disorder, bipolar II, cyclothymia, and dysthymia, but had lower prevalence of substance abuse than the relatives of the bipolar probands without panic disorder in kindred with a heavy loading for bipolar disorder. Additionally, preliminary results from the Otago Familial Bipolar Genetic Study found that 27.3% met DSM-IV criteria for panic disorder and subthreshold panic disorder. Taken together with epidemiological data, these studies suggest the testable hypothesis that comorbid panic disorder is a marker of genetic heterogeneity in bipolar disorder.

DEVELOPMENTAL CONTINUITY OF ANXIETY DISORDERS IN THE LIFE CYCLE

Inferences about the developmental sequence of anxiety disorders have relied primarily on retrospective data, although one prospective study of individuals diagnosed with separation anxiety disorder in childhood found that these children were at risk for subsequent emergence of panic disorder and agoraphobia (Gittleman & Klein, 1984). Compared with the expense of longitudinal studies, a family/genetic approach offers a cost-effective method for the assessment of the developmental continuity of related disorders. This genetic/epidemiological approach has been utilized successfully as part of the Massachusetts General Hospital Family Study conducted by Rosenbaum, Biederman, Kagan, and colleagues (Rosenbaum et al., 1992, 2000). These investigators examined the prevalence of various psychiatric disorders among two groups of children, one selected through parents diagnosed with panic disorder and another control group of parents who did not have panic disorder. In comparison to the control group, offspring of parents with panic disorder were found to have significantly higher rates of anxiety disorder. Twenty-five percent of these children were diagnosed with two or more anxiety disorders, while 7% had panic disorder. The study demonstrated that the offspring of parents with panic disorder were at higher risk for separation anxiety disorder, agoraphobia, social phobia, and overanxious disorder. From a developmental point of view, because panic disorder, agoraphobia, and social phobia have been found to co-occur, and are not uncommonly found among adults in clinical samples of adult psychiatric patients, it is quite possible that this association represents a developmental continuity over the life cycle.

TEMPERAMENTAL TRAITS AS PRECURSORS TO LATER PSYCHIATRIC ILLNESS

Kagan, Reznick, and Snidman (1988) have found that shyness or behavioral inhibition represents an enduring trait or feature of temperament that is associated with a specific physiological substrate *in utero* and in infancy, including more rapid fetal heart rates at several weeks before birth and at 2 weeks of age. Additionally, at a later age, shy children exhibit a greater acceleration of heart rate and pupillary dilation when exposed to stressors in comparison to control subjects. These children were more fearful during the first days of school, and experienced marked separation anxiety as well as avoidant behaviors.

These findings prompted Kagan to hypothesize that behaviorally inhibited children have a low threshold for arousal when exposed to unfamiliar or novel events. Given the observed relationship between shyness and a propensity for fearful, anxious responses developmentally, Rosenbaum and colleagues (2000) examined the young offspring of parents diagnosed with panic disorder and agoraphobia, and found a higher risk for behavioral inhibition among their children compared to offspring of parents without panic disorder. Additionally, the presence of behavioral inhibition was found to predict higher rates of anxiety disorders 3 years later.

A recent retrospective study of parental reports of chronological symptom development in children later diagnosed with bipolar disorder found that 42% of the sample had prodromal separation anxiety disorder, 55% reported arousal disorders of sleep (night terrors, restless leg syndrome, bruxism), and 70% reported marked sensitivity to sensory stimuli in infancy and early childhood (Papolos, Fann, Tresker, & Papolos, 2002). Since panic disorder is highly comorbid with adult bipolar disorder, taken together the foregoing studies suggest, that, if indeed the temperamental trait of behavioral inhibition represents a low threshold for arousal, and separation anxiety disorder in children is a precursor to both panic disorder and bipolar disorder, it is possible that both trait and several DSM-IV conditions may share a common genetic diathesis with variations on a theme. Examining the offspring of bipolar disorder parents comorbid for panic disorder to determine whether these children also have behavioral inhibition would be a specific test of this hypothesis.

QUESTIONS AND CAVEATS

One clear problem is how can we begin to separate bipolar disorder as an independent clinical entity from all of these other conditions with overlapping symptoms? Is it distinguishable? If so, what are its defining features? A number of questions remain to be answered before we can bring clarification to the current diagnostic criteria now being used by the field to define childhood-onset bipolar disorder:

1. Does bipolar disorder occur simultaneously with other psychiatric disorders, making it possible for a child to actually have three or four separate diagnoses, as is also now reported in adolescent and adult epidemiological samples?
2. Are the clusters of symptoms that suggest distinct disorders merely early precursors on a developmental continuum that eventually expresses itself as a full-blown bipolar disorder?
3. Is early-onset bipolar disorder a distinct subtype of the adult form of bipolar disorder with co-occuring conditions in childhood predisposing to specific variants in their adult manifestations—for example, an ultra-ultra rapid cycling variant, bipolar disorder/obsessive–compulsive disorder, bipolar disorder/obsessive–compulsive disorder/panic disorder, bipolar disorder/conduct disorder/substance abuse, bipolar disorder/attention-deficit/hyperactivity disorder/conduct disorder/substance abuse—perhaps forming specific subtypes that may be defined genetically?

BEHAVIORAL GENETIC METHODS IN THE STUDY OF COMORBIDITY: FIRST STEPS TOWARD A NEW DIAGNOSTIC NOSOLOGY

While bipolar disorder exhibits some familiarity, the illness does not appear to be inherited according to Mendelian rules, and it is well known that complex traits or diseases that show no simple Mendelian pattern of inheritance are unlikely to yield simple genetic answers. Unlike simple Mendelian disorders caused by highly penetrant but rare functional polymorphisms (mutations) in a single gene, the genetic component of complex psychiatric disorders is more likely to be associated with low penetrance but common functional variations in a number of susceptibility genes. In such a model, multiple genes with small effects may contribute to a predisposition for bipolar disorder in an affected individual. These multiple gene effects can contribute additively and interchangeably, like risk factors, to the vulnerability for a disorder (Plomin, 2000; Plomin & Rutter, 1998). Combined groups of symptoms from different but related disorders may be the expression of genotypic variation that may account for the genetic influence in bipolar disorder. Twin-pair, family aggregation, and comorbidity studies provide information that can help to discriminate between overlapping symptomatology and validate that comorbid conditions diagnosed in the proband do in fact have a common genetic diathesis.

Given the confusion over diagnostic boundaries in our current nosological system, twin-pair studies may be one of the most parsimonious and direct strategies to address some of the questions raised by comorbid conditions, and may help to tease apart the weight of various symptoms within diverse diagnostic constructs and determine their degree of heritability in terms of co-occurance.

Although previous family and twin studies have examined the relationship between the genetic and environmental risk factors for pairs of psychiatric disorders, the interrelationship between these classes of risk factors for a broad range of psychiatric disorders remains largely unknown. Kendler and colleagues (1995) were the first to examine the structure of the genetic and environmental risk factors for a group of major psychiatric disorders in twins. Using an epidemiological sample of 1,030 female–female twin-pairs with known zygosity, ascertained from the Virginia Twin Registry, these investigators assessed lifetime history of phobia, generalized anxiety disorder, panic disorder, bulimia nervosa, major depression, and alcoholism. Their multivariate twin analysis suggested the following:

1. Each major risk factor domain (genes, family environment, and individual-specific environment) influenced comorbidity between these disorders in a distinct manner with genetic influences on these disorders most parsimoniously explained by two factors, the first loading heavily on phobia, panic disorder, and bulimia nervosa, and the second loading on major depression and generalized anxiety disorder.
2. The anxiety disorders were not, from a genetic perspective, found to be etiologically homogeneous.
3. Most of the genetic factors that influenced vulnerability to alcoholism in women did not alter the risk for development of other common psychiatric disorders.

These results should be interpreted in the context of both the strengths and limitations of multivariate twin analysis. This important study informs us that gender may play a significant role in the developmental sequences of some of the conditions that are commonly comorbid with bipolar disorder.

Using this same twin-pair method, Willcutt, Pennington, and DeFries (2000) examined the relationship between genetic and environmental risk factors using a dimensional approach. Rather than examining the interrelationship between classes of risk factors for a range of psychiatric disorders, they focused on the relationship of specific measurable deficits within the broader category of learning disabilities by examining the interrelationship between inattention and hyperactivity/impulsivity in a community sample of 3,738 18-year-old twin-pairs in which at least one twin exhibited a history of learning disabilities. They found that extreme hyperactivity/impulsivity scores were almost entirely attributable to genetic influences, as were extreme inattention scores whether or not the proband exhibited extreme hyperactivity/impulsivity scores. In contrast, the heritability of extreme hyperactivity/impulsivity increased as a linear function of the number of inattention symptoms exhibited by the proband. This finding suggests that extreme hyperactivity/impulsivity may be attributable to different etiological influences in individuals with and without extreme inattention, and that hyperactivity/impulsivity symptoms exhibited by individuals with combined type attention-deficit/hyperactivity disorder and predominantly hyperactivity/impulsivity type attention-deficit/hyperactivity disorder may be attributable to different etiological influences.

Further studies such as the foregoing by Kendler and colleagues (1995) and Willcutt and colleagues (2000) may eventually allow the field to reconceptualize diagnostic boundaries along lines that more closely resemble the presentation of psychiatric disorders within nature. Testing such a view may require eschewing criteria as they are currently specified in DSM-IV for diagnosing bipolar disorder, and instead attempting to determine whether linkage to a set of genes exists between a related group of disorders, in addition to specific behavioral traits, and possibly, temperamental features common to bipolar spectrum disorders—for example, high levels of hyperactivity/impulsiveness, easy arousability, prominent cyclic switches in energy and activity levels with diurnal pattern, pronounced separation anxiety during childhood, periodic sweet and carbohydrate cravings with episodic binging, the predisposition for sleep/wake reversals, seasonal variation in symptoms, or a deficit in the capacity to modify the expression of aggressive behaviors (Papolos & Papolos, 1999).

Temperamental features such as behavioral inhibition (shyness) or hyperthymic temperament may also be important factors to include in this dimensional diagnostic nosology, as the work of Rosenbaum, Biederman, Kagan, and colleagues (Rosenbaum et al., 1992, 2000) would attest. The importance of enduring temperamental features and their relationship to course of illness has long been articulated by Akiskal (Akiskal et al., 2000). This quite different view of the problem would lead to the question, Can a unique genetic predisposition influence a rather specific group of behaviors, traits, or temperamental features that have some developmental program, and are associated with bipolar spectrum disorders? This question differs from another: Is a single gene associated with a common group of symptoms?

Variable expression appears to be a common feature of familial psychiatric disorders. The biological relatives of bipolar probands are at high risk for attention-deficit/hyperactivity disorder, major depression, panic disorder, and alcoholism. As genes linked to behavioral dimensions and disorders are identified, genetic studies can be used to answer questions about psychopathological patterns, environmental risk, and etiology. Questions on psychopathological patterns address comorbidity (Are gene–behavior associations diagnosis-specific?), heterogeneity (Do gene–behavior associations apply to specific symptom constellations or to separate components representing risk or protective factors?), as well as the relationship between behavioral syndromes and temperamental features (Does a gene-behavior association for a disorder extend to related dimensions of normal variation?).

The following clinical case report documents the evolution of psychiatric symptoms and behaviors in an 11-year-old boy. This case represents a common presentation of childhood bipolar disorder, and illustrates its multiple comorbidities, temperamental features, and possible developmental sequence.

THE CASE OF AN 11-YEAR-OLD BOY WHO WAS PAINFULLY SHY AS WELL AS AGGRESSIVE AND DISRUPTIVE

- *Age 2–3.* At second birthday party Jeffrey runs from some group activities; group situations overstimulate him. Becomes very insulted/embarrassed if reprimanded, quick to anger, has trouble calming down. Often acts very silly and clown-like to make people laugh.
- *Age 3–4.* Severe separation anxiety going to preschool all year. On immediate joining with the group, he demonstrates severe, painful shyness, yet once he is more comfortable Jeffrey exhibits loud disruptive behavior when he does not get his way. He is described as often being angry and unable to tolerate criticism. In his first summer program, he experienced severe separation anxiety and shyness. Each morning that he entered the building, he refused to go in to his group's room, staying alone in the hall most mornings. The first psychiatric evaluation reported that Jeffrey was angry and required therapy.
- *Diagnosis: Separation anxiety disorder*

- *Age 4–5.* During preschool Jeffrey is extremely shy, yet paradoxically loud and disruptive. He develops a quasi-motor tic (licking/circling lips with tongue). Second consultation with child psychologist reports that on Parent Behavior Rating Scales Jeffrey is "high maintenance," with behavioral difficulties (96th%), restless and disorganized behavior (93rd%), anxious/shy symptoms (97th%), significant behavioral problems as to frequency (97th percentile), and severity (91st percentile). Psychologist reports Jeffrey is strong-willed but sweet and engaging, acutely sensitive to insult and embarrassment, and has difficulty calming down after becoming angry.

- *Diagnosis: Generalized anxiety disorder*

- *Age 5–6.* In kindergarten Jeffrey is described by teachers as silly, disruptive, and hard to manage. Anxiety, shyness, silly clown-like behavior, and anger are prevalent features of his personality. During summer camp program, Jeffrey runs from counselors/group whenever reprimanded.

- *Age 6–7.* In first grade Jeffrey is described by teachers as disruptive, hard to manage, and grandiose. He acts silly and goofy at times, and continues as the class clown. He is not able or does not know when/how to stop when asked to, and is angry when reprimanded by teachers. At times he has to be physically removed from class by the principal, but is then calm, staying quietly in principal's office. He continues to be easily overstimulated in crowded, noisy situations, and typically becomes anxious and misreads social cues. Tic-like mouth licking persists. Second psychiatric consultation:

- *Diagnosis: Generalized anxiety disorder, rule out Tourette's syndrome.* Clonidine is prescribed, which causes daytime sedation—he consistently falls asleep at his desk at school. Parents discontinue the drug after several months. Jeffrey begins group therapy once a week, and continues with the group for 2 years. Noise, sights, and smells overexcite him, and parents consult occupational therapist.

- *Diagnosis: Sensory integration disorder.* Sensory integration therapy initiated. Chewing crunchy foods reported to calm him, as does brushing therapy.

- *Age 7–8.* Second grade: Increase in Tourette's-like tics, throat clearing, and eye turning; the tics alternate periodically. Some irritable moods with raging anger alternating with silly, goofy, giddy mood states, at which times he can become grandiose, telling tall tales about himself. These occur multiple times within a day. Obsessive–compulsive disorder symptoms begin. Jeffrey will not use silverware/glasses, only new plastic tableware. During summer camp Jeffrey is disruptive, and is unable to get along with his peers in group activities.

- *Age 8–9.* Third grade: Teachers describe Jeffrey as disruptive, raging in class, cursing, throwing chairs. When reprimanded he runs away from teacher/principal outside the school building. Obsessive–compulsive disorder symptoms intensify. By winter, Jeffrey is often raging and out of control. Third psychiatric consultation:

- *Diagnosis: Obsessive–compulsive disorder.* Low-dose paroxetine is prescribed at 10 mg/day, which causes pronounced rages and increased aggression and behavioral activation. Paroxetine is rapidly discontinued. Psychiatrist observes mood instability, volatility.

• *Diagnosis: Bipolar disorder, not otherwise specified.* Olanzapine at 2.5 mg/day is prescribed. It is highly sedating, and causes significant weight gain. Olanzepine is discontinued after about 45 days, and Depakote at 250 mg twice a day started (level below 0.60). During Christmas vacation, Jeffrey is raging and cursing, By January, he is suspended from school and transferred to another school. Obsessive–compulsive symptoms persist, but tic-like behaviors are no longer evident.

• *Age 9–10.* Midsummer, in addition to Depakote at 250 mg twice a day, 25 mg of Zoloft is prescribed, and increased to 50 mg for treatment of obsessive–compulsive symptoms. Obsessive–compulsive symptoms lessened on Zoloft, but within first days of school he is clowning and more disruptive. When teacher attempts to maintain classroom order, Jeffrey sees her as a screamer, yelling and punishing. He misreads the situation, personalizing it, blowing it out of proportion. Parents and teachers note signs of paranoid ideation. Jeffrey appears to have an inaccurate perception of situations, and becomes easily angered for no apparent reason. Zoloft is discontinued after about 30 days, as the following psychotic-like behaviors developed as reported by teachers subsequent to its introduction:

1. He leaves class to go to the bathroom, and ends up lying down in the hall, "playing dead."
2. When the principal walks him to his classroom to retrieve his lunch and book bag, he bolts into the classroom and climbs out the window in front of the whole class.
3. He lies to his teacher and his principal, making up fanciful, grandiose tales.
4. He sits under his desk at school all morning, and scratches his arms to the point of self-injury. When asked about these behaviors, Jeffrey reports that there is a little voice in his head that tells him to do bad things, a voice he doesn't hear so much as feel.

Unable to function in school, Jeffrey is removed from school by his parents.

Jeffrey starts private day-treatment school. Lithium carbonate at 150 mg twice a day is prescribed, and slowly increased to 600 mg/day. Depakote is increased to achieve adequate therapeutic levels. Eventually, Jeffrey adapts to the school program, his rages decrease (although for several months he remains hypersensitive to criticism), and his sensory overstimulation also decreases. He completes fourth grade on a much better note in all areas. Jeffrey is now on two mood stabilizers: Depakote (0.92 mg/ml) and lithium carbonate (1.20 mEq/L); his mood swings have stabilized; he is less agitated and anxious; and his psychotic symptoms have remitted. He is able to attend school for the remainder of the year as well as a 4-week summer program without incident.

• *Impression.* Jeffrey's history is quite compatible with a diagnosis of early-onset bipolar disorder. His protracted temper tantrums, severe separation anxiety, and abrupt, rapid mood swings during the day, alternating between irritability and silly, goofy, giddy behaviors and withdrawal, as well as the psychotic symptoms (auditory hallucinations and paranoid delusions) are all classical signs of childhood-onset bipolar disorder. The step-wise progression of diagnosis from age 3–4 separation anxiety disorder to age 4–5 generalized anxiety disorder, to age 7–8 obsessive–compulsive disorder may represent a developmental sequence associated with the condition. Additionally, he responded to a selective serotonin reuptake inhibitor (SSRI) with agitation and increased aggression, as well as with paranoid ideation, not uncommon adverse effects to antidepressant treatment of childhood-onset bipolar disorder.

It was only when lithium carbonate at sufficiently high enough serum levels (1.20 mEq/L) to have a significant effect on the mixed, ultra-ultra rapid cycling states of childhood bipolar disorder, and after a second mood stabilizer, Depakote, was raised to high therapeutic levels, that the condition was brought under control.

The temperamental feature of extreme shyness and the associated anxiety disorders that were diagnosed, coupled, paradoxically, with the manifestation of loud, aggressive, and disruptive behaviors, is of interest given the possibility of a developmental sequence that involves behavioral inhibition as a temperamental precursor.

Is it possible that a pattern of co-occuring disorders will serve to establish new clinical diagnostic entities that cross current boundaries of classification—diagnostic entities possibly with specific treatment indications and contraindications, perhaps even clinical entities with a constellation of symptoms and behaviors on a developmental continuum that correspond to specific genotypes not identifiable through contemporary linkage analysis studies because of the restrictive psychiatric phenotypes that rely on categorical diagnosis rather that a lifetime perspective that might incorporate dimensions of temperament such as behavioral inhibition in childhood predisposing to various possible iterations over the course of a lifetime.

It will, no doubt, be many years before the complex issues that these questions raise can be fully resolved, yet the answers are likely to have major consequences for the field of behavioral genetics, as well as for clinical psychiatry. In the meantime, the impact of day-to-day clinical diagnostic and treatment decisions continues to have far-reaching effects on patients and their families. The emerging evidence merits wider attention and should sound a cautionary note in pharmacological approaches to a number of childhood psychiatric disorders, in particular those that have high rates of comorbidity with childhood-onset bipolar disorder.

COMORBIDITY AND THE CLINICAL VIEW

Drawing from the information that is now available to us from clinical, epidemiological, and family/genetic studies, there are several observations that should inform clinical diagnoses and treatment decisions in the pediatric population with behavioral disorders that are comorbid with bipolar disorder.

1. According to most recent studies, childhood-onset bipolar disorder has high rates of comorbidity with attention-deficit/hyperactivity disorder, conduct disorders, and obsessive–compulsive disorder, and significant but lesser rates of comorbidity with Tourette's syndrome and pervasive developmental disorders. These comorbidities with more easily identifiable disorders have led to long latencies between the emergence of bipolar disorder symptoms in childhood and its clinical diagnoses.

2. Because of overlapping symptoms between current DSM-IV diagnostic categories, incomplete and misleading criteria for the diagnosis of childhood-onset bipolar disorder, as well as a long-standing bias against the diagnosis in childhood, many individuals are commonly first diagnosed with one or another of the co-occuring conditions before childhood-onset bipolar disorder is considered.

3. Longitudinal observations and recent prospective studies strongly support the view that patients with very-early-onset depression are at extremely high risk for bipolar disorder. Recent epidemiological and clinical studies have found that the rate of switching from unipolar depression to bipolar disorder ranges between 48% and 61% in the juvenile population (Geller et al., 2000; Lewinsohn et al., 1995; Papolos & Papolos 1999).

4. A number of clinical reports (Briscoe, Harrington, & Prendergast, 1995; Go, Malley, Birmaher, & Rosenberg, 1998; Soeda, Terao, & Nakamura, 1999; Strober, 1998) have observed manic induction or increased cycling in children and adolescents exposed to antidepressant drugs of various classes who were originally diagnosed with other conditions known to be comorbid with bipolar disorder. High rates of onset of bipolarity and of switching to mania while patients were on tricyclic antidepressants was reported in a treatment study of prepubertal depression (Geller, Fox, & Fletcher, 1993). In a recent retrospective survey of parents

of children with bipolar disorder (n = 120), Papolos and Papolos (1999) found that 65% of those who were treated with stimulants and 85% of those treated with antidepressants of all classes, switched into mania, rapid-cycling agitated states, or psychosis, and many expressed violent and suicidal ideas. While these studies require replication, their preliminary observations will hopefully lead to greater caution, and inform treatment decisions in children diagnosed with any condition now known to co-occur with bipolar disorder, particularly where there is a family history of bipolar disorder.

CLINICAL IMPACT OF COMORBID CONDITIONS: OBSCURING DIAGNOSTIC RECOGNITION OF BIPOLAR DISORDER

In the case of comorbid conditions, if childhood-onset bipolar disorder is diagnosed first, the condition would be treated with mood-stabilizing agents, either lithium or an anticonvulsant, often with the addition of a neuroleptic agent. If attention-deficit/hyperactivity disorder were diagnosed first, and the childhood-onset bipolar disorder was present, but not detected, a stimulant would likely be prescribed. In the case of major depression and obsessive–compulsive disorder, antidepressant treatment would likely be instituted, most commonly with an SSRI.

With outdated and incomplete criteria being used to diagnose bipolar disorder in youth by the majority of mental health practitioners around the country, coupled with the burgeoning administration of stimulants and antidepressants to the general pediatric population, the potential for adverse effects in children with bipolar disorder who go unrecognized is high. It behooves pediatricians, pediatric neurologists, child psychiatrists, and other mental health professionals alike to become more aware of this area of diagnostic confusion and controversy. It will be very important to take into account in their diagnostic practice and treatment approaches the emerging evidence that demonstrates high rates of overlapping symptoms and comorbidity between childhood-onset bipolar disorder and the more commonly diagnosed childhood psychiatric disorders, high rates of switching from unipolar to bipolar depression, and the potential for serious adverse effects of stimulants and antidepressants in this group of patients.

ACKNOWLEDGMENTS

This work was supported by a NARSAD Independent Investigator Award. I would like to thank Ross J. Baldessarini, MD, for reviewing the manuscript, and contributing helpful comments and suggestions.

REFERENCES

Adams, F. (1856). *The extant works of Artaeus, the Cappadocian.* London: Syndenham Society.

Akiskal, H. S., Bourgeois, M. L., Angst, J., Post, R., Moller, H., & Hirschfeld, R. (2000). Reevaluating the prevalence of and diagnostic composition within the broad clinical spectrum of bipolar disorders. *Journal of Affective Disorders, 59*(Suppl. 1), S5–S30.

Akiskal, H. S., Maser, J. D., Zeller, P. J., Endicott, J., Coryell, W., Keller, M., Warshaw M., Clayton, P., & Goodwin, F. (1995). Switching from "unipolar" to bipolar II: An 11 year prospective study of clinical and temperamental predictors in 559 patients. *Archives of General Psychiatry, 52*(2), 114–123.

Baldessarini, R. J., Tohen, M., & Tondo, L. (2000). Maintenance treatment in bipolar disorder. *Archives of General Psychiatry, 57*(5), 490–492.

Baron, M., Freimer, N. F., Risch, N., Lerer B, Alexander, J. R., Straub, R. E., Asokan, S., Das, K., Peterson, A., Amos, J., et al. (1993). Diminished support for linkage between manic depressive illness and X-chromosome markers in three Israeli pedigrees. *Nature Genetics, 3*(1), 49–55.

Biederman, J., Faraone, S. V., Chu, M. P., & Wozniak, J. (1999). Further evidence of a bidirectional overlap between juvenile mania and conduct disorder in children. *Journal of the American Academy of Child and Adolescent Psychiatry, 38*(4), 468–476.

Biederman, J., Faraone, S. V., Hatch, M., Mennin, D., Taylor, A., & George, P. (1997). Conduct disorder with and without mania in a referred sample of ADHD children. *Journal of Affective Disorders, 44*(2–3), 177–188.

Biederman, J., Faraone, S. V., Hirshfeld-Becker, D. R., Friedman, D., Robin, J. A., & Rosenbaum, J. F. (2001). Patterns of psychopathology and dysfunction in high-risk children of parents with panic disorder and major depression. *American Journal of Psychiatry, 158*(1), 49–57.

Biederman, J., Faraone, S., Mick, E., Wozniak, J., Chen, L., Ouellette, C., Marrs, A., Moore, P., Garcia, J., Mennin, D., & Lelon, E. (1996). Attention-deficit hyperactivity disorder and juvenile mania: An overlooked comorbidity? *Journal of the American Academy of Child and Adolescent Psychiatry, 35*(8), 997–1008.

Biederman, J., Faraone, S. V., Milberger, S., Jetton, J. G., Chen, L., Mick, E., Greene, R. W., & Russell, R. L. (1996). Is childhood oppositional defiant disorder a precursor to adolescent conduct disorder?: Findings from a four-year follow-up study of children with ADHD. *Journal of the American Academy of Child and Adolescent Psychiatry, 35*(9), 1193–1204.

Biederman, J., Faraone, S. V., Wozniak, J., & Monuteaux, M. C. (2000). Parsing the association between bipolar, conduct, and substance use disorders: A familial risk analysis. *Biological Psychiatry, 48*(11), 1037–1044.

Biederman, J., Mick, E., Faraone, S. V., Spencer, T., Wilens, T. E., & Wozniak, J. (2000). Pediatric mania: A developmental subtype of bipolar disorder? *Biological Psychiatry, 48*(6), 458–466.

Biederman, J., Russell, R., Soriano, J., Wozniak, J., & Faraone, S. V. (1998). Clinical features of children with both ADHD and mania: Does ascertainment source make a difference? *Journal of Affective Disorders, 51*(2), 101–112.

Biederman, J., Wilens, T., Mick, E., Faraone, S. V., Weber, W., Curtis, S., Thornell, A.,

Pfister, K., Jetton, J. G., & Soriano, J. (1997). Is ADHD a risk factor for psychoactive substance use disorders?: Findings from a four-year prospective follow-up study. *Journal of the American Academy of Child and Adolescent Psychiatry, 36*(1), 21–29.

Biederman, J., Wozniak, J., Kiely, K., Ablon, S., Faraone, S., Mick, E., Mundy, E., & Kraus, I. (1995). CBCL clinical scales discriminate prepubertal children with structured interview-derived diagnosis of mania from those with ADHD. *Journal of the American Academy of Child and Adolescent Psychiatry, 34*(4), 464–471.

Briscoe, J. J., Harrington, R. C., & Prendergast, M. (1995). Development of mania in close association with tricyclic antidepressant administration in children: A report of two cases. *European Journal of Child and Adolescent Psychiatry, 4*(4), 280–283.

Carlson, G. A. (1998). Mania and ADHD: Comorbidity or confusion. *Journal of Affective Disorders, 51*(2), 177–187.

Chen, Y. W., & Dilsaver, S. C. (1995a). Comorbidity for obsessive–compulsive disorder in bipolar and unipolar disorders. *Psychiatry Research, 59*(1–2), 57–64.

Chen, Y. W., & Dilsaver, S. C. (1995b). Comorbidity of panic disorder in bipolar illness: Evidence from the Epidemiologic Catchment Area Survey. *American Journal of Psychiatry, 152*(2), 280–282.

Coolidge, F. L., Thede, L. L., & Young, S. E. (2000). Heritability and the comorbidity of attention deficit hyperactivity disorder and behavioral disorders and executive function deficits: A preliminary investigation. *Developmental Neuropsychology, 17*(3), 273–287.

Coryell, W., Endicott, J., Maser, J. D., Keller, M. B., Leon, A. C., & Akiskal, H. S. (1995). Long-term stability of polarity distinctions in the affective disorders. *American Journal of Psychiatry, 152*(3), 385–390.

DeLong, G. R. (1999). Autism: new data suggest a new hypothesis. *Neurology, 52*(5), 911–916.

Egeland, J. A. (1988). A genetic study of manic–depressive disorder among the old order Amish of Pennsylvania. *Pharmacopsychiatry, 21*(2), 74–75.

Egeland, J. A., Hostetter, A. M., Pauls, D. L., & Sussex, J. N. (2000). Prodromal symptoms before onset of manic–depressive disorder suggested by first hospital admission histories. *Journal of the American Academy of Child and Adolescent Psychiatry, 39*(10), 1245–1252.

Faedda, G. L., Baldessarini, R. J., Suppes, T., Tondo, L., Becker, I., & Lipschitz, D. S. (1995). Pediatric-onset bipolar disorder: A neglected clinical and public health problem. *Harvard Review of Psychiatry, 3*, 171–95.

Faraone, S. V., Biederman, J., Jetton, J. G., & Tsuang, M. T. (1997). Attention deficit disorder and conduct disorder: Longitudinal evidence for a familial subtype. *Psychological Medicine, 27*(2), 291–300.

Faraone, S. V., Biederman, J., Mennin, D., & Russell, R. (1998). Bipolar and antisocial disorders among relatives of ADHD children: Parsing familial subtypes of illness. *American Journal of Medical Genetics, 81*(1), 108–116.

Faraone, S. V., Biederman, J., Mennin, D., Wozniak, J., & Spencer, T. (1997). Attention-deficit hyperactivity disorder with bipolar disorder: A familial subtype? *Journal of the American Academy of Child and Adolescent Psychiatry, 36*(10), 1378–1387; discussion, 1387–1390.

Geller, B., Fox, L. W., & Clark, K. A. (1994). Rate and predictors of prepubertal bipolarity during follow-up of 6- to 12-year-old depressed children. *Journal of the American Academy of Child and Adolescent Psychiatry, 33*(4), 461–468.

Geller, B., Fox, L. W., & Fletcher, M. (1993). Effect of tricyclic antidepressants on switching to mania and on the onset of bipolarity in depressed 6- to 12-year-olds. *Journal of the American Academy of Child and Adolescent Psychiatry, 32*(1), 43–50.

Geller, B., Warner, K., Williams, M., & Zimerman, B. (1998). Prepubertal and young adolescent bipolarity versus ADHD: Assessment and validity using the WASH-U-KSADS, CBCL and TRF. *Journal of Affective Disorders, 51*(2), 93–100.

Geller, B., Williams, M., Zimerman, B., Frazier, J., Beringer, L., & Warner, K. L. (1998). Prepubertal and early adolescent bipolarity differentiate from ADHD by manic symptoms, grandiose delusions, ultra-rapid or ultradian cycling. *Journal of Affective Disorders, 51*(2), 81–91.

Geller, B., Zimerman, B., Williams, M., Bolhofner, K., Craney, J. L., Delbello, M. P., & Soutullo, C. A. (2000). Diagnostic characteristics of 93 cases of a prepubertal and early adolescent bipolar disorder phenotype by gender, puberty and comorbid attention deficit hyperactivity disorder. *Journal of Child and Adolescent Psychopharmacology, 10*(3), 157–164.

Geller, D. A., Biederman, J., Griffin, S., Jones, J., & Lefkowitz, T. R. (1996). Comorbidity of juvenile obsessive–compulsive disorder with disruptive behavior disorders. *Journal of the American Academy of Child and Adolescent Psychiatry, 35*(12), 1637–1646.

Gittelman, R., & Klein, D. F. (1984) Relationship between separation anxiety and panic and agoraphobic disorders. *Psychopathology, 17*(Suppl. 1), 56–65.

Go, F. S., Malley, E. E., Birmaher, B., & Rosenberg, D. R. (1998). Manic behaviors associated with fluoxetine in three 12- to 18-year-olds with obsessive–compulsive disorder. *Journal of Child and Adolescent Psychopharmacology, 8*(1), 73–80.

Hazell, P. L., Lewin, T. J., & Carr, V. J. (1999). Confirmation that Child Behavior Checklist clinical scales discriminate juvenile mania from attention deficit hyperactivity disorder. *Journal of Paediatric Child Health, 35*(2), 199–203.

Joyce, P. R. Oakley-Browne, M. A., Wells, J. E., Bushnell, J. A., & Hornblow A. R. J. (1990). Birth cohort trends in major depression: Increasing rates and earlier onset in New Zealand. *Journal of Affective Disorders, 18*(2), 83–89.

Kagan, J., Reznick, J. S., & Snidman, N. (1988). Biological basis of childhood shyness. *Science, 240,* 167–171.

Kasanin, J. (1931). The affective psychoses in children. *American Journal of Psychiatry, 10,* 897–926.

Kelsoe, J. R., Ginns, E. I., Egeland, J. A., Gerhard, D. S., Goldstein, A. M., Bale, S. J., Pauls D. L., Long. R. T., Kidd, K. K., Conte, G., et al. (1989). Re-evaluation of the linkage relationship between chromosome 11p loci and the gene for bipolar affective disorder in the Old Order Amish. *Nature, 342*(6247), 238–243.

Kendler, K. S., Walters, E. E., Neale, M. C., Kessler, R. C., Heath, A. C., & Eaves, L. J. (1995). The structure of the genetic and environmental risk factors for six major psychiatric disorders in women: Phobia, generalized anxiety disorder, panic disorder, bulimia, major depression, and alcoholism. *Archives of General Psychiatry, 52*(5), 374–383.

Kerbeshian, J., Burd, L., & Klug, M. G. (1995). Comorbid Tourette's disorder and bipolar disorder: An etiologic perspective. *American Journal of Psychiatry, 152*(11), 1646–1651.

Kessler, R. C., McGonagle, K. A., Zhao, S., Nelson, C. B., Hughes, M., Eshleman. S., & Wittchen, H. U., & Kendler, K. S. (1994). Lifetime and 12–month prevalence of DSM-III-R psychiatric disorders in the United States: Results from the National Comorbidity Survey. *Archives of General Psychiatry, 51*(1), 8–19.

Kovacs,M., & Pollock, M. (1995). Bipolar disorder and comorbid conduct disorder in childhood and adolescence. *Journal of the American Academy of Child and Adolescent Psychiatry, 34*(6), 715–723.

Kraepelin, E. (1921). *Manic–depressive insanity and paranoia* (M. Barclay, Trans.). Edinburgh, Scotland: Livingstone.

Kruger, S., Cooke, R. G., Hasey, G. M., Jorna, T., & Persad, E. (1995). Comorbidity of obsessive–compulsive disorder in bipolar disorder. *Journal of Affective Disorders, 34*(2), 117–120.

Lavori, P. W., Klerman, G. L., Keller M. B., Reich T., Rice J., & Endicott, J. (1987). Age-period-cohort analysis of secular trends in onset of major depression: Findings in siblings of patients with major affective disorder. *Journal of Psychiatric Research, 21*(1), 23–35.

Lewinsohn, P. M., Klein, D. N., & Seeley, J. R. (1995). Bipolar disorders in a community sample of older adolescents: Prevalence, phenomenology, comorbidity, and course. *Journal of the American Academy of Child and Adolescent Psychiatry, 34*(4), 454–463.

Loeber, R., Green, S. M., Keenan, K., & Lahey, B. B. (1995). Which boys will fare worse?: Early predictors of the onset of conduct disorder in a six-year longitudinal study. *Journal of the American Academy of Child and Adolescent Psychiatry, 34*(4), 499–509.

MacKinnon, D. F., McMahon, F. J., Simpson, S. G., McInnis, M. G., & DePaulo, J. R. (1997). Panic disorder with familial bipolar disorder. *Biological Psychiatry, 42*(2), 90–95.

Maier, W., Lichtermann, D., Minges, J., Delmo, C., & Heun, R. (1995). The relationship between bipolar disorder and alcoholism: A controlled family study. *Psychological Medicine, 25*(4), 787–796.

Maier, W., & Merikangas, K. (1996). Co-occurrence and contransmission of affective disorders and alcoholism in families. *British Journal of Psychiatry, 30*(Suppl.), 93–100.

Papolos, D. F., Fann, C., Tresker, S., & Papolos, J. D. (2002). *Pediatric mania: Prodromal symptoms and antecedent conditions.* Manuscript submitted for publication.

Papolos, D. F., & Papolos, J. D. (1999). *The bipolar child: The definitive and reassuring guide to one of childhood's most misunderstood disorders.* New York: Broadway Books.

Pauls, D. L., Gerhard, D. S., Lacy, L. G., Hostetter, A. M., Allen, C. R., Bland, S. D., LaBuda, M. C., & Egeland, J. A. (1991). Linkage of bipolar affective disorders to markers on chromosome 11p is excluded in a second lateral extension of Amish pedigree 110. *Genomics, 11*(3), 730–736.

Perugi, G., Akiskal, H. S., Pfanner, C., Presta, S,. Gemignani, A., Milanfranchi, A., Lensi, P., Ravagli, S., & Cassano, G. B. (1997). The clinical impact of bipolar and unipolar affective comorbidity on obsessive–compulsive disorder. *Journal of Affective Disorders, 46*(1), 15–23.

Pliszka, S. R., Sherman, J. O., Barrow, M. V., & Irick, S. (2000). Affective disorder in juvenile offenders: A preliminary study. *American Journal of Psychiatry, 157*(1), 130–132.

Plomin, R. (2000). Genes and behaviour. *Annals of Medicine, 27*(5), 503–505.

Plomin, R., & Rutter, M. (1998). Child development, molecular genetics, and what to do with genes once they are found. *Child Development, 69*(4), 1223–1242.

Reeves, J. C., Werry, J. S., Elkind, G. S., & Zametkin, A. (1987). Attention deficit, conduct, oppositional, and anxiety disorders in children: Part 2. Clinical characteristics. *Journal of the American Academy of Child and Adolescent Psychiatry, 26*(2), 144–155.

Regier, D. A., Farmer, M. E., Rae, D. S., Locke, B. Z., Keith, S. J., Judd, L. L., & Goodwin, F. K. (1990). Comorbidity of mental disorders with alcohol and other drug abuse: Results from the Epidemiologic Catchment Area (ECA) Study. *Journal of the American Medical Association, 264*(19), 2511–2518.

Rey, J. M. (1993). Oppositional defiant disorder. *American Journal of Psychiatry, 150*(12), 1769–1778.

Rosenbaum, J. F., Biederman, J., Bolduc, E. A., Hirshfeld, D. R., Faraone, S. V., & Kagan, J. (1992). Comorbidity of parental anxiety disorders as risk for childhood-onset anxiety in inhibited children. *American Journal of Psychiatry, 149*(4), 475–481.

Rosenbaum, J. F., Biederman, J., Hirshfeld-Becker, D. R., Kagan, J., Snidman, N., Friedman, D., Nineberg, A., Gallery, D. J., & Faraone, S. V. (2000). A controlled study of behavioral inhibition in children of parents with panic disorder and depression. *American Journal of Psychiatry, 157*(12), 2002–2010.

Sachs, G. S., Baldassano, C. F., Truman, C. J., & Guille, C. (2000). Comorbidity of attention deficit hyperactivity disorder with early- and late-onset bipolar disorder. *American Journal of Psychiatry, 157*(3), 466–468.

Savino, M., Perugi, G., Simonini, E., Soriani, A., Cassano, G. B., & Akiskal, H. S. (1993). Affective comorbidity in panic disorder: is there a bipolar connection? *Journal of Affective Disorders, 28*(3), 155–163.

Schurhoff, F., Bellivier, F., Jouvent, R., Mouren-Simeoni, M. C., Bouvard, M., Allilaire, J. F., & Leboyer, M. (2000). Early and late onset bipolar disorders: Two different forms of manic-depressive illness? *Journal of Affective Disorders, 58*(3), 215–221.

Soeda, S., Terao, T., & Nakamura, J. (1999). The influence of clomipramine-induced mania on rapid cycling affective disorder. *Journal of UOEH, 21*(4), 309–315.

Sonne, S. C., & Brady, K. T. (1999). Substance abuse and bipolar comorbidity. *Psychiatric Clinics of North America, 22*(3), 609–627.

Strober, M. (1998). Mixed mania associated with tricyclic antidepressant therapy in prepubertal delusional depression: Three cases. *Journal of Child and Adolescent Psychopharmacology, 8*(3), 181–185.

Szatmari, P., Boyle, M., & Offord, D. R. (1989). ADDH and conduct disorder: Degree of diagnostic overlap and differences among correlates. *Journal of the American Academy of Child and Adolescent Psychiatry, 28*(6), 865–872.

Todd, R. D., Geller, B., Neuman, R., Fox, L. W., & Hickok, J. (1996). Increased prevalence of alcoholism in relatives of depressed and bipolar children. *Journal of the American Academy of Child and Adolescent Psychiatry, 35*(6), 716–724.

Weller, E. B., Weller, R. A., & Fristad, M. A. (1995). Bipolar disorder in children:

Misdiagnosis, underdiagnosis, and future directions. *Journal of the American Academy of Child and Adolescent Psychiatry, 34*(6), 709–714.

Wender, P. H. (1998). Attention-deficit hyperactivity disorder in adults. *Psychiatric Clinics of North America, 21*(4), 761–774.

Wilens, T. E., Biederman, J., Millstein, R. B., Wozniak, J., Hahesy, A. L., & Spencer, T. J. (1999). Risk for substance use disorders in youths with child- and adolescent-onset bipolar disorder. *Journal of the American Academy of Child and Adolescent Psychiatry, 38*(6), 680–685.

Willcutt, E. G., Pennington, B. F., & DeFries, J. C. (2000). Twin study of the etiology of comorbidity between reading disability and attention-deficit/hyperactivity disorder. *American Journal of Medical Genetics, 96*(3), 293–301.

Winokur, G., Coryell, W., Akiskal, H. S., Endicott, J., Keller, M., & Mueller, T. (1994). Manic-depressive (bipolar) disorder: The course in light of a prospective ten-year follow-up of 131 patients. *Acta Psychiatrica Scandinavica, 89*(2), 102–110.

Winokur, G., Tsuang, M. T., & Crowe, R. R. (1982). The Iowa 500: Affective disorder in relatives of manic and depressed patients. *American Journal of Psychiatry, 139*(2), 209–212.

Wozniak, J., & Biederman, J. (1997). Childhood mania: Insights into diagnostic and treatment issues. *Association of Academic Minority Physicians, 8*(4), 78–84.

Wozniak, J., Biederman, J., Kiely, K., Ablon, J. S., Faraone, S. V., Mundy, E., & Mennin, D. (1995). Mania-like symptoms suggestive of childhood-onset bipolar disorder in clinically referred children. *Journal of the American Academy of Child and Adolescent Psychiatry, 34*(7), 867–876.

Wozniak, J., Biederman, J., Mundy, E., Mennin, D., & Faraone, S. V. (1995). A pilot family study of childhood-onset mania. *Journal of the American Academy of Child and Adolescent Psychiatry, 34*(12), 1577–1583.

5

Offspring Studies in Child and Early Adolescent Bipolar Disorder

KIKI CHANG and HANS STEINER

Offspring of parents with bipolar disorder represent a rich resource for study. They may present researchers with a window into prodromal forms of bipolar disorder and allow for early intervention to prevent the full onset of a bipolar disorder.

"Bipolar offspring," for the purposes of this chapter, will refer to children and adolescents with at least one biological parent with bipolar disorder. We do not include here the few studies of adult children of parents with bipolar disorder, as they cover somewhat different issues from studies of still-developing children. This chapter provides an overview of the significance of bipolar offspring studies, methodological difficulties in studying bipolar offspring, results of bipolar offspring studies completed to date, and future directions for this field of study.

SIGNIFICANCE OF OFFSPRING STUDIES

Many studies have been conducted regarding the phenomenology, biology, and treatment of adult forms of bipolar disorder. These studies are necessary to address the needs for treatment of millions of people worldwide who suffer from bipolar disorder, a typically chronic and debilitating disorder. However, not as much attention has been focused on *prevention* studies of bipolar disorder. As with other examples of preventative medicine, theoretically, by intervening before the onset of full-blown bipolar disorder, the disorder may be prevented or at least ameliorated in its severity, necessitating less treatment later in life and preventing high morbidity and poor social and vocational functioning. This idea is not dissimilar to the goals of prevention in other fields of medicine. For example, in families with familial hypercholesterolemia it is recommended to modify diet and exercise regimens as early in life as possible to prevent later cardiovascular disease.

The concept of *kindling*, proposed in affective disorders by Post (1992), argues for the need for early intervention in children at risk for bipolar disorder. The kindling theory suggests that mood disorders are created by an interplay between a susceptible genetic diathesis and environmental stressors, which causes actual biological changes at the genetic level that over time lead to the crossing of a neurobiological threshold for a mood episode. With the onset of each successive episode of mania or depression, these biological changes are reinforced, leading to more frequent and spontaneous episodes. This kindling theory has been supported by animal epilepsy studies and human retrospective mood charting. However, longitudinal prospective studies of populations at risk are required to fully investigate this phenomenon. Bipolar offspring are the natural choices for such studies.

However, risk factors for developing bipolar disorder have not been as well delineated as, for example, risk factors for developing diabetes or atherosclerosis. Currently, a family history of bipolar disorder appears to be a generally agreed-upon risk factor for developing bipolar disorder. Among psychiatric disorders, bipolar disorder vies with schizophrenia as being most tied to genetic causes. Studies have shown an approximately 67% concordance rate of bipolar disorder for monozygotic twins and a 25% concordance rate for dizygotic twins (Kelsoe, 1997). These twin studies would indicate that bipolar disorder is a highly heritable disorder, albeit not one with complete genetic penetrance.

Having any close relative with bipolar disorder does not in itself create an overly significant risk. Having a first-degree relative with bipolar disorder may confer a 6.5% risk of developing bipolar disorder, and a 10% risk for developing a major depressive episode, compared to 1% and 5%, respectively, for controls (individuals without a first-degree relative with bipolar disorder) (Kelsoe, 1997). However, as will be discussed later in this chapter, having a biological *parent* with bipolar disorder may confer much greater risk, with perhaps up to 27% of such offspring developing bipolar disorder (Gershon et al., 1982). Again, a 27% chance of illness still does not confer an automatic presumption of eventual development of the disorder. There are certainly also cases of patients with bipolar disorder who have no or only a very distant family history of mood disorders. Therefore, factors other than genetics that may identify those at high risk for development of bipolar disorder, need to be delineated. These additional risk factors may be phenomenological, neurobiological, or environmental in nature.

In a questionnaire sent to adult members of the National Depressive and Manic Depressive Association, Lish and colleagues inquired as to when these members with bipolar disorder first developed significant symptoms of bipolar disorder (Lish, Dime-Meenan, Whybrow, Price, & Hirschfeld, 1994). Of 245 responses, 31% described experiencing psychiatric symptoms before the age of 15 years, with 17% reporting symptoms occurring before 10 years of age. These symptoms consisted mostly of depressed mood, hyperactivity, suicidality, and manic behavior. Respondents further reported on average a 10-year interval between experiencing these symptoms and receiving a diagnosis of bipolar disorder with subsequent treatment. The sensitivity, specificity, and positive predictive value of these symptoms are unclear, but these data point again to the potential of early intervention. If this cohort had been identified as at risk for bipolar disorder upon presentation of their first childhood symptoms, could intervention have been made and progression of the disorder halted? However, isolated symptoms of depression or mania in a child are not by themselves specific to prodromal bipolar disorder. To accurately identify those at high risk for bipolar disorder, it is necessary to further delineate the presentation of prodromal bipolar disorder in children and adolescents.

Child and adolescent bipolar offspring may represent the most fruitful cohort to study in order to shed light on the development of bipolar disorder. First, as a population at high risk for developing bipolar disorder, they may serve to demonstrate early symptoms of prodromal bipolar disorder. Second, with longitudinal observation and assessment, they may reveal the nature of the natural progression of bipolar disorder, especially childhood-onset bipolar disorder. Third, they may represent a group of at-risk subjects who have not yet had significant drug or alcohol use, which may confound or change the presentation of bipolar disorder in later adolescence and adulthood. Fourth, these children are unique in having been raised by and/or exposed to a parent with bipolar disorder. The environmental effects of having a parent with bipolar disorder can therefore be studied as well, although it is difficult to separate out environmental from genetic factors. One last natural extension of studying bipolar offspring is the possibility of studying various interventions and their efficacy in preventing the onset of full bipolar disorder.

CHALLENGES IN STUDYING BIPOLAR OFFSPRING

Despite the attractiveness of studying children who are at high risk for developing bipolar disorder, researchers face a fair number of challenges when studying bipolar offspring. In order to conduct valid and useful research, certain variables should be taken into consideration. First, what aspects of bipolar offspring should be studied? The possibilities include phenomenology, presence of psychiatric symptoms, temperament, family environment, psychosocial functioning, academic ability, or biological factors. Also, is a control population needed? To study the uniqueness of bipolar offspring, one may need to include such a population. Depending on what factors are being studied, one might choose among various control groups, such as offspring of parents with schizophrenia, offspring of parents with chronic medical illness, or offspring of parents without any psychiatric illness at all.

Deciding on recruitment criteria for families with a bipolar parent may pose some challenges as well. As is being rapidly reported in the literature, there is growing evidence for a wide spectrum of bipolar disorders among adults (Akiskal & Pinto, 1999). Which types of bipolar disorder (bipolar I, bipolar II, antidepressant-induced mania, bipolar disorder not otherwise specified) allowed in included parents may affect the specificity and generalizability of the study as well as the actual likelihood of bipolar outcome in the offspring. The presence of comorbid psychiatric symptoms or diagnoses, such as anxiety or personality disorders, in the affected parent may also affect the outcome for their offspring. The psychiatric status of the parent without bipolar disorder also needs to be assessed and entered into the equation. One might argue that inclusion of families with one parent who has unipolar depression would serve to "dilute" the study. For example, it would be unclear if a symptomatic child of a parent with bipolar disorder and a parent with depression would be expressing a prodromal bipolar state or expressing the genetic contribution of the unipolar parent. Due to the incidence of assortative mating in affective disorders (Baron, Mendlewicz, Gruen, Asnis, & Fieve, 1981; Dunner, Fleiss, Addonizio, & Fieve, 1976), this type of parenting couple may be fairly prevalent. Therefore, it might be ideal to include only families in which *both* parents have bipolar disorder, but these type of couples may be much less prevalent. There is the additional question of whether to recruit only fathers or only mothers with bipolar disorder, or to recruit equal cohorts of each. Since the legal system tends to award mothers in divorce cases with child custody, it may prove more difficult to recruit fathers with bipolar disorder from separated families. Finally, there is the specter of needing to determine true paternity or maternity through blood testing. The frequent presence of impulsivity and hypersexuality in adult manic states may make this testing all the more necessary.

If one chooses to assess psychiatric symptoms and diagnoses in bipolar offspring, semistructured interviews are necessary to provide reliable data based on a widely agreed-upon diagnostic standard, such as the *Diagnostic and Statistical Manual of Mental Disorders* (DSM-IV; American Psychiatric Association, 1994). Which interview to use would depend on the level of complexity one wishes to engage in. For example, the Diagnostic Interview Schedule for Children (DISC; Fisher et al., 1993; Shaffer et al., 1993) would allow a fairly quick and thorough screening, but using the Washington University Kiddie Schedule for Affective Disorders and Schizophrenia (WASH-U-KSADS) (Geller, Williams, Zimerman, & Frazier, 1996; Geller et al., 2001) would provide another level of symptom assessment more specific for childhood bipolar disorder and allow for documentation of cycling patterns of mood. Since, as argued earlier in this book, diagnostic criteria from DSM-IV for childhood bipolar disorder require retooling, it may be prudent to use an interview that is wide in its breadth and fairly deep in its probing, so as to allow for both new findings in symptomatology and the possibility of rediagnosis based on later established criteria.

There are also developmental confounds in studying bipolar offspring, as studies in children at one time point are inherently cross-sectional. This narrow focus presents challenges in child studies, for children are still developing rapidly in social and emotional domains. Thus, the child diagnosed with an adjustment disorder at one time point may actually have a gradually developing major depressive episode, or the child with attention-deficit/hyperactivity disorder (ADHD) at one assessment may develop criteria for bipolar disorder a few years later. This developmental confound argues for longitudinal studies in bipolar offspring studies, for as long a time as possible to cover the development into adulthood. Longitudinal studies themselves contain many challenges, among them subject attrition and changes in diagnostic criteria. The age range of subjects when beginning a longitudinal study must also be considered. The range needs to be broad enough to include the historically typical age of onset (15–19 years) (Goodwin & Jamison, 1990) as well as earlier ages that would precede onset. The ideal study would begin at birth and extend through adulthood, but such a long and inclusive study would most likely be prohibitive temporally and financially.

Finally, interpreting data from phenomenological studies of bipolar offspring may be difficult. One challenge is separating out the environmental component of having a parent with bipolar disorder from the genetic component. According to the kindling theory on the development of mood disorders (Post, 1992), individuals may have a certain genetic predisposition to mood disorders, but environmental stress is the other factor that interfaces with this predisposition to cause a destabilization of mood. As the genes involved in bipolar disorder are unknown, there is no current blood screen that can quantify genetic risk for bipolar disorder. Similarly, as environmental stress contains a multitude of factors (e.g., parenting style, school environment, safety of neighborhood, etc.), there is no well-established method for quantifying environmental risk. Therefore, it is difficult to know how much weight each factor, genes and environment, carries to determine psychiatric outcome.

It appears that the ideal study of bipolar offspring would begin at birth and extend through early adulthood. Both biological parents would be diagnosed through structured interviews, and either one or both would have bipolar disorder, possibly only bipolar I disorder with no comorbid disorders. Investigators would directly interview children and parents using semistructured interviews specific for mood-related symptoms in children. A control group, such as children of healthy or of medically ill parents, would also be included, and raters of both subjects and controls would be blinded to parental status. Family environmental and biological data would be collected and correlated with psychopathology. Such a study would likely be prohibitive financially and temporally. However, the phenomenological studies of bipolar offspring presented in the next section should be considered with this prototypical study in mind (Table 5.1).

BIPOLAR OFFSPRING STUDIES: PHENOMENOLOGY

A family history of bipolar disorder has long been considered a risk factor for development of bipolar disorder, at least since Emil Kraeplin published his tome *Manic–Depressive Insanity and Paranoia* (Kraeplin, 1921). In this work, Kraeplin noted that patients with recurrent depressive episodes tended to have family members with alcoholism and manic–depressive illness (Akiskal & Pinto, 1999). This idea was revisited in 1960, when Anthony and Scott (1960) included evidence of a positive family history of bipolar disorder as one of the 10 criteria important in diagnosing childhood bipolar disorder. In 1979, Davis set forth the idea of a "manic–depressant variant of childhood," with one of the criteria being a family history of affective disorder. However, prior to the 1970s no formal studies of children with manic–depressive parents were conducted. Also in 1979, Kestenbaum reported on 13 children with a bipolar parent. These children were found to have a preponderance of temper tantrums, dysphoric symptoms, obsessive and compulsive tendencies, hyperactivity, mood lability, and impulsivity. McKnew and colleagues (McKnew, Cytryn, Efron, Gershon, & Bunney, 1979) reported on children of 14 inpatients with affective disorder (unipolar or bipolar). Over half of the 30 children were noted to be depressed, either at baseline or at 4-month follow-up, without any other diagnoses reported. These studies marked the advent of clinicians and researchers suspecting that bipolar offspring were highly susceptible to mood and behavioral difficulties.

A recent meta-analysis (Lapalme, Hodgins, & LaRoche, 1997) analyzed 17 studies of bipolar offspring published between 1983 and 1993 (Decina et al., 1983; Gershon et al., 1985; Grigoroiu-Serbanescu et al., 1989; Hammen, Burge, Burney, & Adrian, 1990; Hammen et al., 1987; Kashani, Burk, Horwitz, & Reid, 1985; Klein, Depue, & Slater, 1985; Kuyler, Rosenthal, Igel, Dunner, & Fieve, 1980; LaRoche et al., 1985; LaRoche, Cheifetz, & Lester, 1981; LaRoche et al., 1987; Nurnberger,

TABLE 5.1. Phenomenological Studies of Bipolar Offspring

First author (year)	n (families)	% with BD	% with ADHD	% with any Dx	Rating	Comments
McKnew (1979)	30 (13)			16	**	Depression was only diagnosis found.
Kuyler (1980)	49 (27)	0	0	22 (45%)	**	
LaRoche (1981)	17 (10)	0	0	0 (0%)	**	
Cytryn (1982)	19 (13)			11/13 familes	*****	Same cohort as McKnew (1979), but with blinded raters and control group.
Decina (1983)	31 (18)	0 (5)	2 (6%)	16 (52%)	****1/2	Children inteviewed with the Mental Health Assessment form.
Gershon (1985)	29	1 (3%)	4 (14%)	21 (72%)	**** control group included, but unclear if blinded interviewers	8 children had "atypical depression," which included cyclothymic disorder.
Kashani (1985)	9 (5)	0	1 (11%)	?	***1/2 Parent not assessed directly	Bipolar offspring not significantly different from unipolar offspring.
Klein (1985)	37 (24)	10 (27%)		16 (43%)	****	Subjects 15 to 21 years old. Parents not interviewed about children.
LaRoche (1985)	39	0	0	9 (23%)	**1/2	13% with "cyclothymic personality traits."
Weintraub (1987)	134 (58)			27 (20%)	***	Subjects assessed at age > 18 years.
Nurnberger (1988)	53 (32)	?	?	38 (72%)	****	Subjects 15 to 25 years old.
Zahn-Waxler (1988)	7 (7)	0	2 (29%)	6 (86%)	****	Children assessed at age 6 years.
Grigoroiu-Serbanescu (1989)	72 (47)	1 (1%)	15 (21%)	44 (61%)	****1/2	Parents interviewed clinically. Controls with 25% psychopathology.
Hammen (1990)	18 (14)	0	1 (6)	13 (72%)	*****	All mothers with BD. 82% of unipolar comparison group with psychopathology.

(continued)

TABLE 5.1. (*continued*)

First author (year)	n (families)	% with BD	% with ADHD	% with any Dx	Rating	Comments
Radke-Yarrow (1992)	44 (22)			(56%)	****1/2	Results from subjects 8 to 11 years old reported here.
Carlson (1993)	128	6/125 (5%)	39 (30%) at baseline	?	*****	Longitudinal follow-up at over age 18 years.
Duffy (1998)	36 (23)	5 (14%)	1 (3%)	19 (53%)	***	Subjects 10 to 25 years old.
Soutullo (1999)	24	12 (50%)	16 (67%)	?	*****	High rate of BP and ADHD in controls (9%, 18%).
Chang (2000)	60 (37)	8 (13%)	16 (27%)	31 (52%)	****	Parents with retrospective ADHD more likely to have offspring with BD.
Wals (2001)	140 (86)	4 (3%)	7 (5%)	61 (44%)	****	Netherlands, ages 12–21, 27% had a mood disorder.

Ratings guidelines: *****Parents and offspring interviewed with semistructured interviews, parents interviewed about children, children directly interviewed, interviewers blinded to parental status, control group assessed; ****parents and offspring interviewed with semistructured interviews, parents interviewed about children, children directly interviewed; ***offspring interviewed with semistructured interviews, parents interviewed about children; **offspring interviewed with semistructured interviews (children directly interviewed); *offspring evaluated by parental/child questionnaires or nonstructured interviews. BP, bipolar spectrum disorders (bipolar I, II, or NOS, or cyclothymia); ADHD, attention-deficit/hyperactivity disorder; Dx, diagnosis; ?, not reported. Blank cells indicate uncertainty whether interview used allowed for possibility of such a diagnosis.

Hamovit, et al., 1988; Radke-Yarrow, Nottelmann, Martinez, Fox, & Belmont, 1992; Waters & Marchenko-Bouer, 1980; Weintraub, 1987; Zahn-Waxler et al., 1988). These studies all used structured diagnostic interviews or DSM-III or DSM-III-R criteria to diagnose the parents who had bipolar disorder. Eleven of these studies also used a comparison group of parents with either no mental disorder or with no "major mental disorder," the specifics of which was not made clear in the review. A total of 772 children with a bipolar parent and 626 children of healthy controls were included in the meta-analysis. Fifty-two percent of these bipolar offspring met criteria for some psychiatric disorder compared to 29% of the children of the control parents. Relative risk analysis revealed that children with a bipolar parent were more than 2.5 times as likely to develop any psychiatric disorder, and 4.0 times more likely to develop an affective disorder compared to the control group. Of bipolar offspring, 5.4% were diagnosed with bipolar disorder, compared to 0% of the control group

(Lapalme et al., 1997). This finding is fairly significant given that all of these studies except three (Carlson & Weintraub, 1993; Hammen et al., 1990; LaRoche et al., 1987) were cross-sectional, and that many of the bipolar offspring would not yet have been at the most common age of onset of bipolar disorder, between 15 and 19 years (Goodwin & Jamison, 1990).

One of the few longitudinal studies in this population was conducted by Carlson and Weintraub (1993). The relatively large sample ($n = 134$) was drawn from the Stony Brook High Risk Project, a longitudinal study of offspring of parents with schizophrenia, bipolar disorder, unipolar depression, or substance abuse. One hundred and eight controls with parents not having psychiatric illness were also followed. This elegant study compared the bipolar offspring to healthy controls, seeking to investigate the relationship of attention or behavioral problems in childhood to future development of affective disorder. Of bipolar offspring, 27.6% had behavioral problems, and 30.4% had attention problems, as defined by various rating scales. Subjects were then reassessed after age 18 years. The authors found behavioral or attention problems in childhood to be associated with development of a mood disorder in young adulthood, but only in bipolar offspring; the control group did not demonstrate this association.

There has been a trend from 1989 to 2001 to probe for externalizing and behavioral problems in bipolar offspring. It is unclear if incidence of these disorders (i.e., oppositional defiant disorder, attention-deficit/hyperactivity disorder, and conduct disorder) are actually increasing, or if researchers are simply more aware of their existence. Over the last two decades, mental health professionals have been regarding these disorders as less of a failing of weak character or bad parenting and more of an intrinsic disorder meriting study. Problems with "conduct" and general "behavior" were observed in bipolar offspring in the 1970s (Davis, 1979; Kestenbaum, 1979), but systematic diagnoses were not done until more recently. Thus, attention-deficit/hyperactivity disorder was not reported present in bipolar offspring until 1983 (Decina et al., 1983) and mostly neglected as a relevant disorder until after 1988. Since 1988, attention-deficit/hyperactivity disorder, or at least significant behavioral or attention problems, has been reported in approximately 27% of bipolar offspring studied (Table 5.1).

It has been suggested that children with attention-deficit/hyperactivity disorder who have a strong history of bipolar disorder may be experiencing a prodromal bipolar state (Faraone, Biederman, Mennin, Wozniak, & Spencer, 1997; Faraone et al., 1997). Thus, it is possible that this increase in the prevalence of attention-deficit/hyperactivity disorder in bipolar offspring may actually reflect an overall increase in early-onset bipolar disorder. Notably, Chang and colleagues found seven out of eight offspring with bipolar disorder to have comorbid attention-deficit/hyperactivity disorder; by retrospective diagnosis, they concluded that all these subjects had symptoms of attention-deficit/hyperactivity disorder before the onset of bipolar disorder (Chang, Steiner, & Ketter, 2000). Furthermore, the investigators found that parents with bipolar disorder who had retrospectively reported a history of attention-deficit/hyperactivity disorder during their own childhood were more likely to have children already with bipolar disorder than bipolar parents without a history of attention-deficit/hyperactivity disorder. The parents of bipolar children also had an earlier onset of their own bipolar disorder compared to parents of nonbipolar children. This finding supports the possibility of attention-deficit/hyperactivity disorder in bipolar offspring as an early nonisomorphic manifestation of a type of bipolar disorder that is familial and presents relatively earlier in life.

Lithium responsivity may represent another subtype of bipolar disorder that is supported by offspring studies. Duffy and colleagues (Duffy, Alda, Kutcher, Fusee, & Grof, 1998) studied children with lithium-responsive bipolar parents versus those with lithium-nonresponsive parents. In this study, bipolar disorder not otherwise specified, was added as a possible diagnosis for the first time in the offspring literature. Children of lithium-nonresponsive parents tended to have a wider range of psychopathology and more comorbid diagnoses compared to children of lithium-responsive parents. Furthermore, the children who had affective disorders in the former group had more chronic cycling and more irritability than the children who had affective disorders in the latter group. This preliminary study ($n = 36$) supports the idea of subtypes of bipolar disorder in adults that may be transmittable to their offspring. However, as this was a cross-sectional study, it is not known how many of the children with varied psychopathology and increased comorbidity would eventually develop a (presumably lithium-nonresponsive) bipolar disorder.

Since 1997, studies have continued to consistently report about a 50% incidence of some psychiatric disorder in cross-sectional assessment of child and adolescent bipolar offspring (Chang et al., 2000; Duffy et al., 1998; Soutullo et al., 1999). Bipolar disorder itself was rarely reported in bipolar offspring before 1983. Since then, however, the spectrum of bipolar disorder has been enlarged over the past 6 years with the inclusion of bipolar disorder not otherwise specified, and bipolar II disorder in DSM-III-R and DSM-IV (American Psychiatric Association, 1994). Thus, Duffy and colleagues reported five of 36 bipolar offspring as having bipolar spectrum disorders, and Chang and colleagues reported nine of 60 offspring as having bipolar I or bipolar II disorder. Soutullo and colleagues recently reported on 24 bipolar offspring, whom they compared to 13 healthy controls. *Fifty percent* of bipolar offspring were found to have a bipolar spectrum disorder (bipolar I, bipolar II, bipolar not otherwise specified, or cyclothymia) and 71% had some mood disorder, compared to 9% and 14%, respectively, for the controls (Soutullo et al., 1999). Again, similar to the phenomenon of increased reporting of attention-deficit/hyperactivity disorder in bipolar offspring, this increase in the reported incidence of bipolar disorder may be due to several possibilities. First, it may reflect the slowly growing acceptance by clinicians of the possibility of children having true bipolar disorder. Second, the widening of the bipolar spectrum may be allowing for more diagnoses of bipolar disorder in children. Third, only recently has the development of structured interviews that specifically assess for pediatric bipolar symptoms allowed for more accurate diagnosis of pediatric bipolar disorder (DelBello & Geller, 2001). Fourth, this increase in diagnosis may actually represent a growing increase in the incidence of childhood bipolar disorder. Theories of genetic anticipation may support a gradually increasing incidence of childhood-onset bipolar disorder (McInnis et al., 1993; Petronis & Kennedy, 1995). Most likely, this increased incidence of bipolar disorder reported in bipolar offspring is a reflection of all four events occurring simultaneously.

One study that bucks this trend involved bipolar offspring in the Netherlands (Wals et al., 2001). The researchers found only 3% of offspring to have a lifetime diagnosis of bipolar disorder and 5% with attention-deficit/hyperactivity disorder. However, 27% did have some type of mood disorder. Furthermore, the study did not include school-age children, possibly accounting for less reporting of past attention-deficit/hyperactivity disorder symptoms. The possibility remains, though, that bipolar offspring in countries outside the United States may have less risk of developing bipolar disorder, whether due to differences in environment, genetics, or differences in medication-prescribing practices. The latter possibility may be relevant, as stimulants and antidepressants are used much more frequently with children in the United States than in the Netherlands, and these medications have been reported to exacerbate or cause mania in children (this topic is discussed later in this chapter).

A few studies of bipolar offspring have used a comparison group of children with a parent with a unipolar depressive disorder (Hammen et al., 1990; Kashani et al., 1985; Radke-Yarrow et al., 1992; Weintraub, 1987). Two studies reported no differences in amount of psychopathology between the unipolar and the bipolar offspring (Kashani et al., 1985; Weintraub, 1987); two others indicated that children with unipolar parents actually had higher rates of psychopathology (Hammen et al., 1990; Radke-Yarrow et al., 1992). Therefore, while bipolar disorder is usually considered to be a more heritable disorder with more morbidity than unipolar depression, the environmental factors of having a parent with a mood disorder cannot be ignored.

Effects of family environment on offspring psychopathology have been studied somewhat. Marital discord and exposure of offspring to parental illness before age 3 years were found to be correlated with offspring psychopathology in one study of 39 bipolar offspring (LaRoche et al., 1985). Mothers with bipolar disorder were found in another study to have more negativity in their interactions with their offspring, compared to depressed or nondisordered mothers (Inoff-Germain, Nottelmann, & Radke-Yarrow, 1992). In a study using the Family Environmental Scale, Chang and colleagues (Chang, Blasey, Ketter, & Steiner, 2001), found families with a bipolar parent to have less cohesion and organization and more conflict than families from a national, unscreened sample. However, no particular family environment profile was correlated with presence or absence of specific psychopathology. Other investigators have suggested correlations between pathological family environments and severity of illness in bipolar offspring (Grigoroiu-Serbanescu et al., 1989; Kuyler et al., 1980). These findings highlight the importance that family environment and parenting technique may have on psychiatric outcome of bipolar offspring.

From these phenomenologically based studies, it is clear that bipolar offspring are at high risk for development of psychiatric disorders, specifically attention-deficit/hyperactivity disorder, depression, and bipolar disorder. It is not clear, though, to which extent genetic and environmental factors each play a role in the development of these conditions. Also, because of the cross-sectional nature of the majority of these studies, we do not have enough data on the eventual outcome in adulthood of bipolar offspring, whether or not they have psychopathology as children. Additional prospective longitudinal studies of phenomenology would provide outcome data that would give perspective to psychiatric presentations of bipolar offspring during childhood.

BIPOLAR OFFSPRING STUDIES: PSYCHOSOCIAL FACTORS AND FUNCTIONING

There are fewer studies examining the psychosocial functioning of child and adolescent bipolar offspring. Zahn-Waxler and colleagues (Zahn-Waxler, Cummings, McKnew, & Radke-Yarrow, 1984) noted in 1984 that 2-year-old children of bipolar parents showed "heightened distress and preoccupation with the conflicts and suffering of others." These children were also noted to have problems socializing appropriately with peers, with less inclination to share and more aggression toward both peers and adults. In a controlled study, child bipolar offspring were found to have a lack of a strong social support group and a notable absence of a "best friend" (Pellegrini et al., 1986). A longitudinal study followed offspring of either a bipolar or a unipolar depressed parent compared to offspring of nondisordered parents (Radke-Yarrow et al., 1992). At 3-year follow-up, significantly more offspring of affectively ill parents had developed depressive and behavioral problems. However, offspring of unipolar depressed parents, but not of bipolar parents, had the earliest onset of these problems.

Similarly, offspring of depressed mothers were shown to have worse overall psychosocial functioning than offspring of bipolar, medically ill, or normal mothers (Anderson & Hammen, 1993). This study included measures of externalizing and internalizing behaviors, school performance, and behavior in class. In a previously mentioned study (Chang et al., 2000), Chang and colleagues noted the mean Global Assessment of Functioning (GAF) of their cohort of bipolar offspring to be 76 +/- 12, which indicates fairly good functioning. Furthermore, scores on the Wide Range Achievement Test—Revision 3 (WRAT-3), an indicator of academic achievement, were all at or slightly above grade level. However, bipolar offspring with psychopathology had significantly lower GAF scores than those without, but academic achievement did not differ between these two groups.

It appears that bipolar offspring are clearly at risk for poor psychosocial and academic functioning. Psychotherapeutic interventions in this population appear to be indicated, but the ideal psychotherapeutic methods and the time at which to apply them have not yet been identified by research.

BIPOLAR OFFSPRING STUDIES: PSYCHOLOGICAL AND BIOLOGICAL MARKERS

Other characteristics of bipolar offspring have been investigated in an attempt to establish biological or psychological markers for risk of bipolar outcome. Through Rorshach testing, bipolar offspring have been found to have higher ratios of color to movement determinants (Decina et al., 1983) and elevated levels of thought disorder, lack of cognitive-mediated affective responses, and a decreased capacity for conventional reception (Osher, Mandel, Shapiro, & Belmaker, 2000) compared to healthy controls. Researchers of this last study, conducted in bipolar offspring over age 15 years, noted that their findings were strikingly similar to the Rorschach profiles of adults with bipolar disorder in their clinic (Osher et al., 2000).

IQ testing of bipolar offspring has also revealed some interesting results. Weintraub (1979, as reported by Kestenbaum, 1980) found Verbal IQ to be significantly higher than Performance IQ in child and adolescent bipolar offspring. Furthermore, bipolar offspring had the highest mean Verbal IQ scores among offspring of schizophrenics, offspring of unipolars, and controls. This finding of relatively elevated Verbal IQ was replicated by Decina and colleagues in 1983, who found Verbal scores to be more than 15 points greater than Performance scores in 39% of 31 bipolar offspring compared to an expected 13% by population norms or to 11% of their control group (Decina et al., 1983). However, naturalistic IQ data gathered in adult bipolar offspring by Waters and colleagues (Waters,

Marchenko-Bouer, & Smiley, 1981) did not support this Verbal–Performance split. In that same study, 29% of bipolar offspring were predominantly left-handed, versus only 6% of controls, a finding that has not since been replicated. A more recent study found bipolar offspring to perform worse than controls in IQ testing and tests of executive function (McDonough-Ryan et al., 2000).

Other studies have failed to establish markers such as differences in eye-tracking abnormalities (Rosenberg et al., 1997) or electrodermal activity (Zahn, Nurnberger, & Berrettini, 1989) in bipolar offspring compared to healthy controls. One interesting study, however, did find differences in melatonin suppression by light between the two groups (Nurnberger, Berrettini, et al., 1988). Twenty-five bipolar offspring, 15 to 25 years old, were compared to 20 healthy controls. These subjects were exposed to bright light from 2:00 A.M. to 4:00 A.M., after which plasma melatonin levels were drawn and compared to baseline melatonin levels. Bipolar offspring showed significantly higher suppression of melatonin levels after bright light exposure compared to controls. Furthermore, the group of seven offspring with two bipolar parents appeared to have the highest percentage of subjects (57%) with melatonin suppression greater than a previously determined cutoff of 0.84 standard deviations above the control mean. Only 21% of controls and 33% of offspring with one bipolar parent had melatonin suppression above this threshold. Ninety-one percent of a sample of euthymic adults with bipolar disorder also were reported to suppress melatonin to this degree (Lewy et al., 1985), suggesting a possible increasing relationship between melatonin suppression and genetic loading for bipolar disorder (Nurnberger, Berrettini, et al., 1988). However, this possible trait marker for bipolar disorder has not since been investigated in bipolar offspring.

Neuroimaging studies of bipolar offspring are currently in progress. DelBello and colleagues (2000) recently found bipolar offspring to have larger hippocampal volumes than healthy controls. Functional MRI and MR spectroscopy studies are also currently being conducted. One MRS study investigated levels of prefrontal N-acetyl aspartate (NAA), a marker of neuronal density, in bipolar offspring who had either fully developed bipolar disorder or mood and behavioral problems short of meeting full criteria for bipolar disorder (Chang, Adelman, Dienes, Reiss, & Ketter, 2001). The investigators noted decreased NAA in the offspring with bipolar disorder, but found that the offspring with putative prodromal bipolar disorder had no differences in NAA from controls. If these subjects were truly prodromal for bipolar disorder, this finding might indicate a prefrontal neurodegenerative process occurring only after bipolar disorder is fully developed. These brain imaging studies show great promise, as they directly study the end organ involved in bipolar disorder, maximizing the chances of providing relevant biological information. However, biological studies of bipolar offspring again need to be conducted in a prospective, longitudinal manner to take full advantage of studying a population that is at high risk for development of bipolar disorder. These type of studies would be more likely than cross-sectional studies to establish trait markers for bipolar disorder that could be detected before the actual onset of the disorder.

PROPHYLAXIS OF BIPOLAR DISORDER

A natural extension of the aforementioned studies of bipolar offspring is to investigate the possibility of preventing the development of bipolar disorder. While there is currently no reliable biological marker that can be used to detect impending bipolar disorder, studying the phenomenology of bipolar offspring allows for the identification of early symptoms that may represent prodromal states of bipolar disorder. In line with the theory of kindling in mood disorders, intervention with appropriate treatment, whether psychotherapeutic or pharmacological, at this juncture may prevent subsequent development of full-blown bipolar disorder.

Identification of prodromal states of bipolar disorder also may eventually allow for more accurate diagnoses and treatment. For example, a child with symptoms of attention-deficit/hyperactivity disorder and mood lability who has a parent with bipolar disorder may actually be in a prodromal state of bipolar disorder. Treatment with stimulants has been reported to trigger manic episodes in children (Biederman, Klein, Pine, & Klein, 1998; Koehler-Troy, Strober, & Malenbaum, 1986), and bipolar offspring may be especially susceptible to this reaction. Therefore, by identification of prodromal bipolar disorder, more appropriate treatment may be initiated. Similarly, bipolar offspring with a major depressive episode may actually be presenting the first mood-related symptoms of a latent bipolar disorder. Recognition of this prodromal bipolar state is important, as antidepressants have been reported to have triggered mania in depressed children, especially those with a family history of bipolar disorder (Achamallah & Decker, 1991; Grubbs, 1997; Kat, 1996; Oldroyd, 1997; Venkataraman, Naylor, & King, 1992). Indeed, a family history of bipolar disorder has been proposed as a risk factor for the development of bipolar disorder in depressed children (Strober & Carlson, 1982), an event that may occur in up to 25% of depressed prepubertal children and 20% of depressed adolescents (Geller, Fox, & Clark, 1994). Intervention with a mood stabilizer would seem potentially more effective and safer than intervention with an antidepressant. However, one study found lithium to be no more effective than placebo in treating 30 prepubertal children with depression (Geller et al., 1998). All of these children had a family history of bipolar disorder, with 40% having a parent with bipolar disorder.

Anticonvulsants have been considered to be antikindling agents (Post, Altshuler, Ketter, Denicoff, & Weiss, 1991; Stoll & Severus, 1996), as they are able to prevent kindling of seizures in laboratory mice given repeated electrical stimuli (Post, 1992). Therefore, it is possible that certain anticonvulsants may serve to prevent the kindling of bipolar disorder as well. Divalproex is an anticonvulsant that is effective in the treatment of mania in adults with bipolar disorder (Bowden et al., 1994) and may be effective in children with bipolar disorder as well (Kowatch et al., 2000; Papatheodorou, Kutcher, Katic, & Szalai, 1995). There are at least two ongoing studies examining the potential of divalproex in treating bipolar offspring with possible prodromal symptoms of full-blown bipolar disorder.

At Stanford University, investigators have studied the use of divalproex in 20 children and adolescents with at least one bipolar parent (Chang, Dienes, Steiner, & Ketter, 2001). Participants were aged from 6 to 18 years (mean = 11.7 years) and were diagnosed with major depression, attention-deficit/hyperactivity disorder, oppositional defiant disorder, dysthymia, and/or cyclothymia. After a 2-week washout period, subjects were begun on open divalproex, and the dose was gradually titrated to achieve serum levels of 50–120 μg/ml (mean dose = 875 mg/day; mean serum level = 88.5 μg/ml). Subjects were monitored weekly for 4 weeks, and then biweekly for the rest of the 12-week trial. Those considered completers finished at least 8 weeks. Primary measure for response was a 2 or 1 on the Clinician Global Impression—Change ("very much improved" or "much improved") at week 8 or week 12. Secondary measures were a 50% decrease from Week 0 to Week 8 or Week 12 in Young Mania Rating Scale or Hamilton Depression scores. Two subjects dropped out after 2 weeks due to continuation or worsening of symptoms. Of the remaining 18 subjects, 11 (61%) were considered responders by primary criteria. By secondary criteria, 12 (67%) were considered responders. Presence of a mood disorder tended to correlate with a positive response to divalproex. These results are limited by the small sample size and open nature of the study. However, many of the responders did not previously respond to standard therapies (stimulants or antidepressants) for their disorders, possibly diminishing the bias of placebo effect. These data are encouraging enough to suggest that blinded, placebo-controlled studies of anticonvulsants in symptomatic bipolar offspring need to be conducted.

At the University Hospitals of Cleveland, Findling and colleagues (Findling, Gracious, McNamara, & Calabrese, 2000) have been conducting a placebo-controlled study of divalproex in bipolar offspring with cyclothymia or bipolar disorder not otherwise specified. Thirty-two subjects have been enrolled and randomized to treatment, with 14 diagnosed with cyclothymia and 18 with bipolar disorder not otherwise specified. Nine of these subjects have discontinued the study secondary to continuing symptoms of depression or mania. This study is currently ongoing and the blind has not been broken yet to reveal efficacy data.

These two studies represent the possibility of early intervention in children at high risk for bipolar disorder. Results from these and similar studies, incorporating control groups with a prospective longitudinal design, will aid in determining the proper treatments for bipolar offspring and the feasibility of preventing bipolar disorder in this population.

CONCLUSIONS AND FUTURE DIRECTIONS

It is evident that child and adolescent bipolar offspring present a great opportunity for examination of the early development of bipolar disorder. Studies of phenomenology of bipolar offspring have already proved that these children are clearly at high risk for psychopathology, especially attention-deficit/hyperactivity disorder, depression, and bipolar disorder. However, many questions regarding the outcome of these children remain. What percentage of bipolar offspring with attention-deficit/hyperactivity disorder will develop bipolar disorder, and what are the risk factors for doing so? Do bipolar offspring with bipolar disorder not otherwise specified or cyclothymia develop criteria as adults for bipolar I disorder? Well-designed and carefully conducted longitudinal studies will tell us the significance of the results from past cross-sectional studies.

Psychological and biological studies of bipolar offspring have thus far revealed scant promising markers for bipolar illness. The advent of MRI as a viable tool to study brain anatomy, chemistry, and function in children provides hope that neuroimaging studies will begin to detect these biological markers. Together with neuroendocrine, genetic, and second messenger-based studies, these studies have the potential for elucidating etiology and pathophysiology of bipolar disorder by studying a population before, during, and after the onset of bipolar disorder.

The ultimate benefit from bipolar offspring studies will be clinical. Discovering risk factors for development of bipolar disorder leads to identifying populations at need for close clinical monitoring. Discovering early bipolar phenomenology leads to early intervention to prevent full-blown bipolar disorder. And finally, discovering etiology rapidly advances treatment options. These studies also point to the great need of many bipolar offspring for clinical care. Bipolar offspring are at high risk for poor psychosocial and academic functioning, chaotic family environments, and development of significant psychopathology. However, clinical intervention needs to be conducted with the high possibility of a bipolar outcome in mind. Is monotherapy with stimulants or antidepressants appropriate treatment for bipolar offspring? What types of psychotherapeutic approaches are most effective in preventing the onset of bipolar disorder in at-risk children? Intervention studies in bipolar offspring will help elucidate the best psychotherapeutic and psychopharmacological treatments for this cohort.

The future holds great promise for bipolar offspring studies to provide this essential information. Prospective, longitudinal studies incorporating phenomenology, neurobiology, family environment, and intervention effects are needed to ensure that this promise is fulfilled.

REFERENCES

Achamallah N. S., & Decker D. H. (1991). Mania induced by fluoxetine in an adolescent patient. *American Journal of Psychiatry, 148*(10), 1404.

Akiskal, H. S., & Pinto, O. (1999). The evolving bipolar spectrum: Prototypes I, II, III, and IV. *Psychiatric Clinics of North America, 22*(3), 517–534, vii.

American Psychiatric Association. (1994). *Diagnostic and statistical manual of mental disorders* (4th ed.). Washington, DC: Author.

Anderson, C. A., & Hammen, C. L. (1993). Psychosocial outcomes of children of unipolar depressed, bipolar, medically ill, and normal women: A longitudinal study. *Journal of Consulting and Clinical Psychology, 61*(3), 448–454.

Anthony, J., & Scott, P. (1960). Manic–depressive psychosis in childhood. *Journal of Child Psychology and Psychiatry, 1*, 53–72.

Baron, M., Mendlewicz, J., Gruen, R., Asnis, L., & Fieve, R. R. (1981). Assortative mating in affective disorders. *Journal of Affective Disorders, 3*(2), 167–171.

Biederman, J., Klein, R. G., Pine, D. S., & Klein, D. F. (1998). Resolved: Mania is mistaken for ADHD in prepubertal children. *Journal of the American Academy of Child and Adolescent Psychiatry, 37*(10), 1091–1096; discussion, 1096–1099.

Bowden, C. L., Brugger, A. M., Swann, A. C., Calabrese, J. R., Janicak, P. G., Petty, F., Dilsaver, S. C., Davis, J. M., Rush, A. J., Small, J. G., et al. (1994). Efficacy of divalproex vs lithium and placebo in the treatment of mania: The Depakote Mania Study Group. *Journal of the American Medical Association, 271*(12), 918–924.

Carlson, G. A., & Weintraub, S. (1993). Childhood behavior problems and bipolar disorder: Relationship or coincidence? *Journal of Affective Disorders, 28*(3), 143–153.

Chang, K. D., Adleman, N., Dienes, K., Reiss, A., & Ketter, T. A. (2001). *¹H-MRS in bipolar offspring with bipolar disorder.* Poster presented at the 40th annual meeting of the American College of Neuropsychopharmacology, Waikaloa, HI.

Chang, K. D., Blasey, C., Ketter, T. A., & Steiner, H. (2001). Family environment of children and adolescents with bipolar parents. *Bipolar Disorders, 2*(3), 68–72.

Chang, K. D., Dienes, K., Steiner, H., & Ketter, T. A. (2001). *Divalproex in bipolar offspring with mood and behavioral disorders.* Paper presented at the meeting of the New Clinical Drug Evaluation Unit, Scottsdale, AZ.

Chang, K. D., Steiner, H., & Ketter, T. A. (2000). Psychiatric phenomenology of child and adolescent bipolar offspring. *Journal of the American Academy of Child and Adolescent Psychiatry, 39*(4), 453–460.

Davis, R. E. (1979). Manic–depressive variant syndrome of childhood: A preliminary report. *American Journal of Psychiatry, 136*(5), 702–706.

Decina, P., Kestenbaum, C. J., Farber, S., Kron, L., Gargan, M., Sackeim, H. A., &

Fieve, R. R. (1983). Clinical and psychological assessment of children of bipolar probands. *American Journal of Psychiatry, 140*(5), 548–553.

DelBello, M. A., & Geller, B. (2001). Review of studies of child and adolescent offspring of bipolar parents. *Bipolar Disorders, 3*(6), 325–334.

DelBello, M. A., Soutullo, C. A., Ryan, P., Graman, S. M., Zimmerman, M. E., Getz, G. E., Lake, K., & Strakowski, S. M. (2000). MRI analysis of children at risk for bipolar disorder. *Biological Psychiatry, 47*(Suppl. 1), 135.

Duffy, A., Alda, M., Kutcher, S., Fusee, C., & Grof, P. (1998). Psychiatric symptoms and syndromes among adolescent children of parents with lithium-responsive or lithium-nonresponsive bipolar disorder. *American Journal of Psychiatry, 155*(3), 431–433.

Dunner, D. L., Fleiss, J. L., Addonizio, G., & Fieve, R. R. (1976). Assortative mating in primary affective disorder. *Biological Psychiatry, 11*(1), 43–51.

Faraone, S. V., Biederman, J., Mennin, D., Wozniak, J., & Spencer, T. (1997). Attention-deficit hyperactivity disorder with bipolar disorder: A familial subtype? *Journal of the American Academy of Child and Adolescent Psychiatry, 36*(10), 1378–1387; discussion, 1387–1390.

Faraone, S. V., Biederman, J., Wozniak, J., Mundy, E., Mennin, D., & O'Donnell, D. (1997). Is comorbidity with ADHD a marker for juvenile-onset mania? *Journal of the American Academy of Child and Adolescent Psychiatry, 36*(8), 1046–1055.

Findling, R. L., Gracious, B. L., McNamara, N. K., & Calabrese, J. R. (2000). The rationale, design, and progress of two novel maintenance treatment studies in pediatric bipolarity. *Acta Neuropsychiatrica, 12,* 136–138.

Fisher, P. W., Shaffer, D., Piacentini, J. C., Lapkin, J., Kafantaris, V., Leonard, H., & Herzog, D. B. (1993). Sensitivity of the Diagnostic Interview Schedule for Children, 2nd edition (DISC-2.1) for specific diagnoses of children and adolescents. *Journal of the American Academy of Child and Adolescent Psychiatry, 32*(3), 666–673.

Geller, B., Cooper, T. B., Zimerman, B., Frazier, J., Williams, M., Heath, J., & Warner, K. (1998). Lithium for prepubertal depressed children with family history predictors of future bipolarity: A double-blind, placebo-controlled study. *Journal of Affective Disorders, 51*(2), 165–175.

Geller, B., Fox, L. W., & Clark, K. A. (1994). Rate and predictors of prepubertal bipolarity during follow-up of 6- to 12-year-old depressed children. *Journal of the American Academy of Child and Adolescent Psychiatry, 33*(4), 461–468.

Geller, B. G., Williams, M., Zimerman, B., & Frazier, J. (1996). *WASH-U-KSADS (Washington University in St. Louis Kiddie Schedule for Affective Disorders and Schizophrenia).* St. Louis, MO: Washington University.

Geller, B., Zimerman, B., Williams, M., Bolhofner, K., Craney, J. L., DelBello, M. P., & Soutullo, C. (2001). Reliability of the Washington University in St. Louis Kiddie Schedule for Affective Disorders and Schizophrenia (WASH-U-KSADS) mania and rapid cycling sections. *Journal of the American Academy of Child and Adolescent Psychiatry, 40*(4), 450–455.

Gershon, E. S., Hamovit, J., Guroff, J. J., Dibble, E., Leckman, J. F., Sceery, W., Targum, S. D., Nurnberger, J. I., Jr., Goldin, L. R., & Bunney, W. E., Jr. (1982). A family study of schizoaffective, bipolar I, bipolar II, unipolar, and normal control probands. *Archives of General Psychiatry, 39*(10), 1157–1167.

Gershon, E. S., McKnew, D., Cytryn, L., Hamovit, J., Schreiber, J., Hibbs, E., & Pellegrini, D. (1985). Diagnoses in school-age children of bipolar affective disorder patients and normal controls. *Journal of Affective Disorders, 8*(3), 283–291.

Goodwin, F. K., & Jamison, K. R. (1990). *Manic–depressive illness*. New York: Oxford University Press.

Grigoroiu-Serbanescu, M., Christodorescu, D., Jipescu, I., Totoescu, A., Marinescu, E., & Ardelean, V. (1989). Psychopathology in children aged 10–17 of bipolar parents: Psychopathology rate and correlates of the severity of the psychopathology. *Journal of Affective Disorders, 16*(2–3), 167–179.

Grubbs, J. H. (1997). SSRI-induced mania. *Journal of the American Academy of Child and Adolescent Psychiatry, 36*(4), 445.

Hammen, C., Burge, D., Burney, E., & Adrian, C. (1990). Longitudinal study of diagnoses in children of women with unipolar and bipolar affective disorder. *Archives of General Psychiatry, 47*(12), 1112–1117.

Hammen, C., Gordon, D., Burge, D., Adrian, C., Jaenicke, C., & Hiroto, D. (1987). Maternal affective disorders, illness, and stress: Risk for children's psychopathology. *American Journal of Psychiatry, 144*(6), 736–741.

Inoff-Germain, G., Nottelmann, E. D., & Radke-Yarrow, M. (1992). Evaluative communications between affectively ill and well mothers and their children. *Journal of Abnormal Child Psychology, 20*(2), 189–212.

Kashani, J. H., Burk, J. P., Horwitz, B., & Reid, J. C. (1985). Differential effect of subtype of parental major affective disorder on children. *Psychiatry Research, 15*(3), 195–204.

Kat, H. (1996). More on SSRI-induced mania. *Journal of the American Academy of Child and Adolescent Psychiatry, 35*(8), 975.

Kelsoe, J. R. (1997). The genetics of bipolar disorder. *Psychiatric Annals, 27*(4), 285–292.

Kestenbaum, C. J. (1979). Children at risk for manic–depressive illness: Possible predictors. *American Journal of Psychiatry, 136*(9), 1206–1208.

Kestenbaum, C. J. (1980). Adolescents at risk for manic–depressive illness. *Adolescent Psychiatry, 8*, 344–366.

Klein, D. N., Depue, R. A., & Slater, J. F. (1985). Cyclothymia in the adolescent offspring of parents with bipolar affective disorder. *Journal of Abnormal Psychology, 94*(2), 115–127.

Koehler-Troy, C., Strober, M., & Malenbaum, R. (1986). Methylphenidate-induced mania in a prepubertal child. *Journal of Clinical Psychiatry, 47*(11), 566–567.

Kowatch, R. A., Suppes, T., Carmody, T. J., Bucci, J. P., Hume, J. H., Kromelis, M., Emslie, G. J., Weinberg, W. A., & Rush, A. J. (2000). Effect size of lithium, divalproex sodium, and carbamazepine in children and adolescents with bipolar disorder. *Journal of the American Academy of Child and Adolescent Psychiatry, 39*(6), 713–720.

Kraeplin, E. (1921). *Manic–depressive insanity and paranoia*. Edinburgh, UK: Livingstone.

Kuyler, P. L., Rosenthal, L., Igel, G., Dunner, D. L., & Fieve, R. R. (1980). Psychopathology among children of manic–depressive patients. *Biological Psychiatry, 15*(4), 589–597.

Lapalme, M., Hodgins, S., & LaRoche, C. (1997). Children of parents with bipolar disorder: A metaanalysis of risk for mental disorders. *Canadian Journal of Psychiatry, 42*(6), 623–631.

LaRoche, C., Cheifetz, P. N., & Lester, E. P. (1981). Antecedents of bipolar affective disorders in children. *American Journal of Psychiatry, 138*(7), 986–988.

LaRoche, C., Cheifetz, P., Lester, E. P., Schibuk, L., DiTommaso, E., & Engelsmann, F. (1985). Psychopathology in the offspring of parents with bipolar affective disorders. *Canadian Journal of Psychiatry. Revue Canadienne de Psychiatrie, 30*(5), 337–343.

LaRoche, C., Sheiner, R., Lester, E., Benierakis, C., Marrache, M., Engelsmann, F., & Cheifetz, P. (1987). Children of parents with manic–depressive illness: A follow-up study. *Canadian Journal of Psychiatry. Revue Canadienne de Psychiatrie, 32*(7), 563–569.

Lewy, A. J., Nurnberger, J. I., Jr., Wehr, T. A., Pack, D., Becker, L. E., Powell, R. L., & Newsome, D. A. (1985). Supersensitivity to light: Possible trait marker for manic–depressive illness. *American Journal of Psychiatry, 142*(6), 725–727.

Lish, J. D., Dime-Meenan, S., Whybrow, P. C., Price, R. A., & Hirschfeld, R. M. (1994). The National Depressive and Manic–depressive Association (DMDA) survey of bipolar members. *Journal of Affective Disorders, 31*(4), 281–294.

McDonough-Ryan, P., Shear, P. K., Ris, D., DelBello, M., Graman, S., Rosenberg, H. L., & Strakowski, S. (2000). IQ and achievement in children of bipolar parents. *Clinical Neuropsychologist, 14*, 248.

McInnis, M. G., McMahon, F. J., Chase, G. A., Simpson, S. G., Ross, C. A., & DePaulo, J. R., Jr. (1993). Anticipation in bipolar affective disorder. *American Journal of Human Genetics, 53*(2), 385–390.

McKnew, D. H., Jr., Cytryn, L., Efron, A. M., Gershon, E. S., & Bunney, W. E., Jr. (1979). Offspring of patients with affective disorders. *British Journal of Psychiatry, 134*, 148–152.

Nurnberger, J. I., Jr., Berrettini, W., Tamarkin, L., Hamovit, J., Norton, J., & Gershon, E. (1988). Supersensitivity to melatonin suppression by light in young people at high risk for affective disorder: A preliminary report. *Neuropsychopharmacology, 1*(3), 217–223.

Nurnberger, J. I., Hamovit, J., Hibbs, E. D., Pelligrini, D., Guroff, J. J., & Maxwell, M. E. (1988). A high-risk study of primary affective disorder: Selection of subjects, initial assessment and 1- to 2-year follow-up. In D. L. Dunner, E. S. Gershon, & J. E. Barrett (Eds.), *Relatives at risk for mental disorder* (pp. 161–177). New York: Raven Press.

Oldroyd, J. (1997). Paroxetine-induced mania. *Journal of the American Academy of Child and Adolescent Psychiatry, 36*(6), 721–722.

Osher, Y., Mandel, B., Shapiro, E., & Belmaker, R. H. (2000). Rorschach markers in offspring of manic–depressive patients. *Journal of Affective Disorders, 59*(3), 231–236.

Papatheodorou, G., Kutcher, S. P., Katic, M., & Szalai, J. P. (1995). The efficacy and safety of divalproex sodium in the treatment of acute mania in adolescents and young adults: An open clinical trial. *Journal of Clinical Psychopharmacology, 15*(2), 110–116.

Pellegrini, D., Kosisky, S., Nackman, D., Cytryn, L., McKnew, D. H., Gershon, E., Hamovit, J., & Cammuso, K. (1986). Personal and social resources in children of patients with bipolar affective disorder and children of normal control subjects. *American Journal of Psychiatry, 143*(7), 856–861.

Petronis, A., & Kennedy, J. L. (1995). Unstable genes—unstable mind? *American Journal of Psychiatry, 152*(2), 164–172.

Post, R. M. (1992). Transduction of psychosocial stress into the neurobiology of recurrent affective disorder. *American Journal of Psychiatry, 149*(8), 999–1010.

Post, R. M., Altshuler, L. L., Ketter, T. A., Denicoff, K., & Weiss, S. R. (1991). Antiepileptic drugs in affective illness: Clinical and theoretical implications. *Advanced Neurology, 55*, 239–277.

Radke-Yarrow, M., Nottelmann, E., Martinez, P., Fox, M. B., & Belmont, B. (1992). Young children of affectively ill parents: A longitudinal study of psychosocial development. *Journal of the American Academy of Child and Adolescent Psychiatry, 31*(1), 68–77.

Rosenberg, D. R., Sweeney, J. A., Squires-Wheeler, E., Keshavan, M. S., Cornblatt, B. A., & Erlenmeyer-Kimling, L. (1997). Eye-tracking dysfunction in offspring from the New York High-Risk Project: Diagnostic specificity and the role of attention. *Psychiatry Research, 66*(2–3), 121–130.

Shaffer, D., Schwab-Stone, M., Fisher, P., Cohen, P., Piacentini, J., Davies, M., Conners, C. K., & Regier, D. (1993). The Diagnostic Interview Schedule for Children—Revised Version (DISC-R): Part 1. Preparation, field testing, interrater reliability, and acceptability. *Journal of the American Academy of Child and Adolescent Psychiatry, 32*(3), 643–650.

Soutullo, C. A., DelBello, M. A., Casuto, L. S., Lake, K., Graman, S. M., McDonough-Ryan, P., McElroy, S. L., Strakowski, S. M., & Keck, P. E. J. (1999, May 15–20). *Psychiatric disorders in children of bipolar patients versus controls: preliminary results.* Paper presented at the annual meeting of the American Psychiatric Association, Washington, DC.

Stoll, A. L., & Severus, W. E. (1996). Mood stabilizers: shared mechanisms of action at postsynaptic signal-transduction and kindling processes. *Harvard Review of Psychiatry, 4*(2), 77–89.

Strober, M., & Carlson, G. (1982). Predictors of bipolar illness in adolescents with major depression: A follow-up investigation. *Adolescent Psychiatry, 10*, 299–319.

Venkataraman, S., Naylor, M. W., & King, C. A. (1992). Mania associated with fluoxetine treatment in adolescents. *Journal of the American Academy of Child and Adolescent Psychiatry, 31*(2), 276–281.

Wals, M., Hillegers, M. H., Reichart, C. G., Ormel, J., Nolen, W. A., & Verhulst, F. C. (2001). Prevalence of psychopathology in children of a bipolar parent. *Journal of the American Academy of Child and Adolescent Psychiatry, 40*(9), 1094–1102

Waters, B. G., & Marchenko-Bouer, I. (1980). Psychiatric illness in the adult offspring of bipolar manic–depressives. *Journal of Affective Disorders, 2*(2), 119–126.

Waters, B. G., Marchenko-Bouer, I., & Smiley, D. (1981). Educational achievement, IQ and affective disorder in the adult offspring of bipolar manic–depressives. *British Journal of Psychiatry, 139*, 457–462.

Weintraub, S. (1987). Risk factors in schizophrenia: The Stony Brook High-Risk Project. *Schizophrenia Bulletin, 13*(3), 439–450.

Zahn, T. P., Nurnberger, J. I., Jr., & Berrettini, W. H. (1989). Electrodermal activity in young adults at genetic risk for affective disorder. *Archives of General Psychiatry, 46*(12), 1120–1124.

Zahn-Waxler, C., Cummings, E. M., McKnew, D. H., & Radke-Yarrow, M. (1984). Altruism, aggression, and social interactions in young children with a manic–depressive parent. *Child Development, 55*(1), 112–122.

Zahn-Waxler, C., Mayfield, A., Radke-Yarrow, M., McKnew, D. H., Cytryn, L., & Davenport, Y. B. (1988). A follow-up investigation of offspring of parents with bipolar disorder. *American Journal of Psychiatry, 145*(4), 506–509.

6

The Role of NMDA Receptor Hypofunction in Idiopathic Psychotic Disorders

NURI B. FARBER and JOHN W. NEWCOMER

Extensive research focusing on the amino acid glutatmate (Glu) has documented the central role played by this compound in both the normal and abnormal functioning of the central nervous system (CNS). Glu is now recognized to be the main excitatory neurotransmitter in the CNS, estimated to be released at up to half of the synapses in the brain.

The Glu receptor family is comprised of two major subfamilies (ionotropic and metabotropic), and within these subfamilies there are many additional subdivisions. The ionotropic receptors are further subdivided into three major categories (Watkins & Evans, 1981), each being named for an agonist molecule to which it is preferentially sensitive (NMDA [N-methyl-D-aspartate], AMPA [amino-3-hydroxy-5-methylisoxazole-4-proprionic acid], and KA [kainic acid]). Within each of these categories, multiple subunits and splice variants have been identified; it is believed that these form heteromeric assemblies, the exact number and types of which remain to be determined.

The most studied and reportedly the most widely and densely distributed of the Glu receptor subtypes is the NMDA receptor (Figure 6.1). Several features of the NMDA receptor distinguish it from other subtypes of Glu receptors. This receptor is linked to a cation channel, which has a much higher calcium conductance than ion channels typically associated with other Glu receptor subtypes, and the NMDA ion channel is subject to a voltage-dependent magnesium blockade. The NMDA receptor is functionally coupled to a strychnine-insensitive glycine receptor and a polyamine receptor where glycine and polyamines, respectively, act to facilitate

EXTRACELLULAR SPACE

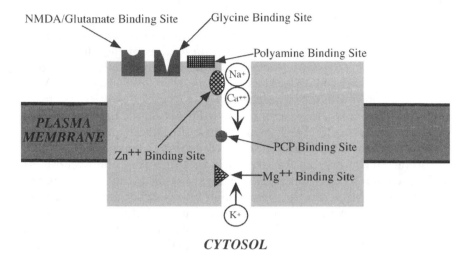

CYTOSOL

FIGURE 6.1. NMDA receptor. The NMDA Glu receptor can be modulated by agents acting at different binding sites. The NMDA receptor is so named because NMDA preferentially binds to this particular Glu binding site. CPP, CPPene, and CGS19755 also preferentially bind to the NMDA/Glu binding site. Since they inhibit Glu's binding, they are termed *competitive antagonists*. D-cycloserine and other glycineric agents bind to the anatomically distinct glycine site. In addition to the Glu and glycine binding sites, the NMDA receptor has multiple other binding sites through which its channel function can be modulated. Binding at the polyamine site facilitates Glu-activated opening of the cation channel. In contrast, binding of zinc or magnesium to their respective sites inhibits NMDA receptor function. PCP, ketamine, and MK-801 all bind to the PCP binding site, which is located inside the ion channel. Once bound, they block the flow of ions through the channel and thus inhibit the functioning of the receptor. Because they interact at a site distinct from the Glu binding site, they do not compete with Glu for binding and are therefore termed *noncompetitive antagonists*. From Farber, Newcomber, & Olney (1999, p. 15). Copyright 1999 by the American Medical Association. Reprinted by permission.

opening of the NMDA ion channel. There is evidence that zinc, acting at a site near the mouth of the NMDA ion channel, acts as an inhibitory modulator of channel function, and there is a site within the ion channel where phencyclidine (PCP) and its analogs (such as MK-801 and ketamine) act to perform an open channel block.

Several decades of work have shown that excessive activation of NMDA receptors plays an important role in the pathophysiology of acute CNS injury syndromes such as hypoxia-ischemia, trauma, and status epilepticus (Choi, 1992; Olney, 1990). More recently it has become apparent that underexcitation of NMDA receptors (NMDA receptor hypofunction [NRHypo]) also has significant consequences for CNS functioning. In particular, NMDA antagonists have been found to produce memory impairments and psychosis in humans, and a myriad of histopathological and neurochemical changes in rodents. Several lines of evidence suggest that these effects are dose-dependent manifestations of the same general process. In brief, progressive increases in the severity of NRHypo within the brain, which can be induced experimentally *in vivo* using NMDA receptor antagonist drugs, can produce a range of clinically relevant effects on brain function. Underexcitation of NMDA receptors, induced by even relatively low doses of NMDA antagonist drugs, can produce specific forms of memory dysfunction. More severe NMDA receptor hypofunction can produce a clinical syndrome that includes core features of psychosis, as well as euphoria and excitation. Finally, sustained and severe underexcitation of NMDA receptors in the adult brain is associated with a form of neurotoxicity, with well-characterized neuropathological features. In this chapter these effects of NMDA antagonists are reviewed. In addition, the possible role of NRHypo in the pathophysiology of idiopathic psychotic disorders are considered.

NMDA RECEPTOR FUNCTION/DYSFUNCTION IN THE ADULT HUMAN BRAIN

In the adult human brain the NMDA transmitter system is thought to have an important role in memory and cognition and in sensory information processing, to name but a few of its many functions. By blocking NMDA receptors, NMDA antagonists produce a NRHypo state that is associated with psychiatric symptoms. PCP and ketamine, two NMDA antagonists, are classified as dissociative anesthetics. Early studies found that with this type of anesthesia adult patients exhibited psychiatric symptoms (referred to as an "emergence reaction"), including maniacal excitation, catatonic signs, euphoria, hallucinations, delusions, and agitation (Camilleri, 1962; Collins, Gorospe, & Rovenstine, 1960; Domino, 1964; Erard, Luisada, & Peele, 1980; Luby, Cohen, Rosenbaum, Gottlieb, & Kelley, 1959; McCarron, Schulze, Thompson, Conder, & Goetz, 1981; Pender, 1971; Reich & Silvay, 1989; White, Wa, & Trevor, 1982). More recent studies employing ketamine in subanesthetic doses have confirmed some of these initial findings but the symptoms produced were milder and not as extensive (Krystal et al., 1994; Malhotra et al., 1996; Newcomer et al., 1999). In these carefully controlled later studies very low doses of ketamine produced selective impairments in explicit/declarative memory in the absence of psychosis. Higher subanesthetic doses of ketamine produced positive symptoms (delusions and hallucinations) and still higher subanesthetic doses produced thought disorder. Because these later studies were appropriately concerned with minimizing symptom severity and protecting human subjects from unpleasant experiences, they did not produce the full range of symptoms seen in the earlier studies using anesthetic doses of PCP and ketamine. However, the dose-dependence of ketamine-induced core schizophrenia-like symptoms suggests that if higher doses of ketamine had been used in the later studies, the full variety and severity of effects seen in earlier studies probably would have been produced. These findings have stimulated interest in the possibility that an NRHypo mechanism could produce cognitive dysfunction and psychotic symptom formation in idiopathic psychotic disorders.

While schizophrenia has received the most attention as the disorder in which an NRHypo state might exist (Duncan, Sheitman, & Lieberman, 1999; Jentsch & Roth, 1999; Lahti, Holcomb, Gao, & Tamminga, 1999; Olney & Farber, 1995), the fact that higher doses of NMDA antagonists can produce maniacal excitation, catatonic signs, and euphoria suggests that such a NRHypo state also could be responsible for some of the signs and symptoms of bipolar disorder and schizoaffective disorder. The possibility that NRHypo is involved in these disorders would be consistent with clinical experience that it is impossible to differentiate a maniform psychosis from a schizophrenic one on cross-sectional examination.

CONSEQUENCES OF NRHYPO IN THE ADULT RODENT BRAIN

To understand the consequences of a NRHypo state several research groups have begun examining the consequences of drug-induced NRHypo in adult rodents, and have shown that one typical consequence is excessive release of Glu (Adams & Moghaddam, 1998; Moghaddam & Adams, 1998; Moghaddam, Adams, Verma, & Daly, 1997; Noguchi, Johnson, & Ellison, 1998) and acetylcholine (ACh [Hasegawa et al., 1993]) (Giovannini, Camilli, Mundula, & Pepeu, 1994; Giovannini, Giovannini, Branchi, Kalfin, & Pepeu, 1997; Giovannini, Mutolo, Bianchi, Michelassi, & Pepeu, 1994; Kim, Price, Olney, & Farber, 1999) in the cerebral cortex. It has been proposed that this excessive release of excitatory transmitters and consequent overstimulation of postsynaptic neurons might explain the cognitive and behavioral disturbances associated with the NRHypo state (Olney & Farber, 1995; Moghaddam et al., 1997).

At doses higher than those needed to produce elevations in neurotransmitter release, NMDA antagonists begin to produce neurotoxicity in adult rodents (Fix et al., 1993; Olney, Labruyere, & Price, 1989). Initially, they induce reversible pathomorphological changes in pyramidal neurons in a region of brain referred to as the *retrosplenial cortex* (RSC [Paxinos & Watson, 1998; Vogt, 1993]). If NMDA receptor blockade is maintained for a prolonged interval, as occurs following a single high dose or repeated treatment with lower doses of an NMDA antagonist, neurons in the RSC and several other cerebrocortical and limbic regions of the adult rat brain undergo irreversible degeneration (Allen & Iversen, 1990; Corso et al., 1997; Ellison, 1994; Ellison & Switzer, 1993; Fix et al., 1993, 1995; Horvath, Czopf, & Buzsaki, 1997; Olney et al., 1991; Wozniak et al., 1998).

The key feature of the circuitry (Figure 6.2) that mediates the NRHypo neurotoxic process is that Glu, acting at NMDA receptors, functions in this circuit as a regulator of inhibitory tone. Glu accomplishes this regulatory function by tonically stimulating NMDA receptors on GABAergic interneurons which, in turn, inhibit excitatory projections that convergently innervate vulnerable cerebrocortical neurons. NMDA receptor antagonists prevent Glu from driving GABAergic inhibitory neurons, and this results in a loss of inhibitory control over two major excitatory projections to the cerebral cortex, one that is cholinergic and originates in the basal forebrain, and one that is glutamatergic and originates in the thalamus (Farber, Kim, Dikranian, Jiang, & Heinkel, 2002; Farber & Olney, unpublished results; Kim et al., 1999). In addition to these basic features, the NRHypo circuitry includes noradrenergic (Farber, Foster, Duhan, & Olney, 1995; Farber et al., 2002; Kim et al., 1999) and serotonergic (Farber, Hanslick, Kirby, McWilliams, & Olney, 1998) neurons that are driven by Glu through NMDA receptors and also perform an inhibitory function so that when NMDA receptors are hypofunctional the inhibitory restraint contributed by these elements is also lost.

One final aspect that may be quite important for understanding how disinhibition of this circuitry can trigger psychotic reactions is that the vulnerable cerebrocortical neurons are glutamatergic neurons that ordinarily control their own firing by activating an NMDA receptor on a GABAergic neuron in an inhibitory feedback loop (Grunze et al., 1996). When the NMDA receptor in this feedback loop is hypofunctional (e.g., blocked by NMDA antagonist drugs), GABAergic inhibition is lost and the cerebrocortical neurons' control over their own firing is lost at the same time that these neurons are being hyperstimulated by disinhibited glutamatergic and cholinergic excitatory inputs. The expected result would be that the cerebrocortical neurons will bombard many other neurons in their projection fields with an abundance of unmodulated noise. This provides an explanation for the psychotomimetic reactions induced by NMDA antagonist drugs, and we propose that a similar NRHypo mechanism could contribute to the psychotic process in idiopathic psychotic disorders.

NMDA antagonists (e.g., MK-801, ketamine, and PCP) also increase metabolism in certain corticolimbic regions (Boddeke, Weiderhold, & Palacios, 1992; Clow, Lee, & Hammer, 1991; Crosby, Crane, & Sokoloff, 1982; Davis, Mans, Biebuyck, & Hawkins, 1988; Duncan, Moy, Knapp, Mueller, & Breese, 1998; Gao, Shirakawa, & Tamminga, 1993; Hammer

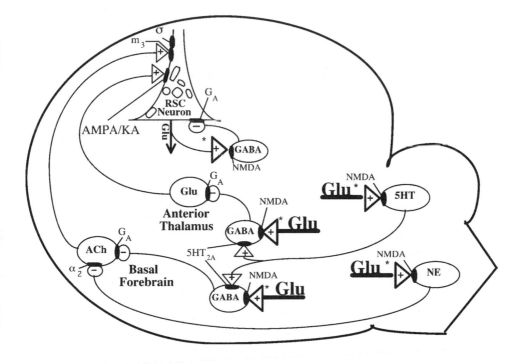

FIGURE 6.2. NRHypo disinhibition circuitry. Glu acting through NMDA receptors on GABAergic, serotonergic, and noradrenergic neurons maintains tonic inhibitory control over two major excitatory pathways that convergently innervate RSC neurons. Systemic administration of an NMDA antagonist blocks NMDA receptors, thereby abolishing inhibitory control over both excitatory inputs to the RSC neuron. The disinhibited excitatory pathways then simultaneously hyperactivate the RSC neuron, which would create chaotic disruption of multiple intracellular signaling systems, thereby causing immediate derangement of cognitive functions subserved by the afflicted neurons (psychotomimetic effects), and reversible or irreversible neuronal injury, depending on how long the disruption lasts. This circuit diagram focuses exclusively on RSC neurons. We hypothesize that a similar disinhibition mechanism and similar but not necessarily identical neural circuits and receptor mechanisms mediate damage induced in other corticolimbic brain regions by sustained NRHypo. +, excitatory input; –, inhibitory input; ACh, acetylcholine; NE, norepinephrine; Glu, glutamate; GABA, γ-aminobutyric acid; 5HT, serotonin; α_2, α_2 subtype of adrenergic receptor; G_A, GABA$_A$ subtype of GABA receptor; m_3, m_3 subtype of muscarinic cholinergic receptor; AMPA/KA, AMPA/KA subtype of Glu receptor; NMDA, NMDA subtype of Glu receptor; σ, sigma site; 5HT$_{2A}$, 5HT$_{2A}$ subtype of serotonin receptor. Asterisks indicate the postulated sites where dopamine inputs may presynaptically regulate Glu release. From Farber, Kim, Dikranian, Jiang, & Heinkel (2002). Copyright 2002 by Nature Publishing Group. Adapted by permission.

& Herkenham, 1983; Hawkins, Hass, & Ransoff, 1979; Kurumaji & McCulloch, 1989; Lund, Miller, & Courville, 1981; Meibach, Glicks, Cox, & Maayani, 1979; Nelsom, Howard, Cross, & Samson, 1980; Oguchi, Arakawa, Nelson, & Samson, 1982; Sharkey, Ritchie, Butcher, & Kelley, 1996). While it is difficult to make specific comparisons across different research groups using different NMDA antagonists and different protocols, in general the corticolimbic regions experiencing hypermetabolism tend to be the same corticolimbic regions that also develop NRHypo neurotoxicity. The increase in metabolism in these corresponding regions could be a reflection of a disinhibition syndrome in which Glu and ACh are excessively released at certain corticolimbic neurons that are injured in the NRHypo neurotoxic syndrome. Consistent with this proposal, clozapine and halothane reverse the hypermetabolism induced by NMDA antagonists (Duncan, Leipzig, Mailman, & Lieberman, 1998; Kurumaji & McCulloch, 1989), just as they reverse NRHypo neurotoxicity (Farber, Foster, Duhan, & Olney, 1996; Ishimaru, Fukamauchi, & Olney, 1995).

In addition to increasing the release of Glu and ACh and producing neurotoxicity, NRHypo also produces several other effects in the CNS. Soon after the original report of neuronal vacuolation, Dragunow and Faull (1990) reported that MK-801 induced the production of c-Fos protein in these same neurons. Subsequent work has found that not only c-Fos but other immediate-early genes (IEG), including c-Jun, Jun-B, NGFI-A (aka zif268, krox-24), NGFI-B, NGFI-C, and Nurr1 (Gao, Hashimoto, & Tamminga, 1998; Gass, Herdegen, Bravo, & Kiessling, 1993; Hughes, Dragunow, Beilhorz, Lawlor, & Gluckman, 1993; Nakao et al., 1996; Nakki, Sharp, Sagar, & Hankaniem, 1996), are activated by NRHypo. In addition, the heat shock stress protein HSP70 (and its mRNA) is also induced in these vulnerable neurons by NRHypo (Olney et al., 1991; Sharp, Jasper, Hall, Noble, & Sagar, 1991). Lastly, NRHypo also induces the expression of brain-derived growth factor (BDNF) mRNA (Castren, Da Phena Berzaghi, Lindholm, & Thoenen, 1993; Hughes et al., 1993).

These additional changes in rodents have been suggested to underlie some of the cognitive and behavioral effects seen with NMDA antagonists in humans. The ability of some of the same pharmacological treatments, which have been shown to prevent NRHypo neurotoxicity, to prevent these other NMDA antagonist-induced responses (Table 6.1) suggests these other responses, when induced by NMDA antagonists, are also likely to be secondary to activation of the same NRHypo disinhibition mechanism. However, IEGs, heat shock proteins, and BDNF also can be induced after a wide variety of other stimuli, including trauma, injury, and neuronal depolarization. Thus, these additional changes, while particularly sensitive to the disruption induced by NRHypo, would not be specific for psychosis or the NRHypo disinhibition mechanism. Since the protein products of these IEGs recognize and bind certain DNA sequences and modify the transcription of target genes (Hughes & Dragunow, 1995), NRHypo-induced pro-

TABLE 6.1. Pharmacological Agents that Prevent NRHypo Neurotoxicity and Other NRHypo-Induced Phenomena

NRHypo-induced phenomenon	Protective agent	Reference
Hypermetabolism	Halothane	Kurumaji & McCulloch (1989)
	Clozapine	Duncan et al. (1998)
HSP70	Antimuscarinics	Olney et al. (1991); Tomitaka et al. (1997)
	GABAergics	Sharp et al. (1994); Nakao et al. (1996)
	Non-NMDA Glu antagonists	Sharp et al. (1995)
	Sigma ligands	Sharp et al. (1992, 1994); Nakki et al. (1996); Sharp & Williams, 1996)
	Clozapine	Sharp et al. (1994)
c-Fos, c-Jun, Jun-B, NGFI-A	GABAergics	Nakao et al. (1996, 1998)
	Antimuscarinics	Hughes et al. (1993)
BDNF	GABAergics	Castren et al. (1993)
	Antimuscarinics	Castren et al. (1993); Hughes et al. (1993)

duction of IEGs might be a clue to understanding the more enduring intracellular and nuclear events that occur in response to the disinhibition syndrome induced by NRHypo.

Thus, in the rodent, NRHypo produces a broad range of effects. Cognizant of the inherent difficulty in comparing results from different model systems, it appears that the NRHypo disinhibition mechanism produces a range of effects, depending on its severity and duration. Mild versions of the NRHypo disinhibition syndrome produce mild elevations in neurotransmitter release, a loss of recurrent feedback inhibition, and elevated metabolism. More moderate degrees would probably begin to produce changes in IEGs and other cellular processes. Finally, even more severe degrees of NRHypo would result in reversible and then irreversible neurotoxicity.

AGE DEPENDENCY OF NRHypo EFFECTS IN RODENTS

The ability of NRHypo to induce these changes in brain is highly dependent on the age of the animal. The reversible vacuolar changes induced by MK-801 or PCP were not found in fetal (embryonic ages 17–19) or postnatal rats at day 15 or at day 30 of life. However, at 45 days of life (onset of puberty) partial susceptibility occurred and this gradually increased to full susceptibility between 90 and 120 days of age (Farber et al., 1995). PCP's induction of c-Fos and HSP70 has a similar age-dependency profile, as does the formation of vacuoles (Sato, Umino, Kaneda, Takigawa, & Nishikawa, 1997; Sharp et al., 1992). Thus, in normal brain, these NRHypo-induced changes appear to occur only in the pubertal and postpubertal period.

NRHYPO DISINHIBITED STATE MIGHT UNDERLIE NRHYPO-INDUCED PSYCHOSIS IN HUMANS

Pharmacological Data

As noted above, the main reason for studying the effects of NRHypo in rodents is to gain clues about the mechanism underlying the psychotomimetic effects of NMDA antagonists in humans. If the NRHypo disinhibited state does underlie the mental effects of NMDA antagonists, then the pharmacological treatments that ameliorate the NRHypo-induced effects in rodents could ameliorate NRHypo-induced psychosis. Information pertaining to this question, although incomplete, provides some interesting correlations. Agents that promote $GABA_A$ neurotransmission prevent the NRHypo state from releasing excessive acetylcholine (Kim et al., 1999) and prevent NRHypo neurotoxicity in the rat cerebral cortex (Olney et al., 1991), and it is well recognized by anesthesiologists that these agents in sufficient dosage attenuate the psychotomimetic actions of ketamine (Magbagbeola & Thomas, 1974; Reich & Silvay, 1989; White et al., 1982). The effect is dose-dependent, with higher dosages more effective than lower dosages. The dose dependency of the effect might account for a reported negative finding of Krystal and colleagues (1998) with lorazepam. α_2-adrenergic agonists prevent the NRHypo state from releasing excessive acetylcholine (Kim et al., 1999) and prevent NRHypo neurotoxicity in the rat cerebral cortex (Farber et al., 1995) by acting in the basal forebrain where cholinergic cell bodies reside (Farber et al., 2002). Furthermore, it was recently shown that an α_2-adrenergic agonist can prevent ketamine from inducing positive schizophrenia-like symptoms in normal human volunteers (Newcomer et al., 1998). Lamotrigine, an agent that inhibits excessive release of Glu, prevents NRHypo neurotoxicity in the rat cerebral cortex (Jevtovic-Todorovic, Olney, & Farber, 1998) and prevents ketamine-induced schizophrenia-like symptoms in human volunteers (Anand et al., 2000). Clozapine is quite potent in blocking NRHypo neurotoxicity in the rat cerebral cortex (Farber et al., 1993), and clozapine has been reported to block ketamine-induced increases in positive symptoms in patients with schizophrenia (Malhotra et al., 1997). Given the difficulties in making cross-species comparisons, we find it rather remarkable that four classes of compounds (GABAergics, α_2-adrenergic agonists, clozapine, lamotrigine) have been found to work in both models.

In addition, haloperidol, when used at its D_2 blocking dose, has been found to be minimally active against ketamine-induced psychosis (Krystal et al., 1999). In rodents, while haloperidol can block NRHypo neurodegeneration, it does so only at a dose that is 10 times greater than its D_2 dose, whereas sulpiride, a D_2 selective antagonist, is ineffective (Farber et al., 1993). These D_2 findings suggest that the D_2 receptor system is not an intrinsic component of the NRHypo disinhibition circuitry and is not directly involved in ketamine's production of psychosis (see below).

Age-Dependency Data

Thus, the pharmacological data reviewed above support the hypothesis that a NRHypo-induced disinhibited state may underlie both the neurotoxic and the psychotomimetic effects of NMDA antagonists. Consistent with this hypothesis, prepubertal rats do not develop NRHypo-induced neurodegeneration (Farber et al., 1995), just as prepubertal humans rarely develop psychosis after exposure to PCP or ketamine (Baldridge & Bessen, 1990; Karp, Kaufman, & Anand, 1980; Reich & Silvay, 1989; Welch & Correa, 1980; White et al., 1982).

Dose–Response Relationship among Different NRHypo Effects

The hypothesis that a similar NRHypo disinhibition syndrome underlies the psychotomimetic effect in humans and the neurotoxic effect in rodents does not mean that the neurotoxicity must exist in brains of people with NRHypo-induced psychosis. Instead, we propose that the severity of the NRHypo state is a critical variable in determining the specific NRHypo effect seen. Specifically, we propose that mild degrees of NRHypo would produce slight elevations in the release of ACh and Glu and slight decrements in local recurrent inhibition. These changes could produce mild derangements in memory function without significant behavioral changes. More moderate degrees of NRHypo would produce greater aberation in the circuit, resulting in more obvious cognitive and behavioral disturbances, but still not producing neurotoxicity. At this stage one might begin to see nuclear and cellular changes, like the production of certain IEGs, as a response to the aberrant functioning of the NRHypo circuit. Only in the case where NRHypo was severe would the NRHypo state produce enough of an increase in transmitter release and in the degree of postsynaptic m_3 and non-NMDA receptor overstimulation to produce first reversible, then irreversible neurotoxicity.

DOPAMINE, NRHYPO DISINHIBITED STATE, AND PSYCHOSIS

The role of dopamine and D_2 receptors in the production and treatment of psychosis has been long established. What, then, is the relationship between the D_2 dopaminergic and the NMDA glutamatergic systems? Based partly upon the well-described ability of NMDA antagonists to increase dopaminergic activity, many have assumed that NMDA antagonists cause an excessive activity at D_2 receptors and that this excessive activity then directly produces psychosis (Grace, 1991; Verma & Moghaddam, 1996). However, the lack of correlation in animals between the time course of NMDA antagonist-induced dopamine release and NMDA antagonist-induced behavioral changes suggests that the increase in dopamine release might not be responsible for the psychosis produced by NMDA antagonist (Adams & Moghaddam, 1998). The inability of D_2 antagonists to reverse ketamine-induced psychosis (Krystal et al., 1999) is consistent with the proposal that changes in activation of D_2 receptors downstream from the NMDA receptor are not involved in the production of psychosis.

There is another role that D_2 receptors may play in the NRHypo model. As indicated above, we have found no evidence that D_2 receptors function internally within the NRHypo disinhibition network, but we postulate that they may be exceedingly important extrinsic regulators of the network. The type of interaction between the dopamine and NMDA systems that might best explain psychotic symptom formation could be one in which the dopamine system wields influence over the NMDA system. Specifically, we postulate that at critical points in the circuitry that mediate NRHypo effects, D_2 receptors may regulate the release of Glu at NMDA receptors. If this is the case, in idiopathic psychotic disorders a genetically determined aberration in the dopamine system causing hyperinhibition of Glu release would result in an NRHypo state, that could explain psychotic symptom formation. Conversely, treatment with a D_2 antagonist could normalize Glu release, relieve the NRHypo state and attenuate psychosis. Paul Greengard and colleagues (Greengard et al., 1998) have recently reported evidence that in many brain systems dopamine receptors do regulate the NMDA receptor system in this way.

NRHYPO DISINHIBITED STATE AND PSYCHIATRIC ILLNESS

We propose that in major psychotic disorders (e.g., schizophrenia, schizoaffective disorder, bipolar disorder) the NRHypo state is instilled in the brain by a pathological event very early in life (e.g., prenatally). Because NRHypo does not produce the disinhibited mechanism or psychosis prior to puberty, the NRHypo state that was created prenatally can remain quiescent throughout childhood. Then, in adolescence, unknown maturational changes occur, causing the NRHypo disinhibited mechanism to become active and symptoms to begin to appear. Since some brain regions and their associated mental functions may be more sensitive to disruption by NRHypo, different symptoms may present at different times even if brain maturation is relatively homogeneous. Alternatively, the maturation process could occur in particular brain regions at different times, so that mental functions subserved by different brain regions would become dysfunctional at different times. In either case, therefore, the full syndrome would unfold over time as each specific clinical sign appears in succession. For example, relatively subtle impairments in cognitive functions such as attention and memory might occur in early adolescence while more obvious psychotic signs might not become present until later in adolescence.

How might an NRHypo lesion be instilled in the developing brain? Genetic abnormalities are known to be etiological factors in the major psychotic disorders. Based upon our knowledge of the NRHypo circuitry, several likely candidates can be identified. Obviously abnormalities in NMDA receptor gene products would be candidates. In addition, various NRHypo "equivalent" conditions could similarly produce the relevant network disturbances. Primary disturbances in the GABAergic system or non-NMDA system would be other likely candidates. A wide variety of environmental factors could delete NMDA receptor-bearing neurons from the brain and render the immature brain into a NRHypo state (see below). Different genetic abnormalities are expected to be associated with different clinical syndromes (e.g., bipolar disorder vs. schizophrenia and schizophrenia spectrum disorders) which tend to aggregate together in families, and these different genetic abnormalities might affect the NRHypo circuit in different ways. In addition, a wide range of nongenetic factors could interact differentially with these disease-related genetic abnormalities, modulating the NRHypo circuit and the clinical presentation of the disorder. The NRHypo state may represent an important final common pathway in the pathophysiology of various psychotic illnesses, explaining some of the clinical overlap between different psychotic syndromes (Kendler & Gardner, 1997; Kendler, Karkowski, & Walsh, 1998; Kendler et al., 1997).

Producing a NRHypo State in the Developing CNS

During a specific stage in development, the *synaptogenesis* stage, neurons with NMDA receptors are exquisitely sensitive to Glu stimulation, and the amount of Glu stimulation must be regulated within narrow bounds, because either too much or too little can be lethal for the NMDA receptor-bearing neuron. Too much Glu stimulation results in *excitotoxic* neurodegeneration (Ikonomidou et al., 1989), and too little Glu stimulation results in *apoptotic* neurodegeneration (Ikonomidou et al., 1999). In either case, the neurons deleted from the brain are neurons that have NMDA receptors on their surface and the deletion of these NMDA receptor-bearing neurons produces an NRHypo state.

Hypoxia/ischemia, which causes excessive amounts of Glu to be released at NMDA receptors, is a prime example of too much Glu stimulation causing an excitotoxic lesion leading to an NRHypo state. We propose that this type of lesion can be triggered in the developing brain by a mechanism as simple as compression of the umbilical cord and could be an etio-logical event for producing idiopathic psychotic disorders.

Exposure of the *in utero* fetus to an NMDA antagonist drug is a prime example of too little Glu stimulation causing apoptotic neurodegeneration leading to an NRHypo state. Exposure of the developing rodent brain *in vivo* to any of several NMDA antagonists (e.g., MK-801, PCP, CPP, ketamine) in doses that maintain blockade of NMDA receptors for 4 or more hours during the synaptogenesis period triggers a massive wave of apoptotic neurodegeneration, deleting millions of neurons from several major regions of the developing brain (all major divisions of the cerebral cortex, several thalamic nuclei, the hippocampus, the caudate nucleus, the globus pallidus, and the nucleus accumbens) (Ikonomidou et al., 1999). In addition, ethanol, which is known to have NMDA antagonist properties, when administered during the synaptogenesis period, induces a pattern of apoptotic neurodegeneration similar to but more extensive than that in-duced by other NMDA antagonist drugs (Ikonomidou et al., 2000; Olney et al., 1999; Price et al., 1999). Doses of ethanol that maintain blood etha-nol levels in the 200 mg percent range for 4 or more hours are sufficient to trigger this neurodegenerative syndrome. These findings support the inter-pretation that developing neurons depend on NMDA receptor stimulation for survival and are programmed to commit suicide (die by apoptosis) if deprived of this stimulation for several consecutive hours during synapto-genesis. Thus, we use the acronym NRD (NMDA receptor deprivation) to refer to this developmental neuropathology mechanism. The adult conse-quence of NRD would be an NRHypo condition that could be an etiologi-cal event for idiopathic psychotic disorders.

Consequences of Instilling an NRHypo State in the Developing Human Brain

Is there any evidence substantiating the hypothesis that the deletion of NMDA receptor-bearing neurons *in utero* is associated with psychosis in adulthood? It is well known that exposure of human fetuses to ethanol can cause neurodevelopmental deficits, termed *fetal alcohol syndrome* (FAS) or *fetal alcohol effects* (FAE), depending on severity. One major mechanism by which ethanol could cause such deficits is by deleting NMDA receptor-bearing neurons from the fetal brain. Thus, the FAE/FAS provides an in-structive example of a human neurodevelopmental brain disorder in which widely distributed NRHypo neuropathology is instilled in the developing brain during synaptogenesis (third trimester of pregnancy).

In a recent study (Famy, Streissguth, & Unis, 1998), a large cohort of human subjects with a childhood diagnosis of FAE/FAS were studied as adults and it was determined that a very high percent (72%) of these indi-viduals required psychiatric care for diverse adult-onset disorders, includ-ing a 40% incidence of psychosis and a 20% incidence of bipolar disorder.

To fully appreciate the potential significance of this observation, one must also factor in the precise time during the synaptogenesis period that the developing CNS is exposed to ethanol. This is important because different neuronal groups become sensitive to the NRD mechanism at different times within the synaptogenesis period (because each group has its own schedule for forming synaptic connections). Therefore, different combinations of neuronal groups will be deleted from the brain by a NRD event, depending on whether the event occurs in the early, mid-, or late phase of the synaptogenesis period. It follows that the NRD mechanism can produce a wide variety of dysfunctional syndromes, each having its own constellation of neurobehavioral disturbances. Presumably, certain patterns of neuronal loss could be more conducive than others to producing a psychotic behavioral outcome. Therefore, in the Famy and colleagues (1998) study it is possible that the large percentage of FAE/FAS individuals who displayed psychotic symptoms as adults were a subgroup who were exposed to ethanol at a time when a psychotogenic combination of NMDA receptor-bearing neurons were at peak vulnerability for being deleted by the NRD mechanism.

Instilling an NRHypo State *in Utero* and Idiopathic Psychotic Disorders

To establish the relevance of these observations to schizophrenia, schizoaffective disorder, or bipolar disorder, it is not necessary to prove that fetal ethanol exposure by itself causes an adult psychotic disorder, mimicking all features of these idiopathic psychotic disorders. It is sufficient to view ethanol as a nongenetic factor that can act in concert with genetic factors to tip the balance and potentially cause a genetic predisposition for the disorder to be clinically expressed (Lohr & Bracha, 1989), or for the expression of a more severe and psychotic presentation of a specific disorder.

Because of the key role played by NMDA receptor-bearing GABAergic neurons in the NRHypo disinhibition circuit, it will be important to determine whether the NMDA receptor-bearing neurons deleted by the NRD mechanism are GABAergic interneurons. The loss of NMDA-receptor bearing GABAergic neurons is of particular interest given that deficiencies in the GABAergic system exist in postmortem brain tissue of patients with schizophrenia, bipolar disorder, and schizoaffective disorder (Benes, 1999; Benes, McSparren, Bird, San Giovanni, & Vincent, 1991; Guidotti et al., 2000; Woo, Whitehead, Melchitzky, & Lewis, 1998). Because the GABAergic neuron in the feedback loop normally regulates the firing pattern of corticolimbic pyramidal neurons and aberrant firing of these neurons could cause considerable mental dysfunction, this population of GABAergic neurons might be differentially abnormal in patients with an idiopathic psychotic disorder. Indeed, an excellent formula for psychosis would be loss of GABAergic inhibition simultaneously in this feedback loop and in any one of the two main excitatory inputs to the pyramidal neuron, since this would cause the pyramidal neuron to be persistently hyperactivated at the same time that it has lost feedback control over its firing on other neurons.

Structural Brain Changes Associated with the NRHypo State

We propose that mildly increased neurotransmitter release and associated overstimulation of postsynaptic neurons can explain cognitive symptoms in idiopathic psychotic disorders. More moderate degrees of NRHypo could produce core psychotic symptoms. In instances where the NRHypo state and associated excitatory transmitter release is unremittingly severe on a chronic basis, neurodegenerative changes would occur and could explain the deterioration seen in some patients. For research purposes, creating a drug-induced NRHypo state in the rodent brain provides a highly effective means of identifying neuronal populations that are at risk of being hyperstimulated and eventually injured or killed as a consequence of the NRHypo state. Findings indicate that a protracted NRHypo state can trigger irreversible degeneration and death of neurons throughout many corticolimbic brain regions (Corso et al., 1997; Ellison, 1994; Horvath et al., 1997). Presumably, any of these hyperstimulated neurons might be instrumental in producing psychotic symptoms.

Regarding glial scarring, although it is accepted as a general rule that neurodegenerative reactions in the adult brain produce scarring, NRHypo-induced neurodegeneration in the adult rat brain is an exception to that rule. Studies employing histochemical stains for glial fibrillary acidic protein (astrocyte stain) or for activated microglia have shown that when a high percentage of the neuronal population in the RSC is destroyed by treatment with an NMDA antagonist drug, there is a transient increase in the markers for these two types of glia lasting for several days and soon thereafter these markers return to normal (Fix, Wightman, & O'Callaghan, 1995). Thus, the observation that structural brain changes in idiopathic psychotic disorders are not associated with evidence for gliosis could signify either that the changes occurred during development or that they occurred by an NRHypo mechanism during adulthood. The NRHypo hypothesis proposes that structural brain changes can occur both during development and in adulthood.

THE NRHYPO HYPOTHESIS: IMPLICATIONS AND CAVEATS

Heterogeneity of Symptoms

An important way in which the adult NMDA antagonist-induced NRHypo model fails to mirror idiopathic psychotic disorders precisely is that

NMDA antagonist drugs render NMDA receptors hypofunctional throughout the brain, and this disrupts every brain circuit containing NMDA receptors, but we assume that in idiopathic psychotic disorders the defect state will be more selective for specific circuits or subcomponents within specific circuits. Heterogeneity of presenting symptoms in clinical disorders may be partially explained by differences in the severity of the network disinhibition, or by differences in the specific corticolimbic circuits that are affected by the NRHypo state.

Because NRD at one stage is associated with one pattern of neuronal degeneration and at another stage is associated with a different pattern of neuronal degeneration, heterogeneity of symptoms may also be explained by the potential of NRD in the developing brain to produce a variety of different neurobehavioral symptom complexes depending on whether this condition occurs during the period of synaptogenesis, and exactly when during this period. Thus, an early occurring NRD event producing a NRHypo state could be involved in a variety of clinically distinct adult presentations that include psychosis. Specific genetic lesions could be instrumental in determining which specific disorder an individual would develop (e.g., bipolar disorder), but the clinical course and the occurrence and/or severity of a psychotic component to the illness could be modified by the occurrence and timing of an early environmental insults responsible for the NRD event.

Role of Dopamine

For many years, promising findings involving dopamine have dominated research in psychosis. The NRHypo hypothesis provides an alternate conceptual framework that offers additional explanatory power, including a possible explanation, in NRHypo terms, of why D_2 antagonists are therapeutically beneficial. As indicated above, we believe that the critical D_2 receptors involved in the production of psychotic symptoms lie just upstream from critical NMDA receptors. Stimulation of these dopamine receptors would result in a suppression of glutamate release at the NMDA receptors—a NRHypo equivalent state. Clinically, these individuals could appear similar to those whose NRHypo state is a consequence of abnormalities in other parts of the circuit (e.g., loss of NMDA receptor-bearing GABAergic neurons). While both categories of individuals could have a similar symptom profile, use of D_2 antagonists would have a preferential effect on those individuals with a hyperactive dopamine system. If this view of the relationship between the D_2 and NMDA receptor systems is correct, it does not depreciate the importance of dopamine but opens new paths for progress toward understanding how dysfunction of dompamine, NMDA, and other transmitter systems may contribute to the pathophysiology of psychotic disorders.

Treatment of Idiopathic Psychotic Disorders

Since clozapine is highly effective in reversing the NRHypo disinhibited state (Duncan et al., 1998; Farber et al., 1993), it would be predicted to be effective in all forms of idiopathic psychotic disorders including those nonresponsive to D_2 antagonists. Olanzapine is also highly effective in reversing the effects of NRHypo, being approximately fivefold stronger than clozapine (Duncan, Miyamoto, Leipzeig, & Lieberman, 2000; Farber et al., 1996). While initial attempts to determine whether olanzapine is effective in treatment-resistant schizophrenia have been unsuccessful (Conley et al., 1998), the dose used was too low based on the animal models. Higher doses will need to be studied in order to test the hypothesis.

It would be predicted from the NRHypo model that Glu agonists by increasing NMDA receptor activity might be effective in ameliorating positive, negative, and cognitive symptoms of schizophrenia. Clearly, if a specific defect in NMDA receptor-mediated neurotransmission were identified, therapy aimed at compensating for that specific defect would be indicated. Theoretically, Glu agonists might also be useful in cases where dopamine hyperactivity is the basic defect and NRHypo occurs secondarily due to excessive inhibition of Glu release at certain NMDA receptors. Introduction of a selective agonist that can act at these NMDA receptors would correct the Glu hypofunctional state even though the dopamine hyperactivity would not be corrected. However, such direct approaches are potentially treacherous because using an agonist of Glu receptors might have excitotoxic side effects. Pharmacotherapies aimed at increasing Glu release or inhibiting Glu uptake would be subject to the same drawback.

In an attempt to bypass this problem, groups have focused on the strychnine-insensitive glycine binding site of the NMDA receptor (Figure 6.1). Both the glycine and Glu/NMDA site must be occupied by their respective agents to trigger opening of the ion channel (Mayer & Westbrook, 1987). If only one or the other site is occupied, the ion channel remains closed. Glu is released from the presynaptic axon terminal into the synaptic cleft and is rapidly taken back up or diffuses away so that the Glu receptor sites are never more than transiently occupied (Lester, Clements, Westbrook, & Jahr, 1990). In contrast, glycine is thought to be present in the cleft at all times, presumably in concentrations sufficient to activate its binding site, although the degree of binding and amount of activation might not be maximal (Danysz & Parsons, 1998; Mayer & Westbrook, 1987; McBain & Mayer, 1994; Supplisson & Bergman, 1997). Given this type of arrangement, would increasing the concentration of glycine (or a glycine agonist) in the synaptic cleft be a safe and effective means of increasing the functional activity of the NMDA receptor ion channel complex? Clearly, adding a glycine agonist would be safer than adding a Glu agonist, but whether adding glycine would be effective depends on whether the glycine sites are fully saturated in the disease state. If glycine levels were slightly submaximal, administering a glycine agonist to patients with schizophrenia might mildly augment NMDA receptor function and cause a mild improvement in some symptoms. On the other hand, if the basic mechanism underlying the schizophrenia disease process is a deficiency in synaptic concentrations of glycine, then administering a glycine agonist would be expected to have a profoundly beneficial effect. The fact that these agents in conjunction with D_2 antagonists have had a moderately beneficial effect at best (Goff et al., 1999; Heresco-Levy et al., 1999; Tsai, Pinchen, Chung, Lange, & Coyle, 1998) is consistent with the proposal that the basic disease mechanism in these patients is not a deficit in synaptic levels of glycine.

Another reason why glycinergic agents might not be more effective for schizophrenia or other psychotic disorders might be because the adult NMDA antagonist-induced NRHypo model fails to mirror idiopathic psychotic disorders precisely, as discussed above. The experimental NRHypo model involves transiently inducing the NRHypo state in the normal adult rodent or human brain and simultaneously reversing this state by co-administration of another drug. This obviously is quite different from permanently instilling an NRHypo state in the developing brain by the depletion of developing neurons, and then 20 years later, after extensive aberrant rewiring has occurred, applying drugs to the altered nervous system to reverse symptoms produced by the initial deletion of developing neurons plus all of the subsequent pathological alterations. Thus, we should not expect all classes of compounds that reverse the transiently induced NRHypo state in the normal CNS to be efficacious in treating idiopathic psychotic disorders.

Based on this analysis, one might conclude that the adult NRHypo model would be most predictive of treatment response in those individuals who had minimal alterations in the neurons that constitute the NRHypo disinhibition circuit. While the field is far from understanding the mechanisms underlying idiopathic psychotic disorders, we are intrigued by the recent findings that glial abnormalities might exist in some individuals with bipolar disorder (Ongur, Drevets, & Price, 1998). In such cases decrements in glial functioning could result in specific neuronal dysfunction, thus creating an NRHypo state. Since the neurons and all the important NRHypo circuitry might, in principle, still be present in these individuals, they might respond to most of the agents that have been found to ameliorate the adult NRHypo state when it is induced in normal brain by NMDA antagonists.

If individuals with bipolar disorder do have more intact NRHypo circuitry than individuals with schizophrenia, one would predict that in general patients with bipolar disorder would have a greater clinical response to agents that have been found to be effective in the acute NMDA antagonist-induced NRHypo disinhibition model. While there have been no formal experiments specifically designed to test this proposal, it is notable that many agents (lamotrigine, GABAergic agents, clozapine, and olanzapine) that are effective in the NRHypo model have been found to be clinically useful in the treatment of bipolar disorder.

The fact that severe and sustained levels of NRHypo can produce neurodegeneration could account for the observation that some individuals with idiopathic psychotic disorders develop behavioral and cognitive deterioration over the course of their illness. If this concept is correct, chronic treatment with certain drugs, including olanzapine, clozapine, lamotrigine, α_2 adrenergic agonists, and perhaps antimuscarinic agents, might be useful based on the evidence that these drugs prevent the neurotoxic process associated with the NRHypo disinhibited state.

THE NRHypo HYPOTHESIS, IDIOPATHIC PSYCHOTIC DISORDERS, AND AGE OF ONSET

All three major idiopathic psychotic disorders typically have an age of onset in late adolescence or early adulthood. In order to account for growing evidence of an early developmental lesion in these disorders, investigators have postulated that maturational events must occur in the brain during adolescence that allows for the expression of symptoms. As discussed above, it has been shown that in normal rodents and humans the NRHypo disinhibited mechanism has a similar age of onset in adolescence, suggesting similar dependence on maturational events. The similarity in the age of onset between idiopathic psychotic illnesses and the drug-induced NRHypo model further supports the proposal that a NRHypo disinhibited mechanism underlies the signs and symptoms of these disorders. Information obtained about the specific changes underlying the age-dependency profile of the drug-induced NRHypo state should also provide clues to the specific events that must occur for the eventual expression of illness in humans.

While psychotic disorders typically have an age of onset after the onset of puberty, these disorders can and do occur in childhood but with a very low prevalence (Geller & Luby, 1997; Nicolson & Rapoport, 1999; Thomsen, 1996). Recent work over the past decade has shown that these childhood-onset disorders have signs and symptoms similar to their adult counterparts, suggesting that they may be more severe forms of the adult disorders (Alaghband-Rad et al., 1995; Geller et al., 2002a, 2002b; Maziade et al., 1996; Nicolson & Rapoport, 1999). Given this perspective, one can hypothesize that the NRHypo disinhibited state could also produces cognitive and behavioral symptoms in these childhood disorders. Understanding the maturational changes that allow for the expression of the NRHypo disinhibited state in adulthood might therefore offer clues into the mechanisms that allow these psychotic disorders to present prior to the onset of puberty in certain individuals.

SUMMARY

We have discussed the NRHypo concept, which explains idiopathic psychotic disorders on the basis of genetic and/or nongenetic mechanisms instilling an NRHypo state with related circuit disinhibition in the developing brain. This state usually remains quiescent until early adulthood when maturational changes in brain circuitry make the brain vulnerable to the psychotogenic and neurotoxic potential of the NRHypo state. This hypothesis assumes that if the NRHypo state is mild or moderate, only cognitive and behavioral signs will be expressed, but if the NRHypo state is particularly severe and of long duration, then cognitive, behavioral, and neurotoxic potential will be expressed. The severe NRHypo state could result in chronic severe symptoms complicated by ongoing structural brain changes and the potential for clinical deterioration. If this concept is correct, chronic treatment with certain protective drugs, including olanzapine, clozapine, lamotrigine, α_2 adrenergic agonists, and perhaps antimuscarinic agents, could be useful based on studies that show that these drugs effectively arrest the neurotoxic process associated with the NRHypo state. In general, the animal model for NRHypo-associated neurotoxicity provides an opportunity to test pharmacological approaches for preventing the NRHypo state from hyperstimulating and injuring neurons. A careful analysis of the pharmacological interventions that are protective can also provide insights into the circuitry and receptor mechanisms that mediate this pathological process.

REFERENCES

Adams, B., & Moghaddam, B. (1998). Corticolimbic dopamine neurotransmission is temporally dissociated from the cognitive and locomotor effects of phencyclidine. *Journal of Neuroscience, 18,* 5545–5554.

Alaghband-Rad, J., McKenna, K., Gordon, C. T., Albus, K. E., Hamburger, S. D., Rumsey, J. M., Frazier, J. A., Lenane, M. C., & Rapoport, J. L. (1995). Childhood-onset schizophrenia: The severity of premorbid course. *Journal of the American Academy of Child and Adolescent Psychiatry, 34,* 1273–1283.

Allen, H. L., & Iversen, L. L. (1990). Phencyclidine, dizocilpine, and cerebrocortical neurons. *Science, 247,* 221.

Anand, A., Charney, D. S., Oren, D. A., Berman, R. M., Hu, X. S., Cappiello, A., & Krystal, J. H. (2000). Attenuation of the neuropsychiatric effects of ketamine with lamotrigine. *Archives of General Psychiatry, 57,* 270–276.

Baldridge, E. B., & Bessen, H. A. (1990). Phencyclidine. *Emergency Medicine Clinics of North America, 8,* 541–550.

Benes, F. M. (1999). Evidence for altered trisynaptic circuitry in schizophrenic hippocampus. *Biological Psychiatry, 46,* 589–599.

Benes, F. M., McSparren, J., Bird, E. D., SanGiovanni, J. P., & Vincent, S. L. (1991). Deficits in small interneurons in prefrontal and cingulate cortices of schizophrenic and schizoaffective patients. *Archives of General Psychiatry, 48,* 996–1001.

Boddeke, H. W., Wiederhold, K. H., & Palacios, J. M. (1992). Intracerebroventricular application of competitive and non-competitive NMDA antagonists induce similar effects upon rat hippocampal electroencephalogram and local cerebral glucose utilization. *Brain Research, 585,* 177–183.

Camilleri, J. G. (1962). The use of phencyclidine (CI-395) in obstetric procedures. *Anaesthesia, 17,* 422–426.

Castren, E., Da Phena Berzaghi, M., Lindholm, D., & Thoenen, H. (1993). Differential effects of MK-801 on brain-derived neurotrophic factor mRNA levels in different regions of the rat brain. *Experimental Neurology, 122,* 244–252.

Choi, D. W. (1992). Excitotoxic cell death. *Journal of Neurobiology, 23,* 1261–1276.

Clow, D. W., Lee, S. J., & Hammer, R. P. (1991). Competitive (AP7) and non-competitive (MK-801) NMDA receptor antagonists differentially alter glucose utilization in rat cortex. *Synapse, 7,* 260–268.

Collins, V. J., Gorospe, C. A., & Rovenstine, E. A. (1960). Intravenous nonbarbiturate, nonnarcotic analgesics: Preliminary studies: Part 1. Cyclohexamines. *Anesthesia and Analgesia, 39,* 302–306.

Conley, R. R., Tamminga, C. A., Bartko, J. J., Richardson, C., Peszke, M., Lingle, J., Hegerty, J., Love, R., Gounaris, C., & Zaremba, S. (1998). Olanzapine compared with chlorpromazine in treatment-resistant schizophrenia. *American Journal of Psychiatry, 155,* 914–920.

Corso, T. D., Sesma, M. A., Tenkova, T. I., Der, T. C., Wozniak, D. F., Farber, N. B., & Olney, J. W. (1997). Multifocal brain damage induced by phencyclidine is augmented by pilocarpine. *Brain Research, 752,* 1–14.

Crosby, G., Crane, A. M., & Sokoloff, L. (1982). Local changes in cerebral glucose utilization during ketamine anesthesia. *Anesthesiology , 56,* 437–443.

Danysz, W., & Parsons, C. G. (1998). Glycine and N-methyl-D-aspartate receptors: Physiological significance and possible therapeutic applications. *Pharmacological Reviews, 50,* 597–664.

Davis, D. W., Mans, A. M., Biebuyck, J. F., & Hawkins, R. A. (1988). The influence of ketamine on regional brain glucose use. *Anesthesiology, 69,* 199–205.

Domino, E. F. (1964). Neurobiology of phencyclidine (Sernyl), a drug with an unusual spectrum of pharmacological activity. *International Review of Neurobiology, 6,* 303–347.

Dragunow, M., & Faull, R. L. M. (1990). MK-801 induces c-fos protein in thalamic and neocortical neurons of rat brain. *Neuroscience Letters, 111,* 39–45.

Duncan, G. E., Leipzig, J. N., Mailman, R. B., & Lieberman, J. A. (1998). Differential effects of clozapine and haloperidol on ketamine-induced brain metabolic activation. *Brain Research, 812,* 65–75.

Duncan, G. E., Miyamoto, S., Leipzig, J. N., & Lieberman, J. A. (2000). Comparison of the effects of clozapine, risperidone, and olanzapine on ketamine-induced alterations in regional brain metabolism. *Journal of Pharmacology and Experimental Therapeutics, 293,* 8–14.

Duncan, G. E., Moy, S. S., Knapp, D. J., Mueller, R. A., & Breese, G. R. (1998). Metabolic mapping of the rat brain after subanesthetic doses of ketamine: Potential relevance to schizophrenia. *Brain Research, 787,* 181–190.

Duncan, G. E., Sheitman, B. B., & Lieberman, J. A. (1999). An integrated view of pathophysiological models of schizophrenia. *Brain Research—Brain Research Reviews, 29,* 250–264.

Ellison, G. (1994). Competitive and non-competitive NMDA antagonists induce similar limbic degeneration. *Neuroreport, 5,* 2688–2692.

Ellison, G., & Switzer, R. C. (1993). Dissimilar patterns of degeneration in brain following four different addictive stimulants. *Neuroreport, 5,* 17–20.

Erard, R., Luisada, P. V., & Peele, R. (1980). The PCP psychosis: Prolonged intoxication or drug-precipitated functional illness? *Journal of Psychedelic Drugs, 12,* 235–251.

Famy, C., Streissguth, A. P., & Unis, A. S. (1998). Mental illness in adults with fetal alcohol syndrome or fetal alcohol effects. *American Journal of Psychiatry, 155,* 552–554.

Farber, N. B., Foster, J., Duhan, N. L., & Olney, J. W. (1995). α_2 adrenergic agonists prevent MK-801 neurotoxicity. *Neuropsychopharmacology, 12,* 347–349.

Farber, N. B., Foster, J., Duhan, N. L., & Olney, J. W. (1996). Olanzapine and fluperlapine mimic clozapine in preventing MK-801 neurotoxicity. *Schizophrenia Research, 21,* 33–37.

Farber, N. B., Hanslick, J., Kirby, C., McWilliams, L., & Olney, J. W. (1998). Serotonergic agents that activate $5HT_{2A}$ receptors prevent NMDA antagonist neurotoxicity. *Neuropsychopharmacology, 18,* 57–62.

Farber, N. B., Kim, S. H., Dikranian, K., Jiang, X. P., & Heinkel, C. (2002). Receptor mechanisms and circuitry underlying NMDA antagonist neurotoxicity. *Molecular Psychiatry, 7,* 32–43.

Farber, N. B., Newcomer, J. W., & Olney, J. W. (1999). Glycine agonists: What can they teach us about schizophrenia? *Archives of General Psychiatry, 56,* 13–17.

Farber, N. B., Price, M. T., Labruyere, J., Nemnich, J., St. Peter, H., Wozniak, D. F., & Olney, J. W. (1993). Antipsychotic drugs block phencyclidine receptor-mediated neurotoxicity. *Biological Psychiatry, 34,* 119–121.

Farber, N. B., Wozniak, D. F., Price, M. T., Labruyere, J., Huss, J., St. Peter, H., & Olney, J. W. (1995). Age specific neurotoxicity in the rat associated with NMDA receptor blockade: Potential relevance to schizophrenia? *Biological Psychiatry, 38,* 788–796.

Fix, A. S., Horn, J. W., Wightman, K. A., Johnson, C. A., Long, G. G., Storts, R. W., Farber, N., Wozniak, D. F., & Olney, J. W. (1993). Neuronal vacuolization and necrosis induced by the noncompetitive N-methyl-D-aspartate (NMDA) antagonist MK(+)801 (dizocilpine maleate): A light and electron microscopic evaluation of the rat retrosplenial cortex. *Experimental Neurology, 123,* 204–215.

Fix, A. S., Wightman, K. A., & O'Callaghan, J. P. (1995). Reactive gliosis induced by MK-801 in the rat posterior cingulate/retrosplenial cortex: GFAP evaluation by sandwich ELISA and immunohistochemistry. *Neurotoxicology, 16,* 229–239.

Fix, A. S., Wozniak, D. F., Truex, L. L., McEwen, M., Miller, J. P., & Olney, J. W. (1995). Quantitative analysis of factors influencing neuronal necrosis induced by MK-801 in the rat posterior cingulate/retrosplenial cortex. *Brain Research, 696,* 194–204.

Gao, X. M., Hashimoto, T., & Tamminga, C. A. (1998). Phencyclidine (PCP) and dizocilpine (MK801) exert time-dependent effects on the expression of immediate early genes in rat brain. *Synapse, 29,* 14–28.

Gao, X. M., Shirakawa, O., Du, F., & Tamminga, C. A. (1993). Delayed regional metabolic actions of phencyclidine. *European Journal of Pharmacology, 241,* 7–15.

Gass, P., Herdegen, T., Bravo, R., & Kiessling, M. (1993). Induction and suppression of immediate early genes in specific rat brain regions by the non-competitive N-methyl-D-aspartate antagonist, MK-801. *Neuroscience, 53,* 749–758.

Geller, B., & Luby, J. (1997). Child and adolescent bipolar disorder: A review of the past 10 years. *Journal of the American Academy of Child and Adolescent Psychiatry, 36,* 1168–1176.

Geller, B., Zimerman, B., Williams, M., Bolhofner, K., Craney, J. L., DelBello, M. P., & Soutullo, C. A. (2002a). Diagnostic characteristics of 93 cases of a prepubertal and early adolescent bipolar disorder phenotype by gender, age, puberty and comorbid attention-deficit/hyperactivity disorder. *Journal of Child and Adolescent Psychopharmacology, 10,* 157–164.

Geller, B., Zimerman, B., Williams, M., Bolhofner, K., Craney, J. L., DelBello, M. P., & Soutullo, C. A. (2002b). Six-month stability and outcome of a prepubertal and early adolescent bipolar disorder phenotype. *Journal of Child and Adolescent Psychopharmacology, 10,* 165–173.

Giovannini, M. G., Camilli, F., Mundula, A., & Pepeu, G. (1994). Glutamatergic regulation of acetylcholine output in different brain regions: A microdialysis study in the rat. *Neurochemistry International, 25,* 23–26.

Giovannini, M. G., Giovannelli, L., Bianchi, L., Kalfin, R., & Pepeu, G. (1997). Glutamatergic modulation of cortical acetylcholine release in the rat: A combined in vivo microdialysis, retrograde tracing and immunohistochemical study. *European Journal of Neuroscience, 9,* 1678–1689.

Giovannini, M. G., Mutolo, D., Bianchi, L., Michelassi, A., & Pepeu, G. (1994). NMDA receptor antagonists decrease GABA outflow from the septum and increase acetylcholine outflow from the hippocampus: A microdialysis study. *Journal of Neuroscience, 14,* 1358–1365.

Goff, D. C., Tsai, G., Levitt, J., Amico, E., Manoach, D., Schoenfeld, D. A., Hayden, D. L., McCarley, R., & Coyle, J. T. (1999). A placebo-controlled trial of D-cycloserine added to conventional neuroleptics in patients with schizophrenia. *Archives of General Psychiatry, 56,* 21–27.

Grace, A. A. (1991). Phasic versus tonic dopamine release and the modulation of dopamine system responsivity: A hypothesis for the etiology of schizophrenia. *Neuroscience, 41,* 1–24.

Greengard, P., Nairn, A. C., Girault, J. A., Ouimet, C. C., Snyder, G. L., Fisone, G., Fienberg, A., & Nishi, A. (1998). The DARPP-32/protein phosphatase-1 cascade: A model for signal integration. *Brain Research—Brain Research Reviews, 26,* 274–284.

Grunze, H. C., Rainnie, D. G., Hasselmo, M. E., Barkai, E., Hearn, E. F., McCarley, R. W., & Green, R. W. (1996). NMDA-dependent modulation of CA1 local circuit inhibition. *Journal of Neuroscience, 16,* 2034–2043.

Guidotti, A., Auta, J., Davis, J. M., Gerevini, V. D., Dwivedi, Y., Grayson, D. R., Impagnatiello, F., Pandey, G., Pesold, C., Sharma, R., Uzunov, D., & Costa, E. (2000). Decrease in reelin and glutamic acid decarboxylase$_{67}$ (GAD$_{67}$) expression in schizophrenia and bipolar disorder. *Archives of General Psychiatry, 57,* 1061–1069.

Hammer, R. P., & Herkenham, M. (1983). Altered metabolic activity in the cerebral cortex of rats exposed to ketamine. *Journal of Comparative Neurology, 220,* 396–404.

Hasegawa, M., Kinoshita, H., Amano, M., Hasegawa, T., Kameyama, T., & Nabeshima, T. (1993). MK-801 increases endogenous acetylcholine release in the rat parietal cortex: A study using brain microdialysis. *Neuroscience Letters, 150,* 53–56.

Hawkins, R., Hass, W. K., & Ransoff, J. (1979). Measurement of regional glucose utilization in vivo using [2-^{14}C] glucose. *Stroke, 10,* 690–703.

Heresco-Levy, U., Javitt, D. C., Ermilov, M., Mordel, C., Silipo, G., & Lichtenstein, M. (1999). Efficacy of high-dose glycine in the treatment of enduring negative symptoms of schizophrenia. *Archives of General Psychiatry, 56,* 29–36.

Horvath, Z. C., Czopf, J., & Buzsaki, G. (1997). MK-801–induced neuronal damage in rats. *Brain Research, 753,* 181–195.

Hughes, P., & Dragunow, M. (1995). Induction of immediate early genes and the control of neurotransmitter-regulated gene expression within the nervous system. *Pharmacological Reviews, 47,* 133–178.

Hughes, P., Dragunow, M., Beilharz, E., Lawlor, P., & Gluckman, P. (1993). MK801 induces immediate-early gene proteins and BDNF mRNA in rat cerebrocortical neurones. *NeuroReport, 4,* 183–186.

Ikonomidou, C., Bittigau, P., Ishimaru, M. J., Wozniak, D. F., Koch, C., Genz, K., Price, M. T., Stefovska, V., Horster, F., Tenkova, T., Dikranian, K., & Olney, J. W. (2000). Ethanol-induced apoptotic neurodegeneration and fetal alcohol syndrome. *Science, 287,* 1056–1060.

Ikonomidou, C., Bosch, F., Miksa, M., Bittigau, P., Vockler, J., Dikranian, K., Stefovska, V., Turski, L., & Olney, J. W. (1999). Blockade of NMDA receptors and apoptotic neurodegeneration in the developing brain. *Science, 283,* 70–74.

Ikonomidou, C., Price, M. T., Mosinger, J. L., Frierdich, G., Labruyere, J., Salles, K. S., & Olney, J. W. (1989). Hypobaric-ischemic conditions produce glutamate-like cytopathology in infant rat brain. *Journal of Neuroscience, 9,* 1693–1700.

Ishimaru, M., Fukamauchi, F., & Olney, J. W. (1995). Halothane prevents MK-801 neurotoxicity in the rat cingulate cortex. *Neuroscience Letters, 193,* 1–4.

Jentsch, J. D., & Roth, R. H. (1999). The neuropsychopharmacology of phencyclidine: From NMDA receptor hypofunction to the dopamine hypothesis of schizophrenia. *Neuropsychopharmacology, 20,* 201–225.

Jevtovic-Todorovic, V., Olney, J. W., & Farber, N. B. (1998). Lamotrigine prevents NMDA antagonist neurotoxicity. *Society for Neuroscience Abstracts, 24,* 745.

Karp, H. N., Kaufman, N. D., & Anand, S. K. (1980). Phencyclidine poisoning in young children. *Journal of Pediatrics, 97,* 1006–1009.

Kendler, K. S., & Gardner, C. O. (1997). The risk for psychiatric disorders in relatives of schizophrenic and control probands: A comparison of three independent studies. *Psychological Medicine, 27,* 411–419.

Kendler, K. S., Karkowski, L. M., & Walsh, D. (1998). The structure of psychosis: Latent class analysis of probands from the Roscommon Family Study. *Archives of General Psychiatry, 55,* 492–499.

Kendler, K. S., Karkowski-Shuman, L., O'Neill, F. A., Straub, R. E., MacLean, C. J., & Walsh, D. (1997). Resemblance of psychotic symptoms and syndromes in affected sibling pairs from the Irish Study of High-Density Schizophrenia Families: Evidence for possible etiologic heterogeneity. *American Journal of Psychiatry, 154*, 191–198.

Kim, S. H., Price, M. T., Olney, J. W., & Farber, N. B. (1999). Excessive cerebro-cortical release of acetylcholine induced by NMDA antagonists is reduced by GABAergic and α_2-adrenergic agonists. *Molecular Psychiatry*, 4, 344–352.

Krystal, J. H., D'Souza, D. C., Karper, L. P., Bennett, A., Abi-Dargham, A., Abi-Saab, D., Cassello, K., Bowers, M. B., Jr., Vegso, S., Heninger, G. R., & Charney, D. S. (1999). Interactive effects of subanesthetic ketamine and haloperidol in healthy humans. *Psychopharmacology, 145*, 193–204.

Krystal, J. H., Karper, L. P., Bennett, A., D'Souza, D. C., Abi-Dargham, A., Morrissey, K., Abi-Saab, D., Bremner, J. D., Bowers, M. B., Jr., Suckow, R. F., Stetson, P., Heninger, G. R., & Charney, D. S. (1998). Interactive effects of subanesthetic ketamine and subhypnotic lorazepam in humans. *Psychopharmacology, 135*, 213–229.

Krystal, J. H., Karper, L. P., Seibyl, J. P., Freeman, G. K., Delaney, R., Bremner, J. D., Heninger, G. R., Bowers, M. B., Jr., & Charney, D. S. (1994). Subanesthetic effects of the noncompetitive NMDA antagonist, ketamine, in humans: Psychotomimetic, perceptual, cognitive, and neuroendocrine responses. *Archives of General Psychiatry, 51*, 199–214.

Kurumaji, A., & McCulloch, J. (1989). Effects of MK-801 upon local cerebral glucose utilisation in conscious rats and in rats anaesthetised with halothane. *Journal of Cerebral Blood Flow and Metabolism*, 9, 786–794.

Lahti, A. C., Holcomb, H. H., Gao, X. M., & Tamminga, C. A. (1999). NMDA-sensitive glutamate antagonism: A human model for psychosis. *Neuropsychopharmacology, 21*(6, Suppl. 2), S158–S169.

Lester, R. A., Clements, J. D., Westbrook, G. L., & Jahr, C. E. (1990). Channel kinetics determine the time course of NMDA receptor-mediated synaptic currents. *Nature, 346*, 565–567.

Lohr, J. B., & Bracha, H. S. (1989). Can schizophrenia be related to prenatal exposure to alcohol?: Some speculations. *Schizophrenia Bulletin, 15*, 595–603.

Luby, E. D., Cohen, B. D., Rosenbaum, G., Gottlieb, J. S., & Kelley, R. (1959). Study of a new schizophrenomimetic drug—Sernyl. *Archives of Neurology and Psychiatry, 81*, 363–369.

Lund, J. P., Miller, J. J., & Courville, J. (1981). [^{3}H]2–deoxyglucose capture in the hippocampus and dentate gyrus of ketamine-anesthetized rat. *Neuroscience Letters, 24*, 149–153.

Magbagbeola, J. A., & Thomas, N. A. (1974). Effect of thiopentone on emergence reactions to ketamine anaesthesia. *Canadian Anaesthetists Society Journal, 21*, 321–324.

Malhotra, A. K., Adler, C. M., Kennison, S. D., Elman, I., Pickar, D., & Breier, A. (1997). Clozapine blunts N-methyl-D-aspartate antagonist-induced psychosis: A study with ketamine. *Biological Psychiatry, 42*, 664–668.

Malhotra, A. K., Pinals, D. A., Weingartner, H., Sirocco, K., Missar, C. D., Pickar, D., & Breier, A. (1996). NMDA receptor function and human cognition: The effects of ketamine in healthy volunteers. *Neuropsychopharmacology, 14*, 301–307.

Mayer, M. L., & Westbrook, G. L. (1987). The physiology of excitatory amino acids in the vertebrate central nervous system. *Progress in Neurobiology, 28*, 197–276.

Maziade, M., Gingras, N., Rodrigue, C., Bouchard, S., Cardinal, A., Gauthier, B.,

Tremblay, G., Cote, S., Fournier, C., Boutin, P., Hamel, M., Roy, M. A., Martinez, M., & Merette, C. (1996). Long-term stability of diagnosis and symptom dimensions in a systematic sample of patients with onset of schizophrenia in childhood and early adolescence: Part 1. Nosology, sex and age of onset. *British Journal of Psychiatry, 169,* 361–370.

McBain, C. J., & Mayer, M. L. (1994). N-methyl-D-aspartic acid receptor structure and function. *Physiological Reviews, 74,* 723–760.

McCarron, M. M., Schulze, B. W., Thompson, G. A., Conder, M. C., & Goetz, W. A. (1981). Acute phencyclidine intoxication: Clinical patterns, complications, and treatment. *Annals of Emergency Medicine, 10,* 290–297.

Meibach, R. C., Glicks, D., Cox, R., & Maayani, S. (1979). Localisation of phencyclidine-induced changes in brain energy metabolism. *Nature, 282,* 625–626.

Moghaddam, B., & Adams, B. (1998). Reversal of phencyclidine effects by a group II metabotropic glutamate receptor agonist in rats. *Science, 281,* 1349–1352.

Moghaddam, B., Adams, B., Verma, A., & Daly, D. (1997). Activation of glutamatergic neurotransmission by ketamine: A novel step in the pathway from NMDA receptor blockade to dopaminergic and cognitive disruptions associated with the prefrontal cortex. *Journal of Neuroscience, 17,* 2921–2927.

Nagata, A., Nakao, S., Miyamoto, E., Inada, T., Tooyama, I., Kimura, H., & Shingu, K. (1998). Propofol inhibits ketamine-induced c-fos expression in the rat posterior cingulate cortex. *Anesthesia and Analgesia, 87,* 1416–1420.

Nakao, S. I., Adachi, T., Murakawa, M., Shinomura, T., Kurata, J., Shichino, T., Shibata, M., Tooyama, I., Kimura, H., & Mori, K. (1996). Halothane and diazepam inhibit ketamine-induced c-fos expression in the rat cingulate cortex. *Anesthesiology, 85,* 874–882.

Nakki, R., Sharp, F. R., Sagar, S. M., & Honkaniemi, J. (1996). Effects of phencyclidine on immediate early gene expression in the brain. *Journal of Neuroscience Research, 45,* 13–27.

Nelsom, S. R., Howard, R. B., Cross, R. S., & Samson, F. (1980). Ketamine-induced changes in regional glucose utilization in the rat brain. *Anesthesiology, 52,* 330–334.

Newcomer, J. W., Farber, N. B., Jevtovic-Todorovic, V., Selke, G., Kelly Melson, A., Hershey, T., Craft, S., & Olney, J. W. (1999). Ketamine-induced NMDA receptor hypofunction as a model of memory impairment in schizophrenia. *Neuropsychopharmacology, 20,* 106–118.

Newcomer, J. W., Farber, N. B., Selke, G., Melson, A. K., Jevtovic-Todorovic, V., & Olney, J. W. (1998). Guanabenz effects on NMDA antagonist-induced mental symptoms in humans. *Society for Neuroscience Abstracts, 24,* 525.

Nicolson, R., & Rapoport, J. L. (1999). Childhood-onset schizophrenia: Rare but worth studying. *Biological Psychiatry, 46,* 1418–28.

Noguchi, K., Johnson, R., & Ellison, G. (1998). The effects of MK-801 on aspartate and glutamate levels in the anterior cingulate and retrosplenial cortices: An in vivo microdialysis study. *Society for Neuroscience Abstracts, 24,* 233.

Oguchi, K., Arakawa, K., Nelson, S. R., & Samson, F. (1982). The influence of droperidol, diazepam and physostigmine on ketamine-induced behavior and brain regional glucose utilization in rat. *Anesthesiology, 57,* 353–358.

Olney, J. W. (1990). Excitotoxic amino acids and neuropsychiatric disorders. *Annual Review of Pharmacology and Toxicology, 30,* 47–71.

Olney, J. W., & Farber, N. B. (1995). Glutamate receptor dysfunction and schizophrenia. *Archives of General Psychiatry*, 52, 998–1007.

Olney, J. W., Labruyere, J., & Price, M. T. (1989). Pathological changes induced in cerebrocortical neurons by phencyclidine and related drugs. *Science*, 244, 1360–1362.

Olney, J. W., Labruyere, J., Wang, G., Wozniak, D. F., Price, M. T., & Sesma, M. A. (1991). NMDA antagonist neurotoxicity: mechanism and prevention. *Science*, 254, 1515–1518.

Olney, J. W., Wozniak, D. F., Price, M. T., Tenkova, T. I., Dikranian, K., & Ikonomidou, C. (1999). Ethanol induces widespread apoptotic neurodegeneration in the infant mouse brain. *Society for Neuroscience Abstracts*, 25, 550.

Ongur, D., Drevets, W. C., & Price, J. L. (1998). Glial reduction in the subgenual prefrontal cortex in mood disorders. *Proceedings of the National Academy of Sciences of the United States of America*, 95, 13290–13295.

Paxinos G., & Watson, C. (1998). *The rat brain in stereotaxic coordinates* (4th ed.). New York: Academic Press.

Pender, J. W. (1971). Dissociative anesthesia. *Journal of the American Medical Association*, 215, 1126–1130.

Price, M. T., Wozniak, D. F., Tenkova, T. I., Dikranian, K., Ikonomidou, C., & Olney, J. W. (1999). Ethanol induces widespread apoptotic neurodegeneration in the fetal guinea pig brain. *Society for Neuroscience Abstracts*, 25, 550.

Reich, D. L., & Silvay, G. (1989). Ketamine: An update on the first twenty-five years of clinical experience. *Canadian Journal of Anaesthesia*, 36, 186–197.

Sato, D., Umino, A., Kaneda, K., Takigawa, M., & Nishikawa, T. (1997). Developmental changes in distribution patterns of phencyclidine-induced c-Fos in rat forebrain. *Neuroscience Letters*, 239, 21–24.

Sharkey, J., Ritchie, I. M., Butcher, S. P., & Kelly, J. S. (1996). Comparison of the patterns of altered cerebral glucose utilisation produced by competitive and noncompetitive NMDA receptor antagonists. *Brain Research*, 735, 67–82.

Sharp, F. R., Butman, M., Koistinaho, J., Aardalen, K., Nakki, R., Massa, S., Swanson, R. A., & Sagar, S. M. (1994). Phencyclidine induction of the hsp70 stress gene in injured pyramidal neurons is mediated via multiple receptors and voltage gated calcium channels. *Neuroscience*, 62, 1079–1092.

Sharp, F. R., Butman, M., Wang, S., Koistinaho, J., Graham, S. H., Sagar, S. M., Noble, L., Berger, P., & Longo, F. M. (1992). Haloperidol prevents induction of the hsp70 heat shock gene in neurons injured by phencyclidine (PCP), MK801, and ketamine. *Journal of Neuroscience Research*, 33, 605–616.

Sharp, F. R., Jasper, P., Hall, J., Noble, L., & Sagar, S. M. (1991). MK-801 and ketamine induce heat shock protein HSP72 in injured neurons in posterior cingulate and retrosplenial cortex. *Annals of Neurology*, 30, 801–809.

Sharp, J. W., Petersen, D. L., & Langford, M. T. (1995). DNQX inhibits phencyclidine (PCP) and ketamine induction of the hsp70 heat shock gene in the rat cingulate and retrosplenial cortex. *Brain Research*, 687, 114–124.

Sharp, J. W., & Williams, D. S. (1996). Effects of sigma ligands on the ability of rimcazole to inhibit PCP hsp70 induction. *Brain Research Bulletin*, 39, 359–366.

Supplisson, S., & Bergman, C. (1997). Control of NMDA receptor activation by a glycine transporter co-expressed in xenopus oocytes. *Journal of Neuroscience,* *17,* 4580–4590.

Thomsen, P. H. (1996). Schizophrenia with childhood and adolescent onset: A nationwide register-based study. *Acta Psychiatrica Scandinavica, 94,* 187–193.

Tomitaka, S. I., Hashimoto, K., Narita, N., Minabe, Y., & Tamura, A. (1997). Regionally different effects of scopolamine on NMDA antagonist-induced heat shock protein HSP70. *Brain Research, 736,* 255–258.

Tsai, G., Pinchen, Y., Chung, L.-C., Lange, N., & Coyle, J. T. (1998). D-Serine added to antipsychotics for the treatment of schizophrenia. *Biological Psychiatry, 44,* 1081–1089.

Verma, A., & Moghaddam, B. (1996). NMDA receptor antagonists impair prefrontal cortex function as assessed via spatial delayed alternation performance in rats: Modulation by dopamine. *Journal of Neuroscience, 16,* 373–379.

Vogt, B. A. (1993). Structural organization of cingulate cortex: areas, neurons, and somatodendritic transmiter receptors. In B. A. Vogt & M. Gabriel (Eds.), *Neurobiology of cingulate cortex and limbic thalamus* (pp. 19–70). Boston: Birkhauser.

Watkins, J. C., & Evans, R. H. (1981). Excitatory amino acid transmitters. *Annual Review of Pharmacology and Toxicology, 21,* 165–204.

Welch, M. J., & Correa, G. A. (1980). PCP intoxication in young children and infants. *Clinical Pediatrics, 19,* 510–514.

White, P. F., Way, W. L., & Trevor, A. J. (1982). Ketamine: Its pharmacology and therapeutic uses. *Anesthesiology, 56,* 119–136.

Woo, T. U., Whitehead, R. E., Melchitzky, D. S., & Lewis, D. A. (1998). A subclass of prefrontal gamma-aminobutyric acid axon terminals are selectively altered in schizophrenia. *Proceedings of the National Academy of Sciences of the United States of America, 95,* 5341–5346.

Wozniak, D. F., Dikranian, K., Ishimaru, M., Nardi, A., Corso, T. D., Tenkova, T. I., Olney, J. W., & Fix, A. S. (1998). Disseminated corticolimbic neuronal degeneration induced in rat brain by MK-801: Potential relevance to Alzheimer's disease. *Neurobiology of Disease, 5,* 305–322.

7

Neuroimaging in Pediatric Bipolar Disorder

Melissa P. DelBello and Robert A. Kowatch

Child and adolescent bipolar disorder is a common psychiatric illness with significant morbidity and mortality. Although the neuropathological basis of early-onset bipolar disorder is poorly understood, recent advances in brain imaging techniques have provided the opportunity to directly examine the neuroanatomy that underlies this disorder (Strakowski, DelBello, Adler, Cecil, & Sax, 2000). Mood instability is the core feature of bipolar disorder. Therefore, the neuroanatomic structures that modulate mood regulation are likely to be involved in bipolar disorder. Indeed, reports of affective instability following focal brain lesions suggest that secondary mania is associated with injuries to the orbitofrontal and temporal cortices, the caudate, the thalamus, and the cerebellum (Cutting, 1976; Ghaziuddin, DeQuardo, Ghaziuddin, & King, 1999; Levisohn, Cronin-Golomb, & Schmahmann, 2000; Sayal, Ford, & Pipe, 2000; Strakowski et al., 1999; Strakowski & Sax, 2000). Moreover, recent studies of healthy volunteers suggest that these brain regions are activated in response to induced mood states. Indeed, investigators have proposed two interconnected brain circuits as the neuroanatomical basis for mood regulation: a limbic (amygdala)–thalamic–prefrontal cortical circuit and a limbic–striatal–pallidal–thalamic circuit (Soares & Mann, 1997). In this chapter, we review currently available neuroimaging techniques, examine how neuroimaging might be utilized to study the neurophysiology of bipolar disorder, and provide an overview of recent neuroimaging studies that included children and adolescents with bipolar disorder.

BRAIN IMAGING TECHNIQUES

Brain imaging techniques available to study mood disorders may be broadly divided into two categories: those that image the *structure* of the central nervous system (CNS), which include computed tomography (CT) and magnetic resonance imaging (MRI), and those that image the *function* of the CNS, which include positron emission tomography (PET), single-photon emission computed tomography (SPECT), magnetic resonance spectroscopy (MRS), and functional magnetic resonance imaging (fMRI).

Both of the techniques that examine brain structure, MRI and CT, are commonly used for clinical diagnostic evaluation of children and adolescents by neurologists and pediatricians. These tools are excellent at identifying gross pathological conditions such as tumors, infarctions, hemorrhages, or demyelinating disorders.

Structural Brain Imaging Techniques

Computed Tomography

CT scanners revolutionized diagnostic medicine when they became available in the early 1970s. Their development permitted clinicians to examine soft tissues. CT was the first tomographic imaging technique, which was later followed by MRI, PET, and SPECT. All of these techniques are based on the creation of two-dimensional views of a tissue slice from a set of one-dimensional projections taken at multiple angles. The contrast in a CT image is based on delineation of the differential attenuation of x-rays by distinct tissue types. CT scanners are made up of a rotating x-ray beam surrounded by a ring of x-ray detectors. Images are acquired in a slice-by-slice fashion. CT creates axial images of brain tissue with a spatial resolution of approximately 1 mm. CT scans can be utilized for evaluating CNS lesions such as tumors, infarction, or gross structural changes. In order to highlight areas of blood–brain barrier breakdown, intravenous contrast agents are sometimes necessary with CT scanning.

There are several limitations to CT scanning:

1. The scanning procedure involves exposure to ionizing radiation.
2. Gray–white matter contrast resolution is poor.
3. Visualization of white matter disease is poor.
4. Visualization of the basotemporal cortex and posterior fossa can be obscured because of susceptibility to artifacts in structures near bone.
5. The contrast agent can cause allergic responses.

CT's main advantages to date have been that in general it is less expensive than MR imaging and it is superior for visualization of bone.

Magnetic Resonance Imaging

MRI is currently the imaging method that provides the highest spatial and contrast resolution for visualizing neuroanatomical structures. Additionally, MRI is not associated with ionizing radiation and has no known biological risks, and therefore is advantageous for *in vivo* examination of brain structures in pediatric populations. Structural MRI is the most common clinical application for magnetic resonance (MR) scanners; however, MR methods can also provide chemical and functional information. These newer techniques, such as magnetic resonance spectroscopy (MRS), diffusion imaging, and functional magnetic resonance imaging (fMRI) offer the potential for providing information that cannot currently be obtained *in vivo* by other methods. These techniques are discussed in more detail later in this chapter.

MR images are created based on the magnetic properties of atoms (most commonly hydrogen), which are amplified and enhanced for detection and visualization. A basic general description of the physical principles involved in the production and detection of an MR signal can provide an intuitive appreciation for the imaging technique and its potential flexibility and power. When elemental atomic nuclei have an odd number of electrons or protons, they are associated with a charge, and this charge induces an inherent spin to the atom. The spinning of the charged molecule creates a minute magnetization—a magnetic dipole. Usually, in the natural state, the randomly oriented dipoles cancel out each other's charges and there is no net magnetization of tissue. However, when the tissue is placed in a magnetic field, the nuclei will achieve their lowest energy state and align parallel to the field. This alignment produces a net positive magnetization of the tissue. MR scanners provide a strong magnetic field to facilitate this alignment. In their natural state, the nuclei spin evenly, but nuclei within a magnetic field spin unevenly like a top, in a process known as *precession*. The precession of the molecules releases energy in the form of a radio frequency. These radio frequencies can be measured and localized by the MR scanner under appropriate conditions. In order to amplify the precession or resonance of the nuclei, the tissue is further excited through the application of an external radio frequency pulse, which shifts the nuclear dipoles out of the plane parallel to the magnetic field. When this radio frequency pulse is removed, the nuclei attempt to return to their lowest energy state, parallel to the magnetic field, in a process known as *relaxation*. Generally, the nuclei are shifted 90 degrees or perpendicular to the plane of magnetization. The receiver antenna detects the rate of relaxation and transforms this signal through a series of mathematical Fourier transformations to generate an MR image. The images can be created in any plane of orientation. The most common clinically used images are in the sagittal, coronal, and axial planes.

MRI offers many advantages compared with CT:

1. MRI lacks radiation exposure.
2. MRI permits acquisition of high-resolution images with excellent gray–white matter contrast in any plane of orientation.
3. MRI provides superior detection for pathologic lesions in the white matter.
4. MRI avoids the boney artifacts associated with CT, and thus is superior for visualizing the temporal lobes, posterior fossa, and brain stem.

Standard clinical MR scanners can achieve a spatial resolution of 1–2 mm and the new high-power MR scanners (3–5 Tesla) can achieve microscopic resolution of approximately 300 μm. Therefore, recent advances in MRI techniques permit high-resolution thin-slice images for more valid quantitative morphometric analyses. *Morphometric analysis* is the process by which specific brain structures can be measured. Thus, investigators can examine whether there are differences in specific brain structure volumes among groups of patients and healthy volunteers. This process can help identify the neuroanatomical substrates that underlie a specific disorder.

Functional Brain Imaging Techniques

Single-Photon Emission Computed Tomography

Single-photon emission computed tomography (SPECT) is a nuclear medicine imaging technique that can measure regional cerebral blood flow (rCBF) or receptor densities *in vivo*. SPECT imaging is based on the principle that there is a close association among rCBF, glucose metabolism, and neuronal activity (Raichle, Grubb, & Gado, 1976; Sokoloff, 1981). During a SPECT study, a patient is injected intravenously with a compound composed of a flow tracer which is "bound" to a radionuclide. The radionuclide used (commonly ^{99m}Tc) emits short-lived gamma rays called *photons*. This combination of a flow tracer like HMPAO with a radionuclide produces a "radiopharmaceutical" capable of measuring either rCBF or receptor densities. SPECT radiopharmaceuticals commonly used for measuring rCBF include ^{123}I IMP (Spectamine), ^{99m}Tc-HMPAO (Ceretec), and ^{99m}Tc-ECD (Neurolite). These radiopharmaceuticals remain stable within the brain for several hours. One of the first brain blood flow markers used for SPECT was the gas ^{133}xenon but, because xenon diffuses out of the brain very rapidly and imaging with it has a spatial resolution of 14–17 mm, xenon is not used as often as the stably distributed radiopharmaceutical agents listed above.

A major advantage of SPECT is that it is widely available within most hospital nuclear medicine departments and relatively affordable. The average cost of a SPECT brain scan is $400–$600/scan because the radioisotopes that are used for SPECT imaging, unlike PET isotopes, do not require a cyclotron for their production and are less expensive.

Cerebral SPECT imaging is used in nuclear medicine to diagnose seizures, tumors, and some developmental abnormalities (O'Tuama & Treves, 1993). In child psychiatry there are no known clinical indications at this time for SPECT imaging. Because of the invasiveness of SPECT, there have been few studies of children and adolescents without psychiatric disorders to utilize SPECT as a diagnostic tool. SPECT may be useful for measuring specific brain receptor densities in patients with pediatric mood disorders.

Positron Emission Tomography

Positron emission tomography (PET) is one of the most powerful brain imaging techniques available in psychiatry today. However, due to the high cost of creating and operating a PET facility, it is also one of the least available and most expensive functional brain imaging methods. PET imaging necessitates a cyclotron to produce isotopes of carbon (^{11}C), nitrogen (^{13}N), oxygen (^{15}O), or fluorine (^{18}F), which emit a short-lived particle called a *positron*. Using these positron-emitting radiopharmaceutcials, PET can measure rCBF, cerebral blood volume, oxygen or glucose metabolism, neuroreceptor binding, or water extraction across the blood–brain barrier. A variety of brain receptors may be imaged using specific PET radioligands, including D_2 dopamine, 5-HT2 serotonon, opiate, glutamate-NMDA, and histamine receptors (Wong & Resnick, 1995).

During PET imaging, the injected radiotracer emits positrons within the brain, which collide with electrons to produce two photons traveling in exactly opposite directions. A detector "coincidence circuit" will recognize this simultaneous ionization and create an image from these events. Spatial resolution for PET is usually in the range of 5–6 mm.

Major advantages of PET are that it has a higher spatial resolution than SPECT and it can measure many specific neuroreceptors, as well as rCBF and glucose metabolism. Also, the dose of radiophararaceuticial used in pediatric PET research studies can be adjusted to be within current U.S. Food and Drug Administration radiation safety guidelines for research in children (Zametkin et al., 1993). Disadvantages of PET scanning are that it is expensive and requires a cyclotron, which limits its availability.

Functional Magnetic Resonance Imaging

Functional magnetic resonance imaging (fMRI) is a newer functional imaging technique that permits study of brain function without the risk of ionizing radiation, making it particularly useful for assessing brain function in children and adolescents. So fMRI is repeatable, noninvasive, and has the advantage of better temporal resolution than either PET or SPECT (5 sec vs. 1–2 min for SPECT and PET). fMRI also has the capability of acquiring many more scans in a single scanning session, which allows for an improved signal-to-noise ratio. fMRI also can be performed on most existing MR scanners, although they usually require the addition of specialized software and hardware.

Images using fMRI are obtained based on the difference in paramagnetic properties of oxy- and deoxyhemoglobin. When synaptic activity is increased, there is an increase in cerebral blood flow into that brain region that exceeds the actual increase in oxygen consumption. This relative excess of blood flow leads to a relative decrease in concentration of deoxyhemoglobin as compared to oxyhemoglobin, which can be detected using MRI. This approach is called the BOLD (blood-oxygen-level-dependent) technique. Since MRI structural scans are obtained concurrently with fMRI brain activation maps, coregistration of regions of interest between activation maps and structural scans is very accurate.

Magnetic Resonance Spectroscopy

Magnetic resonance spectroscopy (MRS) is a noninvasive neuroimaging technique that allows *in vivo* measurement of brain neurochemistry. MRS can be used to study a wide variety of isotopes, including hydrogen (proton ^{1}H), lithium (^{7}Li), carbon (^{13}C), fluorine (^{19}F), sodium (^{23}Na), and phosphorous (^{31}P). Of these, lithium, proton, and phosphorous spectroscopies have been used to study mood disorders. Proton MRS is most commonly used and provides a measure of cellular chemical activity by studying neurotransmitters and amino acids. The major components observed in a proton spectrum of the brain are N-acetylaspartate (NAA), glutamate/glutamine/GABA (Glx), creatine (Cr), choline (Cho), and *myo*-inositol (mI) (Strakowski et al., 2000). Spectroscopy generally examines metabolites at 1–10mM levels, as compared to conventional MRI, which measures water concentrations over 100M. Therefore, in order to improve signal-to-noise ratios in MRS, extended scan times of large heterogeneous tissue volumes are needed to obtain an adequate signal. Extended scanning times obviously introduce the risk of patient movement, which results in artifact. Nonetheless, MRS is a unique and powerful imaging technique for measuring membrane and neuronal chemistry.

NEUROBEHAVIORAL PROBES

The use of "neurobehavioral probes" in conjunction with functional imaging techniques like PET or fMRI provides for greater sensitivity and specificity in identifying the neural correlates of mood disorders than the majority of resting studies discussed above. According to Gur, Erwin, and Gur (1992), neurobehavioral probes involve the administration of tasks during measurement of physiologic activity. However, the application of these probes in conjunction with functional neuroimaging techniques involves a number of design challenges to ensure valid experimental results. Task development may be conceptualized as involving the following stages:

1. Selection of a unitary behavioral dimension for measurement.
2. Selection of tasks that tap into the chosen behavioral dimension and that have been validated within the constraints of experimental imaging paradigms.
3. Application of the chosen task with healthy subjects to determine which brain areas are involved in the processing required by the neurobehavioral probe.
4. Application of the neurobehavioral probe to well-characterized neuropsychiatric samples and matched healthy control subjects. (Gur, Erwin, & Gur, 1992)

Two of the cardinal symptoms of bipolar disorder are dysfunction of attention and emotional regulation. Several brain regions, including the prefrontal cortex, thalamus, striatum, amygdala, and cerebellar vermis have been shown to modulate attention and emotional processes. Indeed, these are the same brain regions that have been implicated in the neurophysiology of bipolar disorder. Therefore, utilizing tasks of attention and emotional regulation as behavioral probes for fMRI investigations might clarify the neurophysiological basis for attentional and emotional dysfunction associated with pediatric bipolar disorder.

Abnormalities in neural networks that control emotional processing and regulation potentially affect both emotional behavior and emotion perception (Yurgelun-Todd, Gruber, Kanayama, Baird, & Young, 2000). One way to examine emotion perception is through studies of facial affect. In the past, only the Ekman Facial Photographs were available for use in functional imaging experiments. Recently, the neuropsychiatry group at the University of Pennsylvania led by Ruben Gur and Roland Erwin (Gur, Erwin, et al., 1992) created a newer set of facial photographs of professional actors and actresses portraying three emotions: happy, sad, and neutral (the "PENN Facial Photographs"). These photographs of faces are symmetrical, lit in a standard way, and devoid of clothing or hair cues.

The Ekman facial recognition paradigm described above, as well as several other facial recognition paradigms, have recently been used to study emotion in functional imaging studies with normal subjects; Table 7.1 summarizes these studies. These studies reveal that a variety of imaging modalities and neurobehavioral probes have been used. The early functional studies used PET or SPECT (e.g., Gur, Skolnick, & Gur, 1994; Morris et al., 1996; Schneider, Gur, Jaggi, & Gur, 1994), while the more recent studies used fMRI (e.g., Baird et al., 1999; Phillips et al., 1997; Schneider et al., 1997; Whalen, Bush, et al., 1998; Whalen, Rauch, et al., 1998).

Table 7.1 demonstrates that a wide variety of facial stimuli, control tasks, and methods of analysis were used in these studies. Some of these studies used faces as stimuli by themselves (e.g., Baird et al., 1999; Phillips et al., 1997; Whalen, Rauch, et al., 1998), while others used the Ekman facial photographs as part of a mood induction paradigm (e.g., Schneider et al., 1997, 1994). Stimulus duration varied from approximately 30 sec/face (Gur, Ragland, Resnick, & Skolnick, 1994) to 200 msec/face (Breiter et al., 1996). In some studies the subjects' responses were recorded with a button press and in other studies the subjects were required to passively view the projected faces. In some studies brain activation during the active task (viewing fearful, happy, sad, and/or angry faces) was compared to brain activation during a resting baseline; in other studies the brain activation during the active task was subtracted from activation while viewing emotionally neutral faces.

Table 7.1 also reveals a wide variation in brain regions thought to be involved in the recognition of facial affect, including the entire right hemisphere (Gur, Skolnick, & Gur, 1994) and the left amygdala (Blair, Morris, Frith, Perrett, & Dolan, 1999). In the majority of these studies, the amygdala appears to be involved in affect recognition. For example, Breiter and colleagues (1996) measured amygdalar activation in 18 healthy men. In two separate experiments, they presented the Ekman facial photographs of either fearful versus neutral faces or happy versus neutral faces while using fMRI to measure signal changes in the amygdala. The amygdala was preferentially activated in response to fearful versus neutral faces, as well as in response to happy versus neutral faces, suggesting a possible generalized response to emotionally valenced stimuli.

To our knowledge, there have only been two studies that have examined brain activation in response to facial affect recognition in normal adolescents. Baird and colleagues (1999) studied 12 healthy adolescents ranging in age from 12 to 17 years (mean = 13.9 years) using a facial discrimination paradigm. Subjects were asked to "discriminate and label" the emotional expressions of six different faces, all with fearful expressions from the Ekman series. They reported a significant increase in signal intensity in *both* amygdalae in response to recognition of fearful facial expressions, but not to the control task of viewing nonsense gray-scale images. However, 26% of the responses given by the subjects did not correctly label the fearful faces. Some of their subjects labeled the fearful faces as angry, confused, surprised, or happy, emphasizing the importance of designing developmentally appropriate tasks. In the second study, Thomas and colleagues (2001) examined amygdala activation in response

TABLE 7.1. Functional Imaging Studies That Used Faces to Study Affect

Author (year)	Subjects' mean ages (yr ± SD)	Imaging modality spatial resolution (mm)/ acquisition parameters	Probes	Control task	Stimuli duration and frequency	Results
Gur, Skolnick, & Gur (1994)	40 normal controls: 21 males (26 ± 8), 19 females (24 ± 6)	^{133}Xenon SPECT probe 10 mm	Facial discrimination using PENN facial photographs: happy–neutral, sad–neutral, age discrimination	Resting baseline	"Self-paced administration over 20 minutes"	All three tasks produced right (R) hemisphere activation. Happy and sad discrimination produced R parietal activations. Happy discrimination produced greater left (L) frontal activation relative to sad discrimination.
Schneider et al. (1994)	12 normal controls (22 ± 1.8): 5 males, 7 females	^{133} Xenon SPECT probe 10 mm	Mood induction with PENN facial photographs: happy, sad, sex discrimination	Resting baseline, eyes open	"Self-paced administration over 20 minutes"	CBF increased during sad and happy inductions relative to sex discrimination and resting states. Sad mood induction activated occipital and temporal cortex.
Morris et al. (1996)	5 normal males (25)	PET ^{15}O water 5–6 mm	Ekman Fearful Faces Ekman Happy Faces 6 levels of intensity	Gender classification	3 sec/face 2 sec/blank 10 faces/scan × 12 scans Happy, balanced, fearful	Fearful–happy: A priori: L amygdala and L periamygdaloid complex activated Post hoc: L cerebellum, L cingulate, R sup. frontal gyrus Happy–fearful: R med. temporal gyrus, R putamen, L sup. parietal lobe, L calcarine sulcus
Breiter et al. (1996)	10 & 8 normal controls; mean age 26.5 yr (22–33): all males	Functional MRI: 1.5T Asymmetric spin echo T2*weighted, TR 3000/2000 msec, TE 50 msec, slice thickness 3.125 mm	Two experiments: Ekman Fearful Faces Ekman Happy Faces	Ekman Neutral Faces	200 msec/face × 60 (72 faces) 36 sec/block	Fear: bilateral amygdala and L fusiform activation Happy: L amygdala activation and fusiform activation Amygdala response showed rapid habituation with both fear and happiness.
Schneider et al. (1997)	12 normal controls (29.7 ± 4.3): 7 males, 5 females	Functional MRI: 1.5T T2*weighted FLASH, TR 240 msec, TE 60 msec, slice thickness 4 mm	Mood induction using PENN facial photographs: happy, sad	Resting baseline, eyes open	1 face/ condition	A significant increase in signal intensity found during sad as well as happy mood induction in the L amygdala.
Blair et al. (1999)	13 normal males: mean age 25 yr	PET ^{15}O water 5–6 mm	Ekman Sad Faces Ekman Angry Faces	6 intensity levels Gender classification	3 sec/face 2 sec/blank 10 photos 12 scans	Increasing intensity of sad facial expression associated with enhanced activity in the L amygdala and R temporal pole. Increasing intensity of angry facial expression associated with enhanced activity in the R orbitofrontal and anterior cingulate cortex.

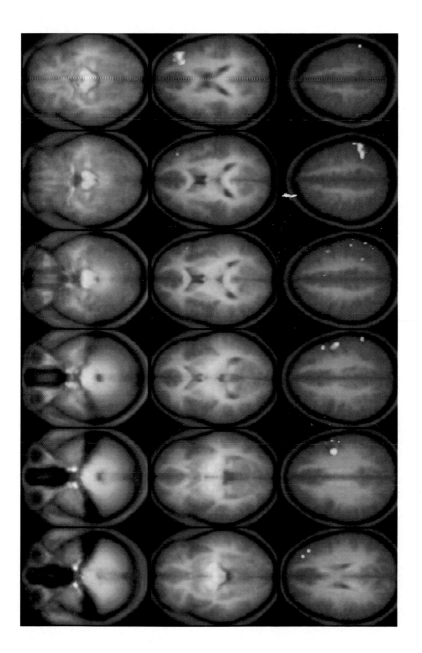

FIGURE 7.1. Areas of brain activation in which healthy volunteer adolescents ($N = 8$) activated more than adolescents with bipolar disorder ($N = 8$) on a task of facial emotional discrimination versus a task of age discrimination include the parietal and dorsolateral prefrontal cortex.

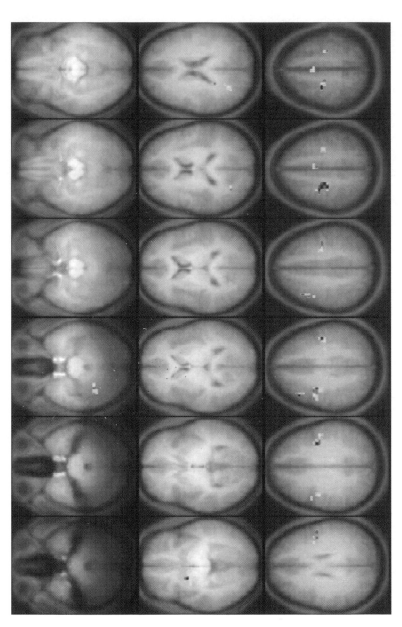

FIGURE 7.2. Areas of brain activation in which healthy volunteer adolescents ($N = 7$) activated more than adolescents with bipolar disorder ($N = 9$) on a task of sustained attention versus a control task of flashing numbers and finger tapping include cerebellar hemisphere, putamen, middle frontal cortex, precentral gyrus, and anterior and posterior cingulate.

Study	Subjects	Method	Stimuli	Task	Timing	Findings
Philips et al. (1997)	7 normal controls: mean age 27 yr; 2 males, 5 females	Functional MRI: 1.5T Echoplanar, TE 40 msec, slice thickness 3 mm	Ekman Disgusted Faces 75% & 150% Ekman Fearful Faces 75% & 150% Ekman Neutral Faces	Gender classification	3 sec/face 0.75 sec interval 8 faces/block 10 blocks	75% Fear: L insula and L amygdala 150% Fear: R putamen and R amygdala 75% Disgust: R insula and R med. front. cortex 150% Disgust: L med. front. cortex L peristriate cortex, R and L insula
Whalen et al. (1998)	10 normal males: mean age 23.8 yr (19–32)	Functional MRI: 1.5T Echoplanar, TE 70 msec, slice thickness 8 mm	Ekman Fearful Faces Ekman Happy Faces	Ekman Neutral Faces	33 msec/face 167 msec Neutral 200 msec block: 28 sec epoch 56 masked, happy, or fearful faces	Masked fearful faces activated bilateral amygdala, substantia innominata, and inferior prefrontal cortex. Fearful and happy faces activated substantia innominata. In the amygdala there was decreased signal intensity in response to happy.
Baird et al. (1999)	12 normal controls; mean age 13.9 yr; 5 males, 7 females	Functional MRI: 1.5T Echoplanar, TE 40 msec, slice thickness 3 mm	Ekman Fearful Faces	3 unique nonsense gray-scale images	10 sec/face 30 sec off 30 sec on	A significant increase in signal intensity found in both amygdala in response to recognition of fearful facial expressions.
Sprengelmeyer et al. (1998)	6 normal controls; mean age 23.5 ± 1.3 yr; 5 female, 2 male	Functional MRI: 2.0 T Echoplanar, TE 50 msec, slice thickness 6 mm	Ekman Fearful Faces Ekman Angry Faces Ekman Disgusted Faces	Ekman Neutral Faces	2.5 sec/face 10 blocks × 4 emotions 8 faces/block Interval 0.5 24 sec/emotion	Disgust: R ant putamen and pallidum, L ant. insula, L inf front. cortex (Brd. 47) Fear: L frontal lobe, R fusiform gyrus Anger: L inf front. cortex, L post. temp lobe, R gyrus cinguli
Blair et al. (1999)	13 normal males; mean age 25 yr	PET ^{15}O water 5–6 mm	Ekman Sad Faces Ekman Angry Faces	6 intensity levels Gender classification	3 sec/face 2 sec/blank 10 photos 12 scans	Increasing intensity of sad facial expression associated with enhanced activity in the L amygdala and R temporal pole. Increasing intensity of angry facial expression associated with enhanced activity in the R orbitofrontal and anterior cingulate cortex.
Yurgelun-Todd et al. (2000)	14 bipolar patients; mean age 31.5 yr; *medicated 10 normal controls	Functional MRI: 1.5T Echoplanar, TE 40 msec, slice thickness 6 mm	Ekman Fearful Faces	Ekman Happy Faces	9.5 sec/face 30 sec off 30 sec on 2 blocks/epoch	A significant increase in signal intensity found in the L amygdala whereas reduction of SI in the R dorsolateral prefrontal cortex in response to recognition of fearful facial expressions.
Thomas et al. (2001)	6 normal control adults 12 normal control children	Functional MRI: 1.5 T, EPI BOLD, TE 40 msec, slice thickness 4 mm	Ekman Fearful Faces Ekman Neutral Faces	Visual fixation	200 msec/face 800 msec interstimulus interval 45 sec of fixation and 42 sec of fearful faces, 42 sec of neutral faces	Adults showed increase in L amygdala activity for fearful relative to neutral faces. Children showed greater amygdala activity with neutral relative to fearful faces.

to fearful and neutral faces in 12 children and six adults. In this study, adults demonstrated increased left amygdala activation in response to fearful faces as compared to neutral faces, whereas children showed greater amygdala activity with neutral as opposed to fearful faces, suggesting that there may be developmental differences in amygdala response to facial affect.

Despite the differences in methods of the studies reviewed in Table 7.1, the following may be concluded about the functional neuroanatomy for the perception of emotions in faces:

- The amygdala appears to be involved whenever fearful, happy, sad, and angry faces are processed.
- Other brain areas involved in facial affect recognition include the insular gyrus, fusiform gyrus, and anterior cingulate.

NEUROIMAGING STUDIES OF PEDIATRIC BIPOLAR DISORDER

Studies of adults with bipolar disorder have used structural MRI, fMRI, PET, SPECT, and MRS to understand the neuropathophysiology of this disorder (reviewed in Strakowski et al., 2000). These studies have revealed structural and functional abnormalities in the amygdala, prefrontal cortex, thalamus, striatum, and cerebellar vermis, as well as periventricular and localized white matter lesions in adults with bipolar disorder. One of the most replicable neuroimaging findings in adults with bipolar disorder is the presence of white matter hyperintensities, although the neurophysiological basis for this finding remains unclear. Investigations involving adults with bipolar disorder suggest enlargement of the amygdala and striatum (Breiter et al., 1996). Additionally, some structural MRI studies suggest reduced prefrontal cortical volumes in bipolar adults.

Functional neuroimaging studies of bipolar adults demonstrate decreased glucose metabolism in the caudate and amygdala as compared to healthy subjects. Functional imaging studies also suggest state-related changes in the prefrontal cortex (e.g., hypoactivity during depression) in patients with bipolar disorder. MRS studies suggest altered membrane phospholipid metabolism in the basal ganglia and prefrontal cortex of bipolar patients. Together, these studies of adults with bipolar disorder suggest abnormalities in prefrontal–subcortical limbic pathways.

In order to validate the neurobiological substrate of the pediatric bipolar phenotype, it is necessary to employ biological studies, such as structural and functional neuroimaging. Despite recent advances permitting high-resolution thin-slice images for more valid morphometric analyses and the development of noninvasive functional methodologies such as fMRI and MRS, there have been few neuroimaging investigations involving children and adolescents with bipolar disorder. Table 7.2 summarizes the published neuroimaging studies of youth with bipolar disorder. Three of these studies examined brain structure. Botteron and colleagues compared children and adolescents with bipolar disorder to healthy subjects using MRI and found reduced structural asymmetry of the cerebral hemispheres (Botteron, Vannier, Geller, Todd, & Lee, 1995). Additionally, four of the eight subjects with bipolar disorder had ventricular abnormalities or deep white matter hyperintensities as compared to one of five control subjects, although the sample size was too small to provide statistical power. To our knowledge, there are only two additional published brain morphometry studies of adolescents with bipolar disorder, both from the same research group (Dasari et al., 1999; Friedman et al., 1999). The studies compared cortical and subcortical brain regions of adolescents with schizophrenia and bipolar disorder and then combined patient groups and compared them to healthy volunteer adolescents. When patient groups were combined, they had significantly reduced intracranial volumes, elevated frontal and temporal fluid fractions, and decreased brain circumferences and thalamic volumes as compared to healthy volunteers; however, there were no differences between patient groups. Furthermore, the authors examined effect sizes for the differences in structures between adolescents with bipolar disorder and healthy controls and found enlarged frontal and temporal fluid and lateral ventricular volumes and decreased intracranial volumes (large effect sizes) in adolescents with bipolar disorder. Because of multiple comparisons, the authors advise caution regarding the interpretability of these results. In summary, these studies suggest that similar to findings from morphometric studies of adults with bipolar disorder, frontal–temporal abnormalities may also be present in adolescents with bipolar disorder. Furthermore, in contrast to study of adults with bipolar disorder, which report enlarged thalamic volumes, adolescents with bipolar disorder demonstrate smaller thalamic volumes. However, the studies to date are methodologically limited in their imaging techniques as well as in their clinical characterization of the patient samples. For example, most of the studies failed to account for previous medications and co-occurring diagnoses. Despite their limitations, these reports suggest that some of the neuroanatomical changes seen in adults with bipolar disorder may also be present in children and adolescents with bipolar disorder.

PET and SPECT studies in adults with bipolar disorder have produced variable results, possibly due to differences in subject selection criteria, diagnostic procedures, severity of illness, medication status, demographic characteristics, imaging techniques, and analytic methods. Since fMRI and MRS are newer functional imaging techniques that do not involve exposure to ionizing radiation and thus are repeatable and noninvasive, these

TABLE 7.2. Neuroimaging Studies of Children and Adolescents with Bipolar Disorder

Study	Number of bipolar subjects (BP)/healthy volunteers (HV)	Age range (years)	Diagnostic instrument	Imaging modality	Results	Limitations
Botteron et al. (1995)	8 BP/5 HV	8–16	K-SADS-P	MRI	4/8 of patients and 1/5 controls displayed ventricular abnormalities. Reduced frontal asymmetry	Small sample size, qualitative assessments.
Dasari et al. (1999)	15 BP/16 HV (also 20 schizophrenics)	10–18	SADS-E	MRI	Decreased thalamic size in patients vs. HV. No difference between patients groups.	Thick MRI slices, only thalamic area (vs. volumes) measured, bipolar and HV not directly compared.
Friedman et al. (1999)	15 BP/16 HV (also 20 schizophrenics)	10–18	SADS-E	MRI	Large effect size for decreased intracranial volume, increased frontal and temporal sulcal size, and enlarged lateral ventricular volumes in BP vs. HV.	Thick MRI slices, did not control for multiple comparisons.
Castillo et al. (2000)	10 BP/10 HV	6–12	K-SADS (version not specified)	Proton MRS	Elevated glutamate/glutamine in both frontal lobes and basal ganglia, elevated lipids in frontal lobes.	Non-age-matched samples, small sample size, poor clinical characterization of the sample, mostly males (9/10).
Davanzo et al. (2001)	11 BP/11 HV	5–18	Mini International Neuropsychiatric Interview for Children and Adolescents (Mini-Kid)	Proton MRS	Acute lithium treatment was associated with a significant reduction in anterior cingulate myo-inositol/creatine. Compared with HV, BP subjects had a trend toward higher myo-inositol/creatine during the manic phase.	BP subjects were receiving concomitant medications.

Note. K-SADS, Kiddie Schedule for Affective Disorders and Schizophrenia; K-SADS-P, Kiddie Schedule for Affective Disorders and Schizophrenia—Present Episode Version; SADS-E, Schedule for Affective Disorders and Schizophrenia—Epidemiological Version; WASH-U-KSADS, Washington University at St. Louis Kiddie Schedule for Affective Disorders and Schizophrenia.

imaging techniques are particularly advantageous for studies involving children and adolescents.

There have been two published studies using MRS in children and adolescents with bipolar disorder. Castillo and colleagues found increased prefrontal and temporal Glx concentrations in children with bipolar disorder, suggesting that in addition to structural abnormalities, neurochemical dysfunction may be present in these brain regions (Castillo, Kwock, Courvoisie, & Hooper, 2000).

Although the exact mechanism by which lithium exerts its antimanic and antidepressant effects is unknown, lithium at therapeutic concentrations is an inhibitor of inositol mono-phosphatase and polyphosphate-1-phosphatase, which are involved in replenishing *myo*-inositol supplies. Thus, it is hypothesized that the therapeutic effects of lithium are mediated through depletion of *myo*-inositol (Davanzo et al., 2001). Davanzo and colleagues compared anterior cingulate *myo*-inositol levels in manic children (*n* = 11) pre- and 1-week postlithium treatment and found that acute lithium treatment was associated with a significant reduction in the *myo*-inositol/Cr ratio, particularly in lithium responders as compared to nonresponders. The authors also reported that at baseline children with bipolar disorder had an elevated *myo*-inositol/Cr ratio as compared to demographically matched healthy subjects. However, many of the children with bipolar disorder were taking several concomitant medications during the study. Nonetheless, to our knowledge, this is the first study of youth with bipolar disorder to provide support for lithium-induced modification of the phosphoinositide cycle.

To our knowledge, there has been only one published fMRI study of adults with bipolar disorder, and it used faces as a probe. In this study, Yurgelun-Todd and colleagues studied 14 adult patients with DSM-IV bipolar disorder and 10 normal controls using a 1.5 Tesla MRI scanner and used the Ekman fearful and happy faces as stimuli (Yurgelun-Todd et al., 2000). They reported that adults with bipolar disorder exhibited a significant increase in signal intensity in the *left* amygdala and a reduction of signal intensity in the *right* dorsolateral prefrontal cortex in response to recognition of fearful facial expressions. While all of their normal controls were able to accurately label 100% of the fearful faces, only 10 of 14 patients with bipolar disorder were able to correctly identify the fearful Ekman faces. These results suggest the presence of fronto–limbic circuitry abnormalities in adults with bipolar disorder as compared to healthy subjects. Although there have been no published fMRI studies of children with bipolar disorder and adolescents with bipolar disorder, preliminary results from our group also indicate frontal–striatal–limbic abnormalities in response to tasks of attention and facial affect recognition in adolescents with mania compared with demographically matched healthy subjects (see Figures 7.1 and 7.2 opposite pp. 166 and 167, respectively).

FUTURE DIRECTIONS

Additional structural and functional neuroimaging investigations are necessary to further validate and characterize the pediatric bipolar phenotype. Future structural MRI studies examining striatal and limbic brain regions with thin-slice quantitative techniques are warranted. With the recent development of a novel MRI technique, diffusion tensor imaging (DTI), it has become feasible to examine white matter tracks and, in combination with fMRI, tissue connectivity. Furthermore, age-appropriate cognitive paradigms for targeting specific behavioral characteristics of pediatric bipolar disorder and specific frontal–striatal–limbic brain regions need to be developed. MRS studies, similar to that of Davanzo and colleagues (2001), examining the neurochemical effects of specific medications will also identify predictors of treatment response, so that in the future more effective treatment interventions can occur. Moreover, combining longitudinal imaging and outcome studies will maximize the interpretability of the imaging data and identify neurobiological predictors of illness course and treatment response.

REFERENCES

Baird, A., Gruber, S., Fein, D., Maas, L., Steingard, R., Renshaw, P., Cohen, B., & Yergelun-Todd, D. (1999). Functional magnetic resonance imaging of facial affect recognition in children and adolescents. *Journal of the American Academy of Child & Adolescent Psychiatry, 38*(2), 195–199.

Blair, R. J., Morris, J. S., Frith, C. D., Perrett, D. I., & Dolan, R. J. (1999). Dissociable neural responses to facial expressions of sadness and anger. *Brain, 122*(Pt. 5), 883–893.

Botteron, K. N., Vannier, M. W., Geller, B., Todd, R. D., & Lee, B. C. (1995). Preliminary study of magnetic resonance imaging characteristics in 8- to 16-year-olds with mania. *Journal of the American Academy of Child and Adolescent Psychiatry, 34*(6), 742–749.

Breiter, H. C., Etcoff, N. L., Whalen, P. J., Kennedy, W. A., Rauch, S. L., Buckner, R. L., Strauss, M. M., Hyman, S. E., & Rosen, B. R. (1996). Response and habituation of the human amygdala during visual processing of facial expression. *Neuron, 17*(5), 875–887.

Castillo, M., Kwock, L., Courvoisie, H., & Hooper, S. R. (2000). Proton MR spectroscopy in children with bipolar affective disorder: Preliminary observations. *American Journal of Neuroradiology, 21*, 832–838.

Cutting, J. (1976). Chronic mania in childhood: A case report of a possible association with a radiological picture of cerebellar disease. *Psychological Medicine, 6*(4), 635–642.

Dasari, M., Friedman, L., Jesberger, J., Stuve, T. A., Findling, R. L., Swales, T. P., & Schulz, S. C. (1999). A magnetic resonance imaging study of thalamic area in adolescent patients with either schizophrenia or bipolar disorder as compared to healthy controls. *Psychiatry Research, 91*(3), 155–162.

Davanzo, P., Thomas, M. A., Yue, K., Oshiro, T., Belin, T., Strober, M., & McCracken, J. (2001). Decreased anterior cingulate myo-inositol/creatine spectroscopy resonance with lithium treatment in children with bipolar disorder. *Neuropsychopharmacology, 24*(4), 359–369.

Friedman, L., Findling, R. L., Kenny, J. T., Swales, T. P., Stuve, T. A., Jesberger, J. A., Lewin, J. S., & Schulz, S. C. (1999). An MRI study of adolescent patients with either schizophrenia or bipolar disorder as compared to healthy control subjects. *Biological Psychiatry, 46*(1), 78–88. (Published erratum appears in *Biological Psychiatry, 46*(4), following 584)

Ghaziuddin, N., Dequardo, J. R., Ghaziuddin, M., & King, C. A. (1999). Electroconvulsive treatment of a bipolar adolescent postcraniotomy for brain stem astrocytoma. *Journal of Child and Adolescent Psychopharmacology, 9*(1), 63–69.

Gur, R. C., Erwin, R. J., & Gur, R. E. (1992). Neurobehavioral probes for physiologic neuroimaging studies. *Archives of General Psychiatry, 49*, 409–414.

Gur, R. C., Erwin, R. J., Gur, R. E., Zwil, A. S., Heimberg, C., & Kraemer, H. C. (1992). Facial emotion discrimination: Part 2. Behavioral findings in depression. *Psychiatry Research, 42*(3), 241–251.

Gur, R. C., Ragland, J. D., Resnick, S. M., & Skolnick, B. E. (1994). Lateralized increases in cerebral blood flow during performance of verbal and spatial tasks: Relationship with performance level. *Brain and Cognition, 24*(2), 244–258.

Gur, R. C., Skolnick, B. E., & Gur, R. E. (1994). Effects of emotional discrimination tasks on cerebral blood flow: Regional activation and its relation to performance. *Brain and Cognition, 25*(2), 271–286.

Levisohn, L., Cronin-Golomb, A., & Schmahmann, J. D. (2000). Neuropsychological consequences of cerebellar tumour resection in children: Cerebellar cognitive affective syndrome in a paediatric population. *Brain, 123*(Pt. 5), 1041–1050.

Morris, J. S., Frith, C. D., Perrett, D. I., Rowland, D., Young, A. W., Calder, A. J., & Dolan, R. J. (1996). A differential neural response in the human amygdala to fearful and happy facial expressions. *Nature, 383*, 812–815.

O'Tuama, L. A., & Treves, S. T. (1993). Brain single-photon emission computed tomography for behavior disorders in children. *Seminars in Nuclear Medicine, 23*(3), 255–264.

Phillips, M. L., Young, A. W., Senior, C., Brammer, M., Andrew, C., Calder, A. J., Bullmore, E. T., Perrett, D. I., Rowland, D., Williams, S. C., Gray, J. A., & David, A. S. (1997). A specific neural substrate for perceiving facial expressions of disgust. *Nature, 389*, 495–498.

Raichle, M. E., Grubb, R. L. J., & Gado, M. H. (1976). Correlation between regional cerebral blood flow and oxidative metabolism: In vivo studies in man. *Archives of Neurology, 33*, 523.

Sayal, K., Ford, T., & Pipe, R. (2000). Case study: Bipolar disorder after head injury. *Journal of the American Academy of Child and Adolescent Psychiatry, 39*(4), 525–528.

Schneider, F., Grodd, W., Weiss, U., Klose, U., Mayer, K. R., Nagele, T., & Gur, R. C. (1997). Functional MRI reveals left amygdala activation during emotion. *Psychiatry Research, 76*(2–3), 75–82.

Schneider, F., Gur, R. C., Jaggi, J. L., & Gur, R. E. (1994). Differential effects of mood on cortical cerebral blood flow: A 133xenon clearance study. *Psychiatry Research, 52*(2), 215–236.

Soares, J. C., & Mann, J. J. (1997). The anatomy of mood disorders: Review of structural neuroimaging studies. *Biological Psychiatry, 41*(1), 86–106.

Sokoloff, L. (1981). Relationships among local functional activity, energy metabolism, and blood flow in the central nervous system. *Federation Proceedings, 40,* 2311.

Sprengelmeyer, R., Rausch, M., Eysel, U. T., & Przuntek, N. (1998). Neural structures associated with recognition of facial expressions of basic emotions. *Proceedings of the Royal Society of London Series B, 265,* 1927–1931.

Strakowski, S. M., DelBello, M. P., Adler, C., Cecil, C. M., & Sax, K. W. (2000). Neuroimaging in bipolar disorders. *Bipolar Disorders, 2,* 148–164.

Strakowski, S. M., DelBello, M. P., Sax, K. W., Zimmerman, M. E., Shear, P. K., Hawkins, J. M., & Larson, E. R. (1999). Brain magnetic resonance imaging of structural abnormalities in bipolar disorder. *Archives of General Psychiatry, 56*(3), 254–260.

Strakowski, S. M., & Sax, K. W. (2000). Secondary mania: A model of the pathophysiology of bipolar disorder? In J. S. S. Gershon (Ed.), *Basic mechanisms and therapeutic implications of bipolar disorder* (pp. 13–30). New York: Marcel-Dekker.

Thomas, K. M., Drevets, W. C., Dahl, R. E., Ryan, N. D., Birmaher, B., Eccard, C. H., Axelson, D., Whalen, P. J., & Casey, B. J. (2001). Amygdala response to fearful faces in anxious and depressed children. *Archives of General Psychiatry, 58*(11), 1057–1063.

Whalen, P. J., Bush, G., McNally, R. J., Wilhelm, S., McInerney, S. C., Jenike, M. A., & Rauch, S. L. (1998). The emotional counting Stroop paradigm: A functional magnetic resonance imaging probe of the anterior cingulate affective division. *Biological Psychiatry, 44*(12), 1219–1228.

Whalen, P. J., Rauch, S. L., Etcoff, N. L., McInerney, S. C., Lee, M. B., & Jenike, M. A. (1998). Masked presentations of emotional facial expressions modulate amygdala activity without explicit knowledge. *Journal of Neuroscience, 18*(1), 411–418.

Wong, D., & Resnick, S. (1995). Neurotransmission. In H. Wagner (Ed.), *Principles of nuclear medicine* (pp. 590–594). Philadelphia: Saunders.

Yurgelun-Todd, D. A., Gruber, S., Kanayama, W., Baird, A., & Young, A. (2000). fMRI during affect discrimination in bipolar affective disorder. *Bipolar Disorders, 2,* 237–248.

Zametkin, A. J., Liebenauer, L. L., Fitzgerald, G. A., King, A. C., Minkunas, D. V., Herscovitch, P., Yamada, E. M., & Cohen, R. M. (1993). Brain metabolism in teenagers with attention-deficit hyperactivity disorder. *Archives of General Psychiatry, 50*(5), 333–340.

8

Affective Neuroscience and the Pathophysiology of Bipolar Disorder

ROBINDER K. BHANGOO, CHRISTEN M. DEVENEY,
and ELLEN LEIBENLUFT

Affective neuroscience can be defined as the study of the neural components of emotional processes (Davidson & Irwin, 1999). Spurred by relevant findings in animals (LeDoux, 1998) and control human subjects (Davidson & Irwin, 1999; Lang, Bradley, & Cuthbert, 1998), researchers are now applying the techniques of affective neuroscience to clinical populations. This work should prove invaluable in increasing our understanding of the pathophysiology of mood disorders. This chapter introduces the relevant concepts of affective neuroscience and discusses how they can be applied to one such clinical disorder: childhood bipolar disorder. After briefly reviewing the most widely accepted definitions and theories of emotion and mood, we will discuss methods that can be used to study these psychological phenomena. In our discussion, we focus on the psychophysiological correlates of emotion that are particularly relevant to the study of early-onset bipolar disorder.

EMOTION AND MOOD

Central to the study of affective neuroscience are the concepts of emotion and mood. Though several definitions exist, *emotions* are generally viewed as responses evoked by environmental stimuli. These environmental stimuli have motivational salience, which can be either negative or positive (Lang et al., 1998). Negative emotions, such as fear, motivate the organism to *withdraw* from, or *avoid*, a situation. Emotions in the positive direction, such as happiness, propel the organism to *approach* a situation. These two aspects of motivation, approach and avoid, are also called the emotional *valence*.

In addition to valence, emotional responses can be classified according to the magnitude of the organism's arousal. *Arousal* is an index of the intensity of the metabolic or neural activation accompanying the negative or positive valence (Lang et al., 1998). The level of arousal reflects the amount of resources mobilized in response to an emotional stimulus, so that more highly arousing situations (either positively or negatively valenced) evoke more intense physiological reactions. These physiological reactions allow the organism to prioritize its responses and to direct its energy and resources toward those situations that are most crucial for its survival. As this discussion demonstrates, the concept of "emotion" includes, in addition to feeling states, the behavioral and physiological responses that are associated with them. Lang (1995) described these different components of emotions as the "database of emotions," which consists of the subjective, physiological, and behavioral components of emotional responses.

Thus, one of the basic tenets of affective neuroscience is that emotions serve an adaptive function in that affectively charged situations motivate the organism to perform behaviors that promote its survival and propagation of the species (Levenson, 1994). In other words, emotions serve to organize the organism's use of its resources, in that the type and urgency of the resources mobilized are influenced by the valence and arousal of the organism's emotional response. A well-known example would be the "fight or flight" response. Here, the fear that one experiences when confronted by a stimulus, such as a large animal, is a negative-valence, high-arousal state accompanied by a set of physiological changes that prepare the organism to fight or to leave the situation quickly. As noted above, emotions with a negative valence, such as fear, typically warn the organism to avoid a situation, and the high arousal attaches more importance to the warning. In addition to mobilizing internal resources, behavioral responses, such as cries and screams, can also draw external resources.

A contrasting example of a positive-valence, high-arousal emotion might involve a hunter returning with his bounty and shouting joyfully for others to join in a feast. A more contemporary example might involve a woman sitting down to a pleasurable meal, feeling contented, smiling and encouraging others to join her, and beginning to experience the physiological changes that initiate the digestive process. Other positively valenced emotional stimuli include the sight of a potential sexual partner or the sound of one's infant cooing. Such positive emotions serve to energize the individual and to promote social and prosocial behavior (Clark & Watson, 1994).

As the discussion indicates, the definition of "emotion" has received considerable attention, and a reasonable degree of consensus has been achieved (Davidson, 1994). Unfortunately, the concept of "mood" has proved considerably more problematic to define. Compared with emotion, *mood* is generally viewed as being less clearly related to an evoking stimulus, more long lasting, more diffuse, and more subjective (Davidson, 1994). Since moods are not necessarily evoked responses, studying them can be a challenge, whereas emotions can be evoked and studied in a research setting. An example of an emotion and a corresponding mood state would be fear (an emotion) versus anxiety (a mood).

Like the definition of mood itself, the interaction between emotions and mood has received little research attention but is of considerable interest to clinicians. The relationship between emotions and moods are clearly bidirectional. For example, Ekman (1994) has proposed that moods can be triggered by a "dense emotional experience," meaning that repetitive experiences of the same emotion at a high intensity without other intervening emotions might produce a more sustained related mood. In addition, it is possible that the presence of an emotional response (e.g., fear) may predispose an individual to a related mood (e.g., anxiety), while a person with an anxious mood may be more likely to experience the corresponding emotion, fear.

Emotions and moods become dysfunctional when they occur in inappropriate situations and when the magnitude of the emotional response (either its valence or its arousal) is out of proportion to the evoking stimulus. When this occurs consistently, a clinician may recognize an anxiety or mood disorder. For example, individuals with panic disorder experience negatively valenced, high-arousal emotional states (Clark & Watson, 1994) in situations not necessitating alarm. Individuals with bipolar disorder experience strong positively valenced, high-arousal emotions (mania) or negatively valenced emotions associated with either low or high arousal (depression or mixed states, respectively) in situations that do not warrant such extreme reactions. So, in contrast to controls, patients with mood disorders experience persistent moods that are in excess of what would be expected and/or that occur in inappropriate contexts.

THE EMOTION/MOOD CIRCUMPLEX

Researchers have used the "emotion circumplex" (see Figure 8.1) to depict and classify emotional states in terms of their valence and arousal. Valence is plotted on the ordinate, with positive valences in the positive region of the ordinate and negative emotions below. Arousal is represented on the abscissa, with the level of arousal increasing as one proceeds from the negative to the positive region of the abscissa. Therefore, positive-valence emotions are plotted above the abscissa, with high-arousal/positive-valence emotions, such as joy and excitement, in the upper right quadrant and low-

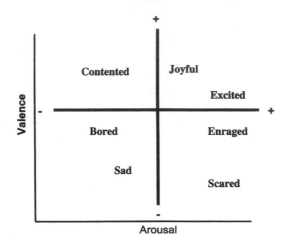

FIGURE 8.1. Normal moods and emotions are plotted on an emotion circumplex. Valence is plotted on the ordinate, with positive valences in the positive region of the ordinate and negative emotions below. Arousal is represented on the abscissa, with the level of arousal increasing as one proceeds from the negative to the positive region of the abscissa.

arousal/positive-valence emotions, such as contentment and calm, in the upper left quadrant. Similarly, negative emotions are plotted below the abscissa, with high-arousal/negative-valence emotions, such as rage and fear, in the lower right quadrant and low-arousal/negative-valence emotions, such as boredom and sadness, in the lower left quadrant.

Lang and colleagues developed a set of standardized emotional stimuli, specifically, a set of over 400 pictures called the International Affective Picture System (IAPS; Attention, 1994) and plotted subjects' responses to them on the emotion circumplex. The IAPS pictures depict a broad range of people, objects, and scenes, and are designed to evoke specific emotions in the viewer, who rates the amount of pleasure and arousal that he or she experiences while viewing the picture. To rate his or her responses, the viewer uses the Self-Assessment Maniken (SAM), a well-validated pictographic device used to record ratings of valence and arousal (Bradley & Lang, 1994). In Figure 8.2, the SAM ratings collected in response to 360 IAPS pictures are plotted on an emotion circumplex. It should be noted that the ratings are not evenly distributed across quadrants, in that negatively valenced responses are disproportionately common in the high-arousal, as compared with the low-arousal, quadrant. This pattern reflects the *negativity bias*, in that negatively valenced stimuli tend to evoke high-arousal responses. Negativity bias has been demonstrated repeatedly using both IAPS pictures and other paradigms (Ito, Larsen, Smith, & Cacioppo, 1998).

One can also apply the emotion circumplex clinically by using it to classify mood disorders and their symptoms (Figure 8.3 on the next page). Depicting depression and mania on such a circumplex allows us to broaden our conceptualization of mood disorders. That is, instead of thinking of depression and mania as existing on opposite ends of a valence spectrum, from elated to depressed, the grid allows us to view these disorders in a more accurate and theoretically based fashion. Specifically, depression and mania are pathological mood states not only because of the extreme, and labile, *valence* of the patient's mood, but also because of the patient's inability to regulate his or her level of *arousal*. This point becomes clear when one plots the symptoms of mania and depression according to whether they stem predominantly from a dysregulation of arousal or of valence (Figure 8.3a). The importance of considering both arousal and valence is further evident when one plots pathological mood states on the emotion circumplex (Figure 8.3b). For example, so-called atypical depres-

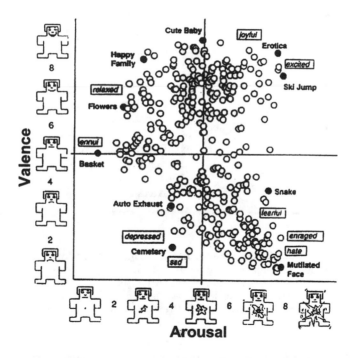

FIGURE 8.2. International Affective Picture System (IAPS; see text) pictures are organized in a two-dimensional space, defined by the judged dimensions of valence and arousal. Specific picture contents are indicated for the images denoted by filled circles. Standardization samples of approximately 100 individuals used the Self-Assessment Manikin (SAM; Bradley & Lang, 1994) to make these judgments. From Lang (1995). Copyright 1995 by the American Psychological Association. Reprinted by permission.

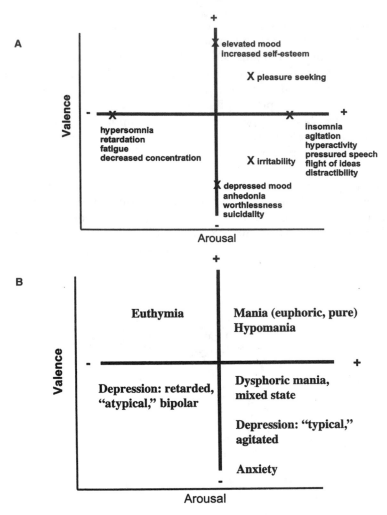

FIGURE 8.3. (A) DSM-IV symptoms of manic and major depressive episodes are plotted on the emotion circumplex according to whether they predominantly represent a dysregulation of valence or of arousal. Note that *pleasure* and *irritability* are plotted in the middle of their respective quadrants because dysregulation of both valence and arousal are pronounced in these symptoms. (B) Pathological mood states are plotted on the emotion circumplex.

sion is plotted in the low-arousal, negative-valence quadrant, reflecting not only the patient's dysphoric feeling state but also his or her psychomotor retardation, fatigue, and hypersomnia. "Typical" depression, on the other hand, is a hyperaroused, negative-valence state in that the patient experiences insomnia and agitation as well as dysphoric mood. Similarly, mania is characterized by an increased state of arousal, as evidenced by hyperactivity, pressured speech, and agitation and either positive-valence (pure mania) or negative-valence (mixed state) moods. Thus, the circumplex allows us to consider both aspects of a mood disorder, valence and arousal, simultaneously. This classification of mood disorders allows us to have a more comprehensive perspective on these disorders and to make more discrete distinctions between different presentations of depression and mania.

Characterizing mood states in terms of valence and arousal may also help to clarify another common clinical problem. Nonspecific symptoms, such as agitation and irritability, can present in several different clinical situations, including mixed states, agitated depressions, and anxiety states. Differentiating between these states clinically can be difficult, precisely because they all fall in the high-arousal, negative-valence quadrant of the emotion circumplex (Figure 8.3b). Thus, the circumplex provides a way to classify mood states in terms of their symptoms, but also within a coherent theoretical system. Such a classification system can be especially useful in childhood psychiatric disorders, where symptoms are frequently nonspecific. For example, one nonspecific symptom that occurs commonly in children is irritability, a high-arousal, negative-valence state. By classifying symptoms using the circumplex, we can view a disorder by its component parts, which may help in identifying target symptoms for treatment.

The emotion circumplex can also be helpful in understanding bipolar disorder and other mood disorders from a developmental perspective. The circumplex is independent of developmental stage, since the same grid is used for all age groups. However, as a mood disorder's presentation changes developmentally, its placement on the circumplex may change. For example, patients with bipolar disorder frequently have histories of both pure and mixed manic episodes and there is some evidence that the proportion of the former to the latter may be lower in children than in adults (Geller et al., 2001). As a result, although manic children sometimes have symptoms that would be plotted on the upper right-hand quadrant, often their symptoms would be plotted in the lower right-hand quadrant. On the other hand, those of manic adults would most often be in the upper right-hand quadrant. In other words, manic children and manic adults both experience high-arousal states, but the valence of their emotions may differ. Indeed, this is consistent with findings indicating that the sine qua non of the manic state is not positive valence, but high arousal (Bauer et al., 1991). If we were to follow longitudinally the symptoms of children with bipolar disorder, measuring both arousal and valence, we could describe the developmental trajectory of the symptoms of the illness. An interesting question is whether, as children with bipolar disorder age, the proportion of pure manic episodes will increase, so that their mood ratings would move from the lower to the upper right-hand quadrants as they mature.

APPLICATIONS OF AFFECTIVE NEUROSCIENCE
TO RESEARCH ON EARLY-ONSET BIPOLAR DISORDER

In addition to providing a conceptually and clinically useful classification system for emotions and moods, the emotion circumplex can be used in conjunction with physiological studies to provide an understanding of the neurobiology underlying bipolar disorder and other mood disorders. As mentioned before, both valence and arousal can be dysregulated in mood disorders, and similar symptoms of dysregulated valence and arousal can exist in a number of DSM-IV disorders. By assessing patients' psychophysiology while they experience abnormal mood states, we can begin to understand if nonspecific symptoms, such as irritability or agitation, have a common physiological basis, or if different presentations of depression have different psychophysiological correlates. In addition, many of the same paradigms that are used to evoke emotion in psychophysiological studies can be used in conjunction with functional neuroimaging in order to ultimately elucidate the neurocircuitry underlying these disorders. For the remainder of the chapter, we focus on the physiological responses evoked by emotional stimuli, and how we can study such responses in order to increase our understanding of the pathophysiology of bipolar disorder in children and adolescents.

Physiological Correlates of Emotional Responses

As described above, subjective emotional states are accompanied by physiological changes that enable the organism to respond appropriately to emotional stimuli. Some of the physiological measures that have been correlated with emotional states include heart rate, skin conductance, corrugator ("frown") and zygomatic ("smile") electromyographic (EMG) activity, the eyeblink response to a startle stimulus, and the P3 component of the evoked potential that occurs in response to a startle stimulus (Lang et al., 1998). For example, Lang and colleagues (1998) demonstrated significant correlations between these physiological measures and subjective measures of valence and arousal ratings in subjects shown the IAPS pictures described above. They found that skin conductance and cortical evoked response potential (ERP) were indicators of arousal states, whereas heart rate and corrugator and zygomatic EMG activity correlated with emotional valence. Specifically, they found that EMG activity was strongly correlated with ratings of pleasantness, in that corrugator EMG activity increased linearly as pictures were rated as more unpleasant ($r = -.90$), and zygomatic EMG activity increased linearly as pictures were rated as more pleasant ($r = .56$) (see Figure 8.4). Heart rate was also correlated with valence, in that heart rate increased linearly when subjects viewed more pleasant pictures and decelerated when subjects viewed unpleasant pictures ($r = .76$) (see Figure 8.4). In contrast, skin conductance, an indicator of au-

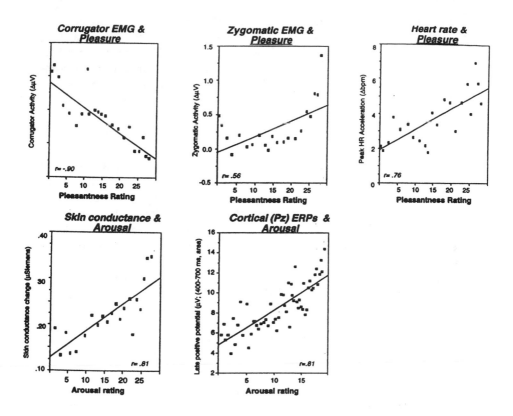

FIGURE 8.4. Covariation of affective judgments of pleasure (top row) or arousal (bottom row) with physiological and behavioral responses to picture stimuli. Corrugator EMG (top left), zygomatic EMG (top middle), and heart rate (top right) each vary consistently with differences in rated pleasure. On the other hand, skin conductance (bottom left) and cortical event-related potentials (ERPs) (bottom right) vary consistently with differences in arousal ratings. In each plot, affective judgments are rank-ordered for each subject; the graphs depict the mean responses at each rank across subjects. From Lang, Bradley, and Cuthbert (1998). Copyright 1998 by the Society of Biological Psychiatry. Reprinted by permission.

tonomic nervous system activity measured through sweat gland activity, was positively correlated with arousal ratings ($r = .81$) (see Figure 8.4), as was the slow cortical (400–700 msec) evoked response potential (cortical ERP), measured at a parietal site (Pz) ($r = .81$) (see Figure 8.4).

Startle Eyeblink

In addition to the physiological measures noted above, the eyeblink response to a startle stimulus can be used to study an organism's response to emotional stimuli. The startle eyeblink reflex, whose magnitude can be measured reliably via obicularis oculi EMG, occurs in response to a standardized negative-valence, high-arousal stimulus. The startle reflex is particulary interesting to affective neuroscientists because, using a technique called *affect-modulated startle*, researchers can index both the prevailing emotional state of the organism and the organism's response to the startle probe itself.

The eyeblink reflex occurs naturally as part of an organism's startle response. When an animal is startled, a set of physiological reactions occur that serve to protect it from harm. Sympathetic changes, such as increased heart rate and increased respirations, are activated to mobilize the organism for fight or flight. Rapid flexor movements occur to protect the animal's internal organs, and rapid eyeblink occurs to protect the eyes (Lang et al., 1998; Ohman, 1997). In rats, scientists measure the whole body reaction (or jump) to the startle stimulus, using a device attached to the cage floor (Hoffman, 1999). In humans, the startle response is assessed by measuring the magnitude of the eyeblink, since electromyography of the obicularis oculi muscle has been noted to be the easiest, most reliable, and most consistent measurement of startle (Landis & Hunt, 1939). Although startle reactions can be elicited by either acoustic (loud noise), visual (flash of light), or cutaneous (airblast, shock) stimuli, here we will focus on the use of acoustic stimuli.

As mentioned earlier, the magnitude of the blink response in response to a startle stimulus is affected by the underlying emotional state of the organism, a phenomenon called *affect-modulated startle*. Classical conditioning studies by Brown, Kalish, and Farber (1951) were among the first to document affective modification of the startle response. These investigators compared a control group of rats that had been exposed to a light and a buzzer to an experimental group that had been exposed to a light and a buzzer with an electric shock. When both groups of rats were exposed to a startle stimulus (in this case, a loud sound), the startle response of the experimental group was significantly greater than that of the control group. Brown and colleagues concluded that the experimental group's conditioned fear state facilitated the startle reaction to the negatively valenced stimulus (i.e.,, the loud sound). This suggests that the startle reflex may be sensitive to emotional valence, in that the startle response is augmented in contexts signaling an aversive situation.

More recent studies have shown that the reverse also occurs, that is, that the startle reflex is inhibited in contexts involving pleasant stimuli. When the magnitude of the eyeblink startle response was measured in subjects viewing pictures from the IAPS series or film clips, the response was smallest when the subjects were viewing pictures they rated as pleasant, largest when they were viewing pictures they rated as negative, and intermediate when they were viewing neutral pictures (Kaviani, Gray, Checkley, Kumari, & Wilson, 1999; Vrana, Spence, & Lang, 1988).

In attempting to understand the neural mechanisms underlying affect-modulated startle, researchers hypothesize that the organism's baseline emotional state reflects a "priming" of neural structures toward either an appetitive or an aversive orientation (Lang, 1995; Lang, Bradley, & Cuthbert, 1990, 1997). Consequently, neural mechanisms are better equipped to produce reactions consistent with the engaged motivational system than with the opposing one. For example, when organisms are appetitively motivated (i.e., experiencing pleasant affect), then their responses to other appetitive cues are primed; at the same time, their responses to aversive cues are reduced or absent. Since an eyeblink startle reaction is a defensive or negative reflex, it follows that this reflex will be potentiated when the organism is in a negative state and inhibited when the organism is in a positive state. Affective modulation is not felt to be a conscious or controlled process, since the rapidity of the response (30–40 msec) after startle probe presentation implies "preattentive processing" (Bradley, Cuthbert, & Lang, 1999), as opposed to intentional mechanisms.

Startle blink responses are modulated not only by the valence of the organism's baseline emotional state, but also by the organism's level of arousal (Lang, 1995). Specifically, Lang and colleagues (1998) demonstrated that the magnitude of a person's eyeblink startle reflex increases as his or her level of arousal increases. They hypothesized that this phenomenon occurs because high arousal states are associated with increased activation in both the appetitive and the aversive motivational systems, as well as increased attention directed toward the stimulus. As we discuss later, the impact of arousal level on startle reflexes may be particularly relevant to studies of childhood bipolar disorder, where high arousal states are especially common.

Only a few studies of affect-modulated startle have been conducted in clinical populations. Allen, Trinder, and Brennan (1999) measured startle eyeblink in a sample of inpatients with major depressive disorder and in age- and gender-matched controls. The subjects viewed pleasant, neutral, and unpleasant pictures from the IAPS series and rated the valence and arousal of their response using the SAM. The control group showed the expected pattern of startle augmentation while viewing negative pictures and startle inhibition while viewing positive pictures, but the depressed group did not. Specifically, when the depressed subjects were divided into three groups according to their ratings on the Beck Depression Inventory (normal/mild, moderate, and severe), an interesting pattern emerged. The normal/mild and moderate groups, like the control group, showed significantly greater eyeblink magnitude when viewing the negative pictures compared to the positive ones. In the severe group, however, the startle eyeblink magnitude was significantly greater when the subjects viewed pleasant, as opposed to unpleasant, pictures (Allen et al., 1999). These data suggest that, in a severely depressed population, pleasant pictures may induce a negatively valenced high-arousal emotional state. The authors suggest that this negatively valenced emotional state may be one of frustrative nonreward, in that the patients are frustrated by their inability to experience positive affect in response to the pictures (Allen et al., 1999).

In a study using another clinical population, Cleckley (1976) compared psychopathic prisoners, nonpsychopathic prisoners, and controls, and found that the nonpsychopathic prisoners and controls showed similar startle reflex potentiation when viewing unpleasant pictures. The psychopathic prisoners, on the other hand, did not show such potentiation, despite the fact that their arousal and valence ratings in response to the pictures were similar to the ratings of the other two groups. Indeed, further analysis revealed that the deficit in startle modification was only observed in psychopathic prisoners who demonstrated emotional indifference and lack of remorse on interview. Thus, this study suggests that stimuli that are viewed negatively by a control population are viewed more neutrally by criminal psychopaths.

Although most of the studies of affect-modulated startle have been in adult populations, there is evidence that startle modification can be elicited in children. Balaban (1995) demonstrated increased startle responses in 5-month-old infants when they were presented with angry, as compared with happy, faces. Using the IAPS pictures, McManis and colleagues (McManis, Bradley, Berg, Cuthbert, & Lang, 2001) examined gender differences in startle modulation in 64 children, ages 7–11 years, and 62 adolescents, ages 12–14 years. The girls showed the predicted pattern of startle augmentation when viewing unpleasant, compared to pleasant, pictures. In boys, there was no significant difference in startle magnitude when viewing unpleasant, compared to pleasant, pictures, although the data tended to be in a direction opposite to that predicted (i.e., decreased startle with unpleasant pictures). This pattern of diminished startle magnitude with negative stimuli has not been seen in adult or children, either male or female. The authors suggest that these findings are consistent with the idea that boys are less reactive to aversive stimuli, as compared with girls.

These studies may indicate that patients with mood and other disorders process emotional stimuli differently than normal controls, suggesting a potential research strategy to address some of the difficulties involved in studying mood and mood disorders. That is, as mentioned above, mood disorders are difficult to study in part because of the methodological problems involved in evoking moods in a standardized way in a research setting. However, also as discussed above, it is likely that the processing of emotions may differ between patients with mood disorders and controls. Thus, one might study the psychophysiology of a mood disorder, such as bipolar disorder, by comparing the responses of patients and controls to standardized emotional stimuli. For example, the authors are studying the responses of children and adolescents with bipolar disorder to emotional stimuli in order to test the hypothesis that their responses to negative emotional stimuli will be more pronounced than those of controls. To test this hypothesis, subjects will be presented with three paradigms designed to elicit either positive or negative emotions and to probe the subjects' underlying emotional state. Two of these paradigms, the lottery game and film clips, are affect-modulated startle paradigms. In the lottery game, subjects either win money (evoking positive emotion) or hear an aversive noise (evoking a negative emotion). The film clip paradigm involves the child watching film clips chosen to evoke positive emotions, such as happiness and laughter, or negative emotions, such as sadness or fear. In the lottery and film clip paradigms, the affect-modulated startle eyeblink response will be used to test the hypothesis that, compared to controls, the children with bipolar disorder will have increased facilitation of startle eyeblink in the negative conditions (i.e., aversive noise condition, fearful film clips). Thus, our hypothesis is that children with bipolar disorder, who are often in an irritable (i.e., high-arousal, negative-valence) state, will be more reactive than controls to aversive stimuli. This hypothesis is supported by the clinical observation that children with bipolar disorder are frequently unable to tolerate negative situations, such as frustration, and therefore exhibit frequent and severe temper tantrums (Wozniak et al., 1995).

Finally, in the last paradigm, called the "affective Posner" paradigm, the child first completes a task in a "neutral" condition (i.e., no contingent reward or punishment), and then "wins" or "loses" money depending on the accuracy and timing of his or her performance on the same task. The program is written so that the child wins and loses a predetermined number of times. In one block of trials, the child loses progressively more money as the game proceeds. This paradigm therefore can elicit positive responses to reward, negative responses to punishment, and frustration. Our hypothesis is that children with bipolar disorder, compared to controls, will have an exaggerated reaction to the addition of contingencies (Derryberry & Reed, 1994). This exaggerated reaction will be manifested behaviorally by a more marked reduction in reaction time as they proceed from the neutral to the reward or punishment conditions. In addition, we predict that the controls will slow their reactions in response to failure, whereas children with bipolar disorder will demonstrate faster responses following failure (Elliott, Sahakian, Herrod, Robbins, & Paykel, 1997; Elliott et al., 1996). We also hypothesize that frustration will elicit more marked behavioral responses in children with bipolar disorder than in controls, including refusal to complete the task, decreased reaction time, and decreased accuracy.

If meaningful patient–control differences are found on these physiological paradigms, subsequent neuroimaging studies could use similar techniques. In such neuroimaging studies, we might expect to find differences between patients and controls in the degree of activation of neuronal structures that have been implicated in animal studies of affect-modulated startle. These structures include limbic areas such as the hippocampus, dorsal striatum, ventral pallidum, medial prefrontal cortex, basolateral amygdala, and nucleus accumbens (Swerdlow, Caine, Braff, & Geyer, 1992). Given that both the amygdala and the medial prefrontal cortex have been implicated in the neurophysiology of bipolar disorder (Strakowski et al., 1999), these regions might mediate any observed differences between patients with bipolar disorder and controls in the affect-modulated startle reflex.

Prepulse Inhibition of Startle Eyeblink

Startle eyeblink magnitude is affected not only by the emotional state of the subject, but also by attentional processes. Specifically, researchers have noted that the amplitude of the startle eyeblink reflex is diminished if a weaker noise precedes the startle probe by 100–600 msec. This finding has been well replicated and forms the basis of what is called prepulse inhibition (PPI). PPI is believed to serve as a protective mechanism for the neural processing of the first, lead stimulus, and therefore has been described by Braff and colleagues as a measure of "sensorimotor gating, reflecting an individual's ability to effectively buffer or screen out the potentially chaotic flow of information and sensory stimuli" (Cadenhead, Geyer, & Braff, 1993, p. 1862).

Investigators studying PPI in psychiatric populations have reported PPI deficits (i.e., potentiated startle magnitude following a weak prepulse, as opposed to the expected inhibition) in patients with schizophrenia, obsessive–compulsive disorder, Huntington's disease, nocturnal enuresis, Tourette's syndrome, and temporal lobe epilepsy with psychosis (Geyer, Swerdlow, Mansbach, & Braff, 1990). In addition, psychotic-prone individuals have also shown PPI deficits (Cadenhead et al., 1993; Cadenhead, Swerdlow, Schaffer, Diaz, & Braff, 2000). These disorders all have in common the presence of gating deficits, in that affected patients are unable to dampen excessive internal or external stimuli effectively. In schizophrenic patients, PPI deficits correlated significantly with neuropsychological measures (perseverative responses on the Wisconsin card sort task), number of psychiatric hospitalizations, chlorpromazine equivalents, and global scores of positive and negative symptoms (Braff, Swerdlow, & Geyer, 1999).

The demonstration of gating deficits in psychotic and psychotic-prone patients is relevant to the study of children and adolescents with bipolar disorder, who have a high rate of psychotic symptoms (Werry, McClellan, & Chard, 1991). In addition, children with early-onset bipolar disorder are often described as being unable to gate internal or external stimuli. For example, distractibility, a common symptom of bipolar disorder, can be viewed as a gating problem, as can behavioral decompensation occurring with overstimulation. These symptoms may be correlated with PPI deficits in this clinical population. Thus, the authors plan to test the hypothesis that children with bipolar disorder will have reduced PPI, compared to age- and gender-matched controls.

SUMMARY

The field of affective neuroscience allows us to examine the concepts of emotion and moods from a perspective that is complementary to the usual one of a clinician. Thus, in addition to involving subjective feeling states, emotions are viewed as complex, biologically based states that can be characterized not only by their valence, but also by their degree of arousal. Both the valence of an emotional state and its arousal level are associated with physiological reactions that can be measured. In addition, using the emotion circumplex, we can characterize pathological mood states in terms of their observed valence and arousal. Classifying emotions and moods in this way provides another approach to understanding the nonspecific symptoms often seen in children, as well as the overlapping symptoms of a number of adult mood and anxiety disorders. This approach might allow us to move beyond subjective descriptions of moods and emotions in disorders such as bipolar disorder in order to better understand the biological underpinnings and etiology of such states.

In animals, much work has been done identifying the neural correlates of emotions. Using this work as a basis, more studies, using both psychophysiological and neuroimaging techniques, can be done in clinical populations. We hope that these studies will ultimately increase our understanding of the pathophysiological mechanisms underlying illnesses such as bipolar disorder in order to further our search for more effective treatments.

REFERENCES

Allen, N. B., Trinder, J., & Brennan, C. (1999). Affective startle modulation in clinical depression: Preliminary findings. *Biological Psychiatry, 46,* 542–550.

Attention, C. f. t. P. S. o. E. a. (1994). *The international affective picture system* (photographic slides). Gainesville: Center for Research in Psychophysiology, University of Florida.

Balaban, M. T. (1995). Affective influences on startle in five-month-old infants: Reactions to facial expressions of emotion. *Child Developement, 66,* 28–36.

Bauer, M. S., Crits-Christoph, P., Ball, W. A., Dewees, E., McAllister, T., Alahi, P.,

Cacciola, J., & Whybrow, P. C. (1991). Independent assessment of manic and depressive symptoms by self-rating: Scale characteristics and implications for the study of mania. *Archives of General Psychiatry, 48*, 807–812.

Bradley, M. M., Cuthbert, B. N., & Lang, P. J. (1999). Affect and the startle reflex. In M. E. Dawson, A. M. Schell, & A. H. Bohmelt (Eds.), *Startle modification: Implications for neuroscience, cognitive science, and clinical science* (pp. 157–183). New York: Cambridge University Press.

Bradley, M. M., & Lang, P. J. (1994). Measuring emotion: The Self-Assessment Manikin and the semantic differential. *Journal of Behavior Therapy and Experimental Psychiatry, 25*, 49–59.

Braff, D. L., Swerdlow, N. R., & Geyer, M. A. (1999). Symptom correlates of prepulse inhibition deficits in male schizophrenic patients. *American Journal of Psychiatry, 156*, 596–602.

Brown, J. S., Kalish, H. I., & Farber, I. E. (1951). Conditioned fear as revealed by magnitude of startle response to an auditory stimulus. *Journal of Experimental Psychology, 41*, 317–328.

Cadenhead, K. S., Geyer, M. A., & Braff, D. L. (1993). Impaired startle prepulse inhibition and habituation in patients with schizotypal personality disorder. *American Journal of Psychiatry, 150*, 1862–1867.

Cadenhead, K. S., Swerdlow, N. R., Schaffer, K. M., Diaz, M., & Braff, D. L. (2000). Modulation of the startle response and startle laterality in relatives of schizophrenic patients and in subjects with schizotypal personality disorder: Evidence of inhibitory deficits. *American Journal of Psychiatry, 157*, 1660–1668.

Clark, L. A., & Watson, D. (1994). Distinguishing functional from dysfunctional affective responses. In P. Ekman & R. J. Davidson (Eds.), *The nature of emotion* (pp. 131–136). New York: Oxford University Press.

Cleckley, H. (1976). *The mask of sanity*. St. Louis, MO: Mosby.

Davidson, R. J. (1994). On emotion, mood, and related affective constructs. In P. Ekman & R. J. Davidson (Eds.), *The nature of emotion: Fundamental questions* (pp. 51–55). New York: Oxford University Press.

Davidson, R. J., & Irwin, W. (1999). The functional neuroanatomy of emotion and affective style. *Trends in Cognitive Sciences, 3*, 11–21.

Derryberry, D., & Reed, M. A. (1994). Temperament and attention: orienting toward and away from positive and negative signals. *Journal of Personality and Social Psychology, 66*, 1128–1139.

Ekman, P. (1994). Moods, emotions, and traits. In P. Ekman & R. J. Davidson (Eds.), *The nature of emotion: Fundamental questions* (pp. 56–58). New York: Oxford University Press.

Elliott, R., Sahakian, B. J., Herrod, J. J., Robbins, T. W., & Paykel, E. S. (1997). Abnormal response to negative feedback in unipolar depression: Evidence for a diagnosis specific impairment. *Journal of Neurology, Neurosurgery, and Psychiatry, 63*, 74–82.

Elliott, R., Sahakian, B. J., McKay, A. P., Herrod, J. J., Robbins, T. W., & Paykel, E. S. (1996). Neuropsychological impairments in unipolar depression: The influence of perceived failure on subsequent performance. *Psychological Medicine, 26*, 975–989.

Geller, B., Craney, J., Bolhofner, K., DelBello, M., Williams, M., & Zimmerman, B. (2001). One-year recovery and relapse rates of children with a prepubertal and early adolescent bipolar disorder phenotype. *American Journal of Psychiatry, 158*, 303–305.

Geyer, M. A., Swerdlow, N. R., Mansbach, R. S., & Braff, D. L. (1990). Startle response models of sensorimotor gating and habituation deficits in schizophrenia. *Brain Research Bulletin, 25*, 485–498.

Hoffman, H. S. (1999). A historical note on the "discovery" of startle modification. In M. E. Dawson, A. M. Schell, & A. H. Bohmelt (Eds.), *Startle modification: Implications for neuroscience, cognitive science, and clinical science* (pp. 1–5). New York: Cambridge University Press.

Ito, T. A., Larsen, J. T., Smith, N. K., & Cacioppo, J. T. (1998). Negative information weighs more heavily on the brain: The negativity bias in evaluative categorizations. *Journal of Personality and Social Psychology, 75*, 887–900.

Kaviani, H., Gray, J. A., Checkley, S. A., Kumari, V., & Wilson, G. D. (1999). Modulation of the acoustic startle reflex by emotionally-toned film clips. *International Journal of Psychophysiology, 32*, 47–54.

Landis, C., & Hunt, W. A. (1939). *The startle pattern.* New York: Farrar & Rinehart.

Lang, P. J. (1995). The emotion probe: Studies of motivation and attention. *American Psychologist, 50*, 372–385.

Lang, P. J., Bradley, M. M., & Cuthbert, B. N. (1990). Emotion, attention, and the startle reflex. *Psychological Review, 97*, 377–395.

Lang, P. J., Bradley, M. M., & Cuthbert, B. N. (1997). Motivated attention: Affect, activation, and action. In P. J. Lang, R. F. Simons, & M. T. Balaban (Eds.), *Attention and orienting: Sensory and motivational processes* (pp. 97–136). Hillsdale, NJ: Erlbaum.

Lang, P. J., Bradley, M. M., & Cuthbert, B. N. (1998). Emotion, motivation, and anxiety: Brain mechanisms and psychophysiology. *Biological Psychiatry, 44*, 1248–1263.

LeDoux, J. (1998). Fear and the brain: where have we been, and where are we going? *Biological Psychiatry, 44*, 1229–1238.

Levenson, R. W. (1994). Human Emotion: A functional view. In P. Ekman & R. J. Davidson (Eds.), *The nature of emotion: Fundamental questions* (pp. 123–130). New York: Oxford University Press.

McManis, M. H., Bradley, M. M., Berg, W. K., Cuthbert, B. N., & Lang, P. J. (2001). Emotional reactions in children: Verbal, physiological, and behavioral responses to affective pictures. *Psychophysiology, 38*, 222–231.

Ohman, A. (1997). As fast as the blink of an eye: Evolutionary preparedness for preattentive processing of threat. In P. J. Lang, R. F. Simons, & M. T. Balaban (Eds.), *Attention and orienting: Sensory and motivational processes* (pp. 165–184). Hillsdale, NJ: Erlbaum.

Strakowski, S. M., DelBello, M. P., Sax, K. W., Zimmerman, M. E., Shear, P. K., Hawkins, J. M., & Larson, E. R. (1999). Brain magnetic resonance imaging of structural abnormalities in bipolar disorder. *Archives of General Psychiatry, 56*, 254–260.

Swerdlow, N. R., Caine, S. B., Braff, D. L., & Geyer, M. A. (1992). The neural substrates of sensorimotor gating of the startle reflex: a review of recent findings and their implications. *Journal of Psychopharmacology, 6*, 176–190.

Vrana, S. R., Spence, E. L., & Lang, P. J. (1988). The startle probe response: A new measure of emotion? *Journal of Abnormal Psychology, 97*, 487–491.

Werry, J. S., McClellan, J. M., & Chard, L. (1991). Childhood and adolescent schizophrenic, bipolar, and schizoaffective disorders: A clinical and outcome study. *Journal of the American Academy of Child and Adolescent Psychiatry, 30,* 457–465.

Wozniak, J., Biederman, J., Kiely, K., Ablon, J. S., Faraone, S. V., Mundy, E., & Mennin, D. (1995). Mania-like symptoms suggestive of childhood-onset bipolar disorder in clinically referred children. *Journal of the American Academy of Child and Adolescent Psychiatry, 34,* 867–876.

9

The Immune System and Bipolar Affective Disorder

OHEL SOTO and TANYA K. MURPHY

The classification of bipolar disorders in children and adolescents is a work in progress. Efforts are being directed toward a better understanding of the phenomenology, in hopes to better understand the neuropatho-physiological mechanisms. Currently, as with many childhood psychiatric disorders, the classification and treatment guidelines are based primarily on adult information. In the past, many believed bipolar disorders to be virtually nonexistent among youth and their mood swings were thought to be part of normal adolescent development. In the last 20 years, research has challenged this notion. Weller, Weller, Tucker, and Fristad (1986) reviewed over 200 articles written between 1809 and 1982 describing prepubertal children with severe psychiatric symptoms and identified 157 cases described that would likely be diagnosed as manic by current diagnostic standards. Bipolar disorder was correctly diagnosed in 48% of these cases. Comorbid psychiatric disorders also contribute to missed diagnoses. Recent research has identified various confounds in diagnosis and emphasized that the recognition of childhood-onset mania should be a priority in order to improve identifying factors associated with illness onset and treatment strategies (National Institute of Mental Health Research Roundtable on Prepubertal Bipolar Disorder, 2001; Weller, Weller, & Fristad, 1995).

In attempts to disentangle the phenomenology of childhood bipolar disorders, phenotypic subtypes are likely to emerge. Grouping children by course of illness (e.g., ultradian cycling) or by the presence/absence of attention-deficit/hyperactivity disorder (Geller et al., 1998) are examples of how subtyping may provide clues to pathophysiology. Interest in the area of immune-mediated pathogenesis of psychiatric disorders leads us to consider an immune-mediated subtype of childhood-onset bipolar disorder. We have correlated the literature on this and other neuropsychiatric conditions to present evidence for an immune-based hypothesis for bipolar affective disorder.

OVERVIEW OF IMMUNOLOGICAL STUDIES

The neuroimmune network of the central nervous system (CNS) is complex and diverse and involves interplay between neuroendocrine and circadian factors, neurotrophic factors, neurotransmitters, and much more. The role of structural brain damage from either mild anoxic injury or prior CNS infection could also theoretically impact the developing immune system. Each individual has a unique genetic vulnerability and immune memory that strongly affects any given immune response. Differential susceptibility of specific neuronal tissues to specific immune insults also likely affect phenotypic expression. The mechanisms of CNS immune-mediated pathophysiology are frequently divided into cell-mediated immunity and humoral immunity. Cell-mediated pathophysiology results from the actions of cytokines, lymphocyte trafficking, and cell death by apoptosis or cytotoxicity. Antibody-mediated illnesses may arise after an infectious illness when the subsequent antibody response is cross-reactive with neuronal tissue or receptors. The end point may be receptor stimulation, blockade, or inflammation and destruction.

Several illnesses or conditions that result from immune dysfunction are known to present with symptoms of mania and/or depression. The most notable are multiple sclerosis, lupus, Lyme disease, HIV infection, and corticosteroid therapy. For example, Heila, Turpeinen, and Erkinjuntti (1995) reported the case of a 15-year-old girl who presented with a 3-day history of hyperactivity, increased talkativeness, insomnia, and delusions. This patient showed immunoactivation by monocytic leukocytosis and elevated IgG in the cerebrospinal fluid, an abnormal electroencephalogram, white matter lesions in magnetic resonance imaging, and abnormalities in single-photon emission computed tomography, which led to a diagnosis of multiple sclerosis. Antibody-mediated neuropsychiatric symptoms, including mania (Khan, Haddad, Montague, & Summerton, 2000; Lahita, 1997), have been reported in patients with lupus.

ASSESSMENT OF CYTOKINES IN BIPOLAR
AFFECTIVE DISORDER AND SCHIZOPHRENIA

For primary psychiatric disorders, the literature often groups major psychiatric disorders when performing comparisons of immune function. The focus of these immune studies has been the measurement of peripheral cytokine profiles, lymphocyte subsets, and antibodies to viruses and self-proteins (see Table 9.1). Because of their role in the viral response and immune activation, interferons and interleukins are the most studied cytokines. Elevations in these cytokines have been observed in the CNS of individuals with schizophrenia and with bipolar affective disorder. In a large study by Mittleman and colleagues (1997), a comprehensive assessment of cerebrospinal fluid type 1 (IL-2, IFN-γ, TNF-β) and type 2 (Il-4, IL-5, IL-10, TNF-α) cytokine levels were performed in subjects with obsessive–compulsive disorder ($n = 24$), schizophrenia ($n = 22$), and attention-deficit/hyperactivity disorder ($n = 42$) ranging from 6 to 22 years of age (see Table 9.2). The most notable finding was that detectable levels of the type 2-cytokine, IL-4, were found in subjects with schizophrenia, but were undetectable in any of the subjects with obsessive–compulsive disorder and attention-deficit/hyperactivity disorder. The authors reported that cytokine profiles skewed toward a type-1 pattern; however, this effect was subtle. Although difficult to obtain, normative data from age- and sex-matched control subjects are needed to better interpret these and other such data. Preble and Torrey (1985) found serum interferon to be elevated in 24% of individuals with schizophrenia; however, this finding has not been replicated. Moises, Schindler, Leroux, and Kirchner (1985) reported that *in vitro* leukocytes from schizophrenics were deficient in the production of interferon. Studies of interleukins have demonstrated that interleukin-2 can be significantly increased, decreased, or remain the same as controls in patients with mental illness (el-Mallakh, Suddath, & Wyatt, 1993; Licinio, Seibyl, Altemus, Charney, & Krystal, 1993; Rapaport, McAllister, Pickar, Nelson, & Paul, 1989). Ganguli, Brar, Solomon, Chengappa, and Rabin (1992) reported an association between decreased IL-2 and autoantibodies in schizophrenia, which suggests a subtype of schizophrenia with autoimmune features. Tsai and colleagues (1999) found that the plasma levels of serum-soluble interleukin-2 receptors (sIL-2R) in individuals with mania were significantly higher than in controls. They also reported increased mitogen-induced lymphocyte proliferation, suggesting T-lymphocyte activation. These elevations were not due to differences in gender, age, or medications. Sourlingas, Issidorides, Havaki, Trikkas, and Sekeri-Pataryas (1998) reported results of an investigation into total histone and histone variant synthesis in the cell cycle of peripheral lymphocytes in patients with bipolar affective disorder and found that the samples correlated with their depressive, manic, or normothymic state. The results showed that in normothymic patients, no difference was observed when compared with controls, while the patients with depressive or manic states showed values consistent with lymphocyte activation. Rapaport, Guylai, and Whybrow (1999) found similar evidence of lymphocyte activation in patients with rapid-cycling bipolar affective disorder. Evidence of immune activation

TABLE 9.1. Important Immunological Definitions

Term	Definition
Antibody	An immunoglobulin molecule that has a specific amino acid sequence by virtue of which it interacts only with the antigen that induced its synthesis in cells of the lymphoid series (especially plasma cells), or with antigen closely related to it.
Antimicrobial	An agent that kills microorganisms or suppresses their multiplication or growth.
Antineuronal antibodies	An immunoglobulin molecule that is reactive or destructive with components of neurons.
Antinuclear antibodies	An immunoglobulin molecule that is reactive or destructive with components of the cell nucleus.
Antiviral	An agent that destroys viruses or suppresses their replication.
Apoptosis	Fragmentation of a cell into membrane-bound particles that are then eliminated by phagocytosis.
Autoantibodies	An antibody (immunoglobulin) formed in response to, and reacting against, one of the individual's own normal antigenic endogenous body constituents.
Autoimmunity	A condition characterized by a specific humoral- or cell-mediated immune response against constituents of the body's own tissues (self-antigens or autoantigens).
Cytokine	Nonantibody proteins released by one cell population (e.g., primed T lymphocytes) on contact with a specific antigen, which act as intercellular mediators, as in the generation of an immune response.
Cytotoxicity	Refers to the lysis of cells by immune phenomena.
Epitope	Antigenic determinant.
Immunoactivation	Acquired immunity attributable to the presence of an antibody or of immune lymphoid cells formed in response to antigenic stimulus.
Immunogenetics	The study of the genetics of the immune response—e.g., the study of immune response genes, the association of HLA antigens with disease susceptibility, or the generation of antibody diversity.
Immunomodulator	An agent that specifically or nonspecifically augments or diminishes immune responses—i.e., an adjuvant, immunostimulant, or immunosuppressant.
Immunoprotectant	An agent capable of causing protectant response.
Immunosuppressive	An agent capable of suppressing immune responses.
Interferon	Any of a family of glycoproteins that exert virus-nonspecific but host-specific antiviral activity by inducing the transcription of cellular genes coding for antiviral proteins that selectively inhibit the synthesis of viral RNA and proteins.
Interleukin	A generic term for a group of protein factors produced by macrophages and T-cells in response to antigenic or mitogenic stimulation and affecting primarily T-cells.
Lymphocyte	Any of the mononuclear, nonphagocytic leukocytes, found in the blood, lymph, and lymphoid tissues, that are the body's immunologically competent cells and their precursors.

Lymphocyte trafficking	A process influenced by cytokines and involving adhesion molecules to promote transmigration of lymphocytes through the vessel walls to the sites of inflammation.
Mitogen	A substance that induces blast transformation; DNA, RNA, and protein synthesis; and proliferation of lymphocytes—e.g., concavalin A, phytohemagglutinin, pokeweed mitogen, or lipopolysacharide.
Neuroplasticity	The capacity of a nervous tissue to restore or build up a lost part.
Neurotrophic	An agent involved in the nutrition and maintenance of tissues as regulated by nervous influence.
Prostaglandin	Any of a group of components derived from unsaturated 20-carbon fatty acids, primarily arachidonic acid, via the cyclooxygenase pathway, that are extremely potent mediators of a diverse group of physiological processes.
Retroviruses	A large group of RNA viruses that includes the leukoviruses and lentiviruses; so called because they carry reverse transcriptase.
Self epitopes	These are small chemical groups on the human antigen molecule that can elicit and react with self-antibodies.

was also described in a study of 14 patients with seasonal affective disorder with no significant change in immune measures following light therapy (Leu, Shiah, Yatham, Cheu, & Lam, 2001). Other studies have suggested that patients with mania as well as those with severe depression have a decreased lymphocyte response to mitogens (Kronfol et al., 1983).

ASSESSMENT OF AUTOANTIBODIES IN BIPOLAR AFFECTIVE DISORDER AND SCHIZOPHRENIA

Studies measuring autoantibodies and microbial antibodies frequently cite alterations in patients with severe psychiatric disorders (Yolken & Torrey, 1995). The presence of antinuclear antibodies in individuals with bipolar affective disorder (Deberdt, Van Hooren, Biesbrouck, & Amery, 1976; Villemain et al., 1988) and schizophrenia (DeLisi, 1996; Ganguli et al., 1992; Sirota, Schild, Elizur, Djaldetti, & Fishman, 1995; Spivak et al., 1991) has been reported. Elevations of antibrain antibodies in patients with mania (Jankovic & Djordjijevic, 1991), schizophrenia (Jankovic & Djordjijevic, 1991; Pandey, Gupta, & Chaturvedi, 1981), and Tourette's syndrome (Singer et al., 1998) have been reported, but other studies have challenged some of these findings (DeLisi, 1986; Schott et al., 1998). Several reports have also noted increases in antibodies to many different viruses, especially retroviruses and Borna virus, in patients with bipolar disorder or schizophrenia (Yolken & Torrey, 1995).

However limited, these studies suggest immune alterations *may* exist in adults with bipolar affective disorder. However, sample sizes are often

TABLE 9.2. Immune Studies in Patients with Schizophrenia and Bipolar Disorder

Reference	Sample characteristics	Type of study	Findings
Kronfol et al. (1983)	Untreated mania (n = 66) and untreated schizophrenics (n = 178)	Total, differential, and absolute blood cell counts	Mania was associated with significantly higher total leukocyte counts, accounted for by a significant increase in the number of neutrophils.
Mittleman et al. (1997)	Childhood-onset schizophrenia (n = 22), OCD (n = 24), and ADHD (n = 42)	CSF IL-2, IFN-γ, TNF-β/LT, IL-4, IL-5, IL-10, and TNF-α	Cytokine profile skewed to type 1 in OCD, type 2 in schizophrenia, intermediate in ADHD.
Leu et al. (2001)	Patients with seasonal affective disorder (n = 15) age-, sex-matched normal controls (n = 15)	Plasma concentrations of IL-6, sIL-6R, and sIL-2R	Patients with SAD had significantly increased IL-6 levels compared to normal controls (p < .0005). No immune parameter changes after 2 wks of successful light therapy.
Licinio et al. (1993)	Neuroleptic-free schizophrenic (n = 10) healthy subjects (n = 10)	Levels of CSF IL-2, IL 1α	Levels of CSF IL-2, but not IL 1α, were found to be higher in schizophrenic patients
Jankovic & Djordjijevic (1991)	Senile dementia (n = 32), Alzheimer's disease (n = 56), with schizophrenia (n = 189), with manic–depressive psychoses (n = 117), other nonorganic psychoses (n = 52), controls (n = 112)	ELISA for autoantibodies to human brain S100 protein, NSE, and MBP	The highest incidence of anti-S100 and anti-NSE antibodies was in Alzheimer's disease and senile dementia, then in manic–depressive and other nonorganic psychoses. MBP autoantibodies found in a very small number of psychiatric patients.
Ganguli et al. (1992)	Schizophrenia (n = 122), normal controls (n = 98)	Mitogen-stimulated IL-2, autoantibodies against seven common antigens	In patients autoantibody-positive, acutely ill patients had significantly lower IL-2 production as compared with other patients and control subjects.
El-Mallakh et al. (1993)	Schizophrenia (n = 28), controls (n = 11)	ELISA of IL 1α, IL-2 in CSF	No significant differences detected, possibly due to low sensitivity of assay.
Pandey et al. (1981)	Schizophrenia (n = 54), controls (n = 27)	Antibrain antibody titers by hemagglutination in sera and CSF	Antibrain antibodies were detected in sera and CSF of 26 schizophrenics but in none of the controls.
Preble et al. (1985)	Caucasian patients with psychotic illness (n = 82), controls (n = 64)	Serum and CSF interferon titers	High titers of interferon were found in serum of 20 patients with psychosis and in two controls. Interferon-positive patients correlated with recent onset or exacerbation of their illness and to be on low-dose or no medication. These findings suggest that there may be immunological abnormalities or viral infections in some patients with psychosis.

TABLE 9.2. (*continued*)

Reference	Sample characteristics	Type of study	Findings
Rapaport et al. (1989)	Treated and untreated schizophrenia (*n* = 30), controls (*n* = 13)	ELISA for sIL-2R in serum	Elevated levels of sIL-2R may be secondary to psychotropic medications or a pathological finding of T-cell activation in schizophrenia.
Rapaport et al. (1999)	Rapid-cycling bipolar patients (*n* = 17), controls (*n* = 18)	Cytokine levels	No correlation between clinical ratings and serum cytokine levels.
Schott et al. (1998)	Major depressive disorder (*n* = 20), paranoid schizophrenia (*n* = 20), schizoaffective psychosis (*n* = 20), controls (*n* = 20)	Antibody in serum to synaptic membranes Western immunoblots and ELISA techniques	No proof of antibrain antibodies in psychiatric patients.
Sirota et al. (1995)	Schizophrenia (*n* = 30), matched controls (*n* = 30)	Spontaneous production of IL-1 and IL-3-LA by PMBC	Cell-mediated immunity measures were found in schizophrenic patients. Significant IL-1 and slightly IL-3 LA in schizophrenic patients compared to controls. Suggests an cell-mediated autoimmune dysfunction in some schizophrenic patients.
Sourlingas et al. (1998)	Female patients with BAD (*n* = 12)	PBMC total histone and histone variant synthesis by electrophoresis/radioactivity	With the histone variant synthesis pattern, lymphocytes of normothymic patients and controls showed similar values to noncycling cells, and depressed or manic patients showed intermediate values to those of resting and cycling cells.
Spivak et al. (1991)	Schizophrenics (*n* = 90), bipolars (*n* = 54), and depressives (*n* = 22)	Peripheral blood for cold agglutinin titration	Cold agglutinin titers in schizophrenic patients but with no direct evidence of pathology at the histologic level but may propose a neurotransmission defect.
Tsai et al. (1991)	Individuals in a manic episode (*n* = 23), matched controls	Lymphocyte proliferation to PHA, Con A, and PWM and plasma levels of sIL-2R and sIL-6R	Acute mania correlated with higher levels of sIL-2R and PHA-induced lymphocyte proliferation.
Villemain et al. (1988)	Schizophrenia (*n* = 51), affective disorders (*n* = 30)	Assays of lupus autoantibodies	Positive antinuclear antibodies and antihistone antibodies were found but unclear if related to bipolar disorder or to their treatment.

Note. CSF, cerebrospinal fluid; IL-2, interleukin-2; sIL-2R, soluble interleukin-2 receptor; sIL-6R, soluble interleukin-6 receptor; PBMC, peripheral blood mononuclear cells; ELISA, enzyme linked immunosorbent assay; PHA, phytohemagglutinin; PWM, pokeweed mitogen; Con A, concanavalin A; NSE, neuron-specific enolase; MBP, myelin basic protein; TNF, tumor necrosis factor; IFN, interferon.

small and the degree to which hypothalamic–pituitary–adrenal alterations and preexisting autoimmunity affected results has yet to be resolved. Another confound is that the presence of immune dysfunction may be temporary. For example, if a subset of patients had infection-triggered CNS pathology or an early-onset autoimmune event, the chance of finding persistent immune alterations in adults has likely diminished. Moreover, factors that play a role in the maintenance of an illness, in comparison to those that play a role in illness onset, are likely to be different. Very few immune indices have been measured in children with neuropsychiatric disorders and few systematic examinations of infection-mediated neuropsychiatric symptoms have been reported.

NEUROPSYCHIATRIC SYMPTOMS TRIGGERED BY GROUP A STREPTOCOCCUS

Sydenham's chorea, originally named "St. Vitus dance" in 1686 by Thomas Sydenham, is a neurological disorder characterized by chorea, tics, hypotonia, dysarthria, and facial grimacing. St. Vitus dance more accurately represented those who succumbed to "dancing mania" or the mass hysterias that began in the eighth century. Over a half century before Sydenham's chorea was linked to group A streptococcus infections, William Osler, in 1894, described irritability, emotionality, and odd behaviors as frequent concomitants of Sydenham's chorea (Osler, 1894). In 1912, Diefendorf provided descriptions of two types of psychiatric symptoms seen in patients with Sydenham's chorea: mild mental symptoms and psychoses. In his description of mild mental symptoms he states, "They become fretful, peevish, fault finding, and change rapidly and without provocation from one mood to another. Hence especially the young patients are hard to please and difficult to manage. They want to get out of bed, tire of restraint, at one moment want some one to read aloud, and at another they wish to be left alone. These emotional changes even lead to passionate outbreaks, when they burst into tears, tear up their books and break playthings." The psychotic state described by Diefendorf is one consistent with delirium, but overlaps symptoms seen in acute mania: "Though they hear false voices, see strange visions and express persecutory and fearful delusions, they cannot express themselves clearly and the delusions never become elaborated. The content of thought as expressed usually consists of disjointed sentences into which are woven incidental observations. The emotional attitude varies; at times the patients are elated and cheerful and at others fearful and anxious." A number of other clinicians later remarked on the psychiatric manifestations of Sydenham's chorea (Bruetsch, 1940; Keeler & Bender, 1952; Wilcox & Nasrallah, 1988), including obsessive–compulsive symptomatology (Chapman, Pilkey, & Gibbons, 1958; Freeman, Aron, Collard, & MacKay, 1965; Grimshaw, 1964). Grimshaw (1964) reported an increased history of Sydenham's chorea in a retrospective review of patients with obsessive–compulsive disorder compared to a nonobsessional control group. Mood symptoms and psychotic symptoms have been described historically in relationship to rheumatic fever and terms such as "rheumatic schizophrenia" were not uncommon. Most studies report that choreic movements occur in close temporal proximity to psychiatric symptoms and that the most severe psychiatric symptoms clear with resolution of the movement disorder. However, many reports of residual changes in personality, stamina, and persistent tics are described. In a large retrospective case–control study, rheumatic fever histories were particularly common in patients with catatonia (Wilcox, 1986). In a follow-up study of children with past diagnosis of Sydenham's chorea, Keeler and Bender (1952) reported that these children developed psychosis, but others developed emotional instability, depressive features, temper tantrums, crying spells, negativism, aggressive outbursts, restlessness, and hyperactivity, along with poor attention and poor concentration in school. These psychiatric symptoms were believed to be due to CNS involvement related to Sydenham's chorea (Keeler & Bender, 1952). The description of these symptoms is similar to that currently seen in childhood and early adolescent bipolar affective disorder and *closely* resembles the non-DSM-IV phenotype outlined by the NIMH Roundtable on Prepubertal Bipolar Disorder (National Institute of Mental Health Research Roundtable on Prepubertal Bipolar Disorder, 2001).

More recently, Swedo and colleagues (Swedo et al., 1993, 1989) conducted several systematic investigations into the neuropsychiatric aspects of Sydenham's chorea. In one study (Swedo et al., 1989), obsessive–compulsive symptoms were assessed and compared in two age- and sex-matched groups of patients with rheumatic fever: one with Sydenham's chorea, another without Sydenham's chorea. The group with Sydenham's chorea had significantly more obsessive–compulsive symptoms. Subsequent studies have shown that over 70% of patients with Sydenham's chorea exhibit obsessive–compulsive symptoms that resemble classic cases of obsessive–compulsive disorder (Asbahr et al., 1998; Swedo, 1994). In one study consisting of 11 children with Sydenham's chorea, concomitant obsessive–compulsive symptomatology, increased emotional lability, motoric hyperactivity, irritability, distractibility, and age-regressed behavior were observed. The children typically demonstrated increased emotional lability, decreased attentiveness, and obsessive–compulsive symptoms shortly before the onset of choreiform movements. The pattern of behavioral changes before the onset of movements and its episodic pattern suggested that these are not just related to stress, but are related to the pathological process underlying the chorea (Swedo et al., 1993). Mercadante and colleagues (2000) examined 20 children with rheumatic fever, 22 with

Sydenham's chorea, and 20 controls (ages 6–16 years) for a diagnosis of obsessive–compulsive disorder and tic disorders. They found that major depressive disorder, tic disorders, and attention-deficit/hyperactivity disorder were more frequent in patients with Sydenham's chorea than in those with rheumatic fever. Symptoms of attention-deficit/hyperactivity disorder appeared to increase the risk of developing Sydenham's chorea in children with rheumatic fever. In contrast to what has been previously described, they found that obsessive–compulsive symptoms were equally found in rheumatic fever and Sydenham's chorea.

During the last decade, a subtype of childhood obsessive–compulsive disorder has been given the acronym PANDAS (pediatric autoimmune neuropsychiatric disorders associated with streptococcus) to delineate children that develop obsessive–compulsive disorder symptoms and other psychiatric disturbances in association with streptococcal infection. The psychiatric symptoms seen in these patients have an episodic or a sawtooth pattern that correlates with exposure to or infection by GAS. Historically, background for PANDAS dates back to 1929 when Selling reported three cases of children with onset and exacerbations of tics in relation to acute sinusitis. In 1993, Kiessling, Marcotte, and Culpepper (1993) described an increased frequency of patients with tics after GAS infections. These children were found to have antineuronal antibodies with similar reactivity to that seen in children with Sydenham's chorea. In 1995, Allen, Leonard, and Swedo reported four cases of apparent infection-triggered obsessive–compulsive disorder. Then, in her comprehensive description of the first 50 cases with PANDAS, Swedo and colleagues (Swedo et al., 1998) proposed criteria for the identification of these patients. The criteria used include full diagnosis of obsessive–compulsive disorder and/or tic disorder, onset between age 3 years and puberty, episodic course of symptoms, documented association with GAS, and neurological abnormalities. Many of the children she described had psychiatric comorbidity. The most prevalent diagnoses were attention-deficit/hyperactivity disorder (40%), affective disorders (42%), and anxiety disorders (32%). Emotional lability was the most common comorbid symptom and always started abruptly, concurrently with onset or worsening of tics and obsessive–compulsive symptoms. In addition to the emotional lability, the exacerbations were frequently accompanied by irritability, personality changes, motor hyperactivity, tactile/sensory defensiveness, choreiform movements, messy handwriting, separation anxiety, and changes in school performance. The correlation to elevated antistreptococcal antibody titers suggests an immunologic response in the pathogenesis of disease. Causation is not explicit, however, as streptococcal infections are frequent in childhood. However, GAS exposure may interplay with developmental and genetic susceptibilities to increase the likelihood of the neuropsychiatric presentation.

The main criterion separating PANDAS from Sydenham's chorea is the lack of signs or findings of rheumatic fever (carditis, arthritis, elevated sedimentation rate, etc.) in children with PANDAS. Recent technology has increased the sensitivity of detecting carditis in patients with Sydenham's chorea to the extent that most with Sydenham's chorea have evidence of at least silent mitral regurgitation (Elevli, Celebi, Tombul, & Gokalp, 1999) compared with normal children, where about 2% have evidence of silent mitral regurgitation (Brand, Dollberg, & Keren, 1992). As of yet, carditis has not been reported in children determined at initial assessment to have PANDAS, although studies to more thoroughly examine this risk are underway at the National Institute of Mental Health. In studies of children with PANDAS and childhood-onset obsessive–compulsive disorder, an association with the rheumatic fever B cell marker D8/17 has been demonstrated (Murphy et al., 1997; Swedo et al., 1997). The significance of this marker in the pathogenesis or its utility as a diagnostic indicator of these illnesses has not been fully characterized.

EVIDENCE FOR OTHER INFECTIOUS TRIGGERS

Although more support exists for GAS in pathogen-triggered neuropsychiatric symptoms, not all cases of infection-triggered obsessive–compulsive disorder have been related to prior GAS infection. While two cases described by Allen and colleagues (1995) were associated with GAS, the other two were associated with a prior viral infection. In these instances, the mechanism of pathophysiology no doubt results directly from the viral process and is not of autoimmune origin. In 1931, Von Economo documented several post-encephalitic syndrome patients whose clinical presentation was remarkable for hyperactivity, tics, and/or obsessive–compulsive symptomatology.

Recently Muller, Riedel, Forderreuther, Blendinger, and Abele-Horn (2000) examined two children with tic exacerbations and found both had evidence of mycoplasma infection after extensive blood work. Both cases were treated with erythromycin, and in 4 weeks the boy no longer had tics and the girl had a marked improvement in her tics but not in her attention-deficit/hyperactivity disorder.

Similarly, secondary mania has been reported following infectious illnesses. Reported cases include Epstein–Barr viral infections (Pavuluri & Smith, 1996), Lyme disease (Fallon, Nields, Parsons, Liebowitz, & Klein, 1993), and HIV infections (Mijch, Judd, Lyketsos, Ellen, & Cockram, 1999). A case report by Pavuluri and Smith (1996) described a 15-year-old adolescent with a 2-year history of chronic active Epstein–Barr viral infection who, after immunotherapy and stabilization, had a recurrence and developed manic–depression. After extensive medical evaluation, she was found to have high levels of prostaglandin -PGE1. They hypothesized that this excess of PGE1 was the causative agent of her mania; after treatment with lithium, her symptoms resolved and her PGE1 precursors were stabilized.

NEUROANATOMIC OVERLAP

Neuroimaging studies have shown that abnormalities in the basal ganglia correlate with the clinical features of Sydenham's chorea, obsessive–compulsive disorder, tics disorders, and PANDAS. In an MRI study of children with Sydenham's chorea compared to controls, the children with Sydenham's chorea had a 10% increase in caudate size and a 7% increase in both putamen and globus pallidus size (Giedd et al., 1995). Evidence for CNS pathology in PANDAS is also suggested by neuroimaging studies. In a case report from the NIMH by Giedd, Rapoport, Leonard, Richter, and Swedo (1996), a child with PANDAS had a baseline MRI scan that demonstrated marked enlargement of the caudate nuclei, bilaterally. Therapeutic plasma exchange reduced his symptoms, and was associated with a 24% reduction in caudate volume, as well as reduction in the size of the putamen (12%) and the globus pallidus (28%). A larger MRI volumetric study of 34 children with PANDAS compared with 82 age- and sex-matched healthy children showed similar basal ganglia volume increases when analyzed blind to subject group (Giedd, Rapoport, Garvey, Perlmutter, & Swedo, 2000). No correlation was found between symptom severity and basal ganglia size.

Although several MRI studies of adults and children suggest increased ventricular abnormalities and deep white matter hyperintensities, neuroimaging studies of bipolar affective disorder have also suggested abnormalities in the basal ganglia (Stoll, Renshaw, Yurgelun-Todd, & Cohen, 2000; Videbech, 1997). Most studies indicate decreased basal ganglia volume in patients with affective disorders, especially those with unipolar depression, but differentiating effects from treatment versus pathology have been unclear. Information obtained from magnetic resonance spectroscopy studies has indicated abnormalities in membrane phospholipid metabolism of the basal ganglia in patients with bipolar affective disorder (Hamakawa, Kato, Murashita, & Kato, 1998; Stoll et al., 2000). Other studies have observed volumetric and metabolic alterations in the basal ganglia and the thalamus in bipolar affective disorder (Baumann et al., 1999; Castillo, Kwock, Courvoisie, & Hooper, 2000; Moore et al., 2000; Noga, Vladar, & Torrey, 2001). Increased glutamate/glutamine levels were found in a MRS study of 10 children with bipolar disorder compared with 10 healthy children (Castillo et al., 2000), suggesting increased neuronal activity. By PET, an increased activity in left dorsal anterior cingulate and left head of caudate was found in five patients with mania compared with six controls (Blumberg et al., 2000). These neuroimaging studies suggest a common anatomical relationship of bipolar affective disorder with PANDAS, obsessive–compulsive disorder, Sydenham's chorea, and tics disorders.

THERAPEUTICS

Medications used to treat neuropsychiatric disorders are believed to exert their primary effect by affecting neurotransmitter functions. Evidence is accumulating, especially through *in vitro* studies, that many of these agents possess some antimicrobial and immunomodulatory properties. Antipsychotics are reported to have immunosuppressive effects (Song, Lin, Kenis, Bosmans, & Maes, 2000), and lithium is reported to have antiviral properties (Rybakowski, 2000). Mild immune activation, observed in patients with rapid-cycling bipolar disorder, was reported to normalize after lithium therapy (Rapaport et al., 1999). Lithium has recently been reputed to possess neuroprotective properties (Manji, Moore, & Chen, 2000). Manji, Moore, Rajkowska, and Chen (2000) propose that mood disorders may result from impairments in neuroplasticity and cellular resilience. Lithium, valproate, and antidepressants indirectly regulate cell survival pathways. Lithium and valproate robustly increase the expression of the cytoprotective protein bcl-2 in the CNS (Chen et al., 1999). Moore, Bebchuk, Wilds, Chen, and Menji (2000) in a small group of patients with bipolar I ($n = 10$) successfully demonstrated the neurotrophic effects of lithium in the human brain *in vivo*. After 4 weeks of treatment with lithium these patients demonstrated a 24 cm^3 increase in total grey matter volume, suggesting that the long-term benefits of lithium are mediated in part by neurotrophic effects. Further development of agents that provide neuroprotection against cytotoxicity and cellular death should prove an interesting avenue for treatment.

Although mood stablilizers are the mainstay therapy for treatment of bipolar affective disorder, other agents have been reported to decrease affective symptoms. Stoll, Locke, Marangell, and Severus (1999) in a preliminary placebo-controlled study of omega-3 fatty acids in the treatment of bipolar affective disorder found significantly increased duration of remission in the treatment group. Omega-3 fatty acids may modulate neuronal signal transduction pathways in a manner similar to that of lithium carbonate and valproate; it may also possess immunoprotectant properties. Many studies support an immunomodulatory effect of the omega-3 fatty acids. Some of the mechanisms that support an anti-inflammatory role for omega-3 fatty acids include competition with omega-6 fatty acids, resulting in decreased levels of the proinflammatory prostaglandin E2, decreased IL-2, increased IL-4, altered cell membrane composition, and decreased lymphocyte proliferation (de Pablo & Alvarez de Cienfuegos, 2000). Medications, such as antiretroviral therapy for HIV, that directly decrease CNS viral load and inflammation have been found to decrease risk for mania (Mijch et al., 1999).

Intravenous immunoglobulin treatments and plasma exchange provided sustained improvements in children with PANDAS at 1-year follow-up. The primary gains were seen in the obsessive–compulsive symptoms, tic severity, global measures of symptom severity, and psychosocial functioning (Perlmutter et al., 1999). A study for antibiotic prophylaxis of obsessive–compulsive disorder/tic exacerbations in children with PANDAS was inconclusive (Garvey et al., 1999), but additional controlled trials are underway. At the time of this writing, research on immune-specific treatments for childhood bipolar disorder has not been performed.

CONCLUSION

Affective symptomatology traverses different neuropsychiatric conditions, like PANDAS, Tourette's syndrome, Sydenham's chorea, obsessive–compulsive disorder, schizophrenia, and other medical conditions like multiple sclerosis, systemic lupus erythematosus, and many others. Many of the immune studies of bipolar affective disorders presented have not been replicated and the samples in children and adolescents are generally too small to be representative. The neuropsychiatric symptoms frequently associated with PANDAS and Sydenham's chorea are acute and sometimes episodic affective symptoms (Table 9.3). These symptoms, predominantly emotional lability/irritability, are prominent features in the diagnosis of bipolar affective disorder in children. This symptom overlap suggests the *possibility* of a common pathophysiological process.

At this juncture, no research provides support of GAS-triggered childhood mania. Affective symptoms in childhood bipolar disorder often have an insidious onset and a chronic course (Wozniak et al., 1995) and would not be consistent with the course seen in PANDAS. However, seasonal fluctuations in affective symptoms and seasonal fluctuations in the incidence of streptococcal infections may suggest that some cases of seasonal affective disorder are streptococcal-related. With as many as 2.4% of prepubertal children endorsing symptoms of seasonal fluctuations of affective symptoms (Swedo et al., 1995), seasonal affective disorder in children may be as common as childhood obsessive–compulsive disorder. The peak of streptococcal illnesses in children is from January to March; historically, rheumatic fever peaks shortly after. The differential diagnosis of children presenting with recurring affective symptoms could be, in theory, classic bipolar illness, seasonal affective disorder, or infection-triggered affective symptoms. A careful history should provide the most compatible diagno-

TABLE 9.3. Comparison of the Clinical Features of Childhood Bipolar Affective Disorder (Wozniak et al., 1995), PANDAS (Swedo et al., 1998), and Sydenham's Chorea (Mercadante et al., 2000)

	Childhood bipolar illness	PANDAS	Sydenham's chorea
GAS relationship	None reported	Proposed	Strong association
Neurological symptoms	High percent with soft neurological signs	"Choreiform"	Definitive
Onset	Insidious, frequently before age 5	Acute, prepubertal	Acute, ages 5–14 years; adult-onset uncommon
Course	Most cases are chronic	Episodic or sawtooth	< 1 year, frequently complete remission
			Recurrences occur, if at all, once or twice
Comorbidity			
ADHD	80%	40%	45%
Anxiety disorders	> 50%	32%	10–15%
Tics	25%	80%	73%
OCD or symptoms	12%	92%	45%
Affective disorder	100%	42%	41%, emotional lability frequently reported
Psychosis	Increased compared to adult bipolar affective disorder	0%	Earlier literature suggests increased
Basal ganglia involvement	Moderate support, but other areas implicated	Nascent support	Strong support, but other areas involved

sis. The clinical picture, however, may be diluted with confounding factors. Many children have subclinical presentations of streptococcal pharyngitis, leading the clinician to presume no streptococcal association unless streptococcal antibodies are measured. A coincidental occurrence of streptococcal infections with affective exacerbations is possible, leading the clinician to make a false association. One case report provides tenuous support that a child with severe recurrent depressive episodes and catatonic features was related to streptococcal pharyngitis. Although documentation by culture or rising titers was lacking, the authors noted rapid symptom improvement following antibiotic therapy (Fernandez-Rivas, Terreros, Ibarmia, Lantaron, & Gonzalez-Torres, 2000). Of interest is the association of rheumatic fever in the histories of those suffering from catatonia (Wilcox,

1986) and the family history of rheumatic fever in this child. Accordingly, immune-based evaluation and treatment guidelines are lacking for clinicians presented with a child with acute mania. In the practice parameters for the assessment and treatment of children and adolescents with bipolar disorder, assessing for the contribution of an infectious process is recommended in the diagnostic phase (American Academy of Child and Adolescent Psychiatry Official Action, 1997). The Jones criteria indicate a high probability of rheumatic fever when previous evidence of streptococcal upper airway infection is detected with two major manifestations (arthritis, carditis, chorea, erythema marginatum, and subcutaneous nodules) or one major and two minor manifestations (fever, arthralgia, high C-reactive protein, or erythrocyte sedimentation rate, prolonged PR interval on electrocardiogram) (Saxena, 2000). Therefore, if a child presents with manic symptoms and/or psychosis *and* has a history of recent illness, rheumatic complaints, or abnormal movements, the child should be appropriately evaluated for rheumatic fever or other immune etiologies.

Bipolar disorder is a condition that has a chronic and intricate nature. Clearly, the role of immune-mediated pathophysiology in childhood bipolar disorder has not been examined and studies on immune function in adult bipolar disorder may not be relevant to children. From a nosological viewpoint, the pathogenesis of PANDAS is postulated to be due to an infection by GAS that triggers an autoimmune state. The immune response to GAS could produce a misreading of self-epitopes. This immunoreactivity may result in exacerbations with repeated GAS infections and possibly other infection agents. Factors contributing to the predisposition to develop PANDAS or bipolar affective disorder need to be elucidated. The primary conjectured risk factor is host susceptibility, and evidence supports that obsessive–compulsive disorder, rheumatic fever, and bipolar affective disorder are familial. Males appear to be at a higher risk, as three-quarters of PANDAS subjects are male (Swedo et al., 1998). Females have a slightly higher risk for developing Sydenham's chorea, suggesting a gender dimorphic vulnerability to GAS. Another factor of susceptibility is age. If we use the rheumatic fever model, rheumatic fever is extremely rare in postpubertal subjects. Environmental influences are also likely contributors, such as the frequency or dose of exposure and the clonotype of the infectious agent. The investigation of susceptibility, triggers, host–pathogen interaction, and neuropathologic process in PANDAS may help not only in the understanding of PANDAS, but also in the understanding of pediatric bipolar affective disorder and other neuropsychiatric presentations. Research in bipolar affective disorder needs to continue, especially in the areas of neuroimmunology and immunogenetics, to improve our preventive measures, diagnostic skills, and treatment strategies in this chronic disorder.

REFERENCES

Allen, A. J., Leonard, H. L., & Swedo, S. E. (1995). Case study: A new infection-triggered, autoimmune subtype of pediatric OCD and Tourette's syndrome. *Journal of the American Academy of Child and Adolescent Psychiatry, 34*(3), 307–311.

American Academy of Child and Adolescent Psychiatry Official Action: Practice Parameters for the Assessment and Treatment of Children and Adolescents with Bipolar Disorder. (1997). *Journal of the American Academy of Child and Adolescent Psychiatry, 36*(1), 138–157.

Asbahr, F. R., Negrao, A. B., Gentil, V., Zanetta, D. M., da Paz, J. A., Marques-Dias, M. J., & Kiss, M. H. (1998). Obsessive-compulsive and related symptoms in children and adolescents with rheumatic fever with and without chorea: A prospective 6-month study. *American Journal of Psychiatry, 155*(8), 1122–1124.

Baumann, B., Danos, P., Krell, D., Diekmann, S., Leschinger, A., Stauch, R., Wurthmann, C., Bernstein, H. G., & Bogerts, B. (1999). Reduced volume of limbic system-affiliated basal ganglia in mood disorders: Preliminary data from a postmortem study. *Journal of Neuropsychiatry and Clinical Neuroscience, 11*(1), 71–78.

Blumberg, H. P., Stern, E., Martinez, D., Ricketts, S., de Asis, J., White, T., Epstein, J., McBride, P. A., Eidelberg, D., Kocsis, J. H., & Silbersweig, D. A. (2000). Increased anterior cingulate and caudate activity in bipolar mania. *Biological Psychiatry, 48*(11), 1045–1052.

Brand, A., Dollberg, S., & Keren, A. (1992). The prevalence of valvular regurgitation in children with structurally normal hearts: A color Doppler echocardiographic study. *American Heart Journal, 123*(1), 177–180.

Bruetsch, W. L. (1940). Chronic rheumatic brain disease as a possible factor in the causation of some cases of dementia precox. *American Journal of Psychiatry, 97*(2), 276–296.

Castillo, M., Kwock, L., Courvoisie, H., & Hooper, S. R. (2000). Proton MR spectroscopy in children with bipolar affective disorder: Preliminary observations. *AJNR American Journal of Neuroradiology, 21*(5), 832–838.

Chapman, A. H., Pilkey, L., & Gibbons, M. J. (1958). A psychosomatic study of eight children with Sydenham's chorea. *Pediatrics, 21*, 582–595.

Chen, G., Zeng, W. Z., Yuan, P. X., Huang, L. D., Jiang, Y. M., Zhao, Z. H., & Manji, H. K. (1999). The mood-stabilizing agents lithium and valproate robustly increase the levels of the neuroprotective protein bcl-2 in the CNS. *Journal of Neurochemistry, 72*(2), 879–882.

de Pablo, M. A., & Alvarez de Cienfuegos, G. (2000). Modulatory effects of dietary lipids on immune system functions. *Immunology and Cell Biology, 78*(1), 31–39.

Deberdt, R., Van Hooren, J., Biesbrouck, M., & Amery, W. (1976). Antinuclear factor-positive mental depression: A single disease entity? *Biological Psychiatry, 11*(1), 69–74.

DeLisi, L. E. (1986). Neuroimmunology: Clinical studies of schizophrenia and other psychiatric disorders. In H. A. Nasrallah & D. R. Weinberger (Eds.), *Handbook of schizophrenia* (Vol. 1, pp. 377–396). Amsterdam: Elsevier Science.

DeLisi, L. E. (1996). Is there a viral or immune dysfunction etiology to schizophrenia?: Re-evaluation a decade later. *Schizophrenia Research, 22*(1), 1–4.

Diefendorf, A. R. (1912). Mental symptoms of acute chorea. *Journal of Nervous and Mental Disease, 39*, 161–172.

Elevli, M., Celebi, A., Tombul, T., & Gokalp, A. S. (1999). Cardiac involvement in Sydenham's chorea: Clinical and Doppler echocardiographic findings. *Acta Paediatrica, 88*(10), 1074–1077.

el-Mallakh, R. S., Suddath, R. L., & Wyatt, R. J. (1993). Interleukin-1 alpha and interleukin-2 in cerebrospinal fluid of schizophrenic subjects. *Progress in Neuropsychopharmacology and Biological Psychiatry, 17*(3), 383–391.

Fallon, B. A., Nields, J. A., Parsons, B., Liebowitz, M. R., & Klein, D. F. (1993). Psychiatric manifestations of Lyme borreliosis. *Journal of Clinical Psychiatry, 54*(7), 263–268.

Fernandez-Rivas, A., Terreros, M. T., Ibarmia, J., Lantaron, G., & Gonzalez-Torres, M. A. (2000). Recurrent depression: Infectious–autoimmune etiology? *Journal of the American Academy of Child and Adolescent Psychiatry, 39*(7), 810–812.

Freeman, J. M., Aron, A. M., Collard, J. E., & MacKay, M. C. (1965). The emotional correlates of Sydenham chorea. *Pediatrics, 35,* 42–49.

Ganguli, R., Brar, J. S., Solomon, W., Chengappa, K. N., & Rabin, B. S. (1992). Altered interleukin-2 production in schizophrenia: Association between clinical state and autoantibody production. *Psychiatry Research, 44*(2), 113–123.

Garvey, M. A., Perlmutter, S. J., Allen, A. J., Hamburger, S., Lougee, L., Leonard, H. L., Witowski, M. E., Dubbert, B., & Swedo, S. E. (1999). A pilot study of penicillin prophylaxis for neuropsychiatric exacerbations triggered by streptococcal infections. *Biological Psychiatry, 45*(12), 1564–1571.

Geller, B., Williams, M., Zimerman, B., Frazier, J., Beringer, L., & Warner, K. L. (1998). Prepubertal and early adolescent bipolarity differentiate from ADHD by manic symptoms, grandiose delusions, ultra-rapid or ultradian cycling. *Journal of Affective Disorders, 51*(2), 81–91.

Giedd, J. N., Kozuch, P., Kaysen, D., Vaituzis, A. C., Hamburger, S. D., Bartko, J. J., & Rapoport, J. L. (1995). Reliability of cerebral measures in repeated examinations with magnetic resonance imaging. *Psychiatry Research, 61*(2), 113–119.

Giedd, J. N., Rapoport, J. L., Garvey, M. A., Perlmutter, S., & Swedo, S. E. (2000). MRI assessment of children with obsessive-compulsive disorder or tics associated with streptococcal infection. *American Journal of Psychiatry, 157*(2), 281–283.

Giedd, J. N., Rapoport, J. L., Leonard, H. L., Richter, D., & Swedo, S. E. (1996). Case study: Acute basal ganglia enlargement and obsessive–compulsive symptoms in an adolescent boy. *Journal of the American Academy of Child and Adolescent Psychiatry, 35*(7), 913–915.

Grimshaw, L. (1964). Obsessional disorder and neurological illness. *Journal of Neurology, Neurosurgery and Psychiatry, 27,* 229–231.

Hamakawa, H., Kato, T., Murashita, J., & Kato, N. (1998). Quantitative proton magnetic resonance spectroscopy of the basal ganglia in patients with affective disorders. *European Archives of Psychiatry and Clinical Neuroscience, 248*(1), 53–58.

Heila, H., Turpeinen, P., & Erkinjuntti, T. (1995). Case study: Mania associated with multiple sclerosis. *Journal of the American Academy of Child and Adolescent Psychiatry, 34*(12), 1591–1595.

Jankovic, B. D., & Djordjijevic, D. (1991). Differential appearance of autoantibodies to human brain S100 protein, neuron specific enolase and myelin basic protein in psychiatric patients. *International Journal of Neuroscience, 60*(1–2), 119–127.

Keeler, W. R., & Bender, L. (1952). A follow-up study of children with behavior disorder and Sydenham's chorea. *American Journal of Psychiatry, 109*, 421–428.

Khan, S., Haddad, P., Montague, L., & Summerton, C. (2000). Systemic lupus erythematosus presenting as mania. *Acta Psychiatrica Scandinavica, 101*(5), 406–408; discussion, 408.

Kiessling, L. S., Marcotte, A. C., & Culpepper, L. (1993). Antineuronal antibodies in movement disorders. *Pediatrics, 92*(1), 39–43.

Kronfol, Z., Silva, J., Greden, J., Dembinski, S., Gardner, R., & Carroll, B. (1983). Impaired lymphocyte function in depressive illness. *Life Sciences, 33*(3), 241–247.

Lahita, R. G. (1997). Effects of gender on the immune system: Implications for neuropsychiatric systemic lupus erythematosus. *Annals of the New York Academy of Science, 823*(1–2), 247–251.

Leu, S., Shiah, I., Yatham, L. N., Cheu, Y., & Lam, R. W. (2001). Immune-inflammatory markers in patients with seasonal affective disorder: Effects of light therapy. *Journal of Affective Disorders, 63*(1–3), 27–34.

Licinio, J., Seibyl, J. P., Altemus, M., Charney, D. S., & Krystal, J. H. (1993). Elevated CSF levels of interleukin-2 in neuroleptic-free schizophrenic patients. *American Journal of Psychiatry, 150*(9), 1408–1410.

Manji, H. K., Moore, G. J., & Chen, G. (2000). Lithium up-regulates the cytoprotective protein Bcl-2 in the CNS in vivo: A role for neurotrophic and neuroprotective effects in manic depressive illness. *Journal of Clinical Psychiatry, 61*(Suppl. 9[5]), 82–96.

Manji, H. K., Moore, G. J., Rajkowska, G., & Chen, G. (2000). Neuroplasticity and cellular resilience in mood disorders. *Molecular Psychiatry, 5*(6), 578–593.

Mercadante, M. T., Busatto, G. F., Lombroso, P. J., Prado, L., Rosario-Campos, M. C., do Valle, R., Marques-Dias, M. J., Kiss, M. H., Leckman, J. F., & Miguel, E. C. (2000). The psychiatric symptoms of rheumatic fever. *American Journal of Psychiatry, 157*(12), 2036–2038.

Mijch, A. M., Judd, F. K., Lyketsos, C. G., Ellen, S., & Cockram, A. (1999). Secondary mania in patients with HIV infection: Are antiretrovirals protective? *Journal of Neuropsychiatry and Clinical Neuroscience, 11*(4), 475–480.

Mittleman, B. B., Castellanos, F. X., Jacobsen, L. K., Rapoport, J. L., Swedo, S. E., & Shearer, G. M. (1997). Cerebrospinal fluid cytokines in pediatric neuropsychiatric disease. *Journal of Immunology, 159*(6), 2994–2999.

Moises, H. W., Schindler, L., Leroux, M., & Kirchner, H. (1985). Decreased production of interferon alpha and interferon gamma in leucocyte cultures of schizophrenic patients. *Acta Psychiatrica Scandinavica, 72*(1), 45–50.

Moore, C. M., Breeze, J. L., Gruber, S. A., Babb, S. M., Frederick, B. B., Villafuerte, R. A., Stoll, A. L., Hennen, J., Yurgelun-Todd, D. A., Cohen, B. M., & Renshaw, P. F. (2000). Choline, myo-inositol and mood in bipolar disorder: A proton magnetic resonance spectroscopic imaging study of the anterior cingulate cortex. *Bipolar Disorder, 2*(3, Pt. 2), 207–216.

Moore, G. J., Bebchuk, J. M., Wilds, I. B., Chen, G., & Menji, H. K. (2000). Lithium-induced increase in human brain grey matter. *Lancet, 356*(9237), 1241–1242.

Muller, N., Riedel, M., Forderreuther, S., Blendinger, C., & Abele-Horn, M. (2000). Tourette's syndrome and mycoplasma pneumoniae infection. *American Journal of Psychiatry, 157*(3), 481–482.

Murphy, T. K., Goodman, W. K., Fudge, M. W., Williams, R. C., Ayoub, E. M., Dalal, M., Lewis, M. H., & Zabriskie, J. B. (1997). B lymphocyte antigen D8/17: A peripheral marker for childhood-onset obsessive–compulsive disorder and Tourette's syndrome? *American Journal of Psychiatry, 154*(3), 402–407.

National Institute of Mental Health Research Roundtable on Prepubertal Bipolar Disorder. (2001). *Journal of the American Academy of Child and Adolescent Psychiatry, 40*(8), 871–878.

Noga, J. T., Vladar, K., & Torrey, E. F. (2001). A volumetric magnetic resonance imaging study of monozygotic twins discordant for bipolar disorder. *Psychiatry Research, 106*(1), 25–34.

Osler, W. (1894). *On chorea and choreiform affections.* Philadelphia: Lewis.

Pandey, R. S., Gupta, A. K., & Chaturvedi, U. C. (1981). Autoimmune model of schizophrenia with special reference to antibrain antibodies. *Biological Psychiatry, 16*(12), 1123–1136.

Pavuluri, M. N., & Smith, M. (1996). A neuroimmune hypothesis for the aetiopathology of viral illness and manic depression: A case report of an adolescent. *Journal of Affective Disorders, 39*(1), 7–11.

Perlmutter, S. J., Leitman, S. F., Garvey, M. A., Hamburger, S., Feldman, E., Leonard, H. L., & Swedo, S. E. (1999). Therapeutic plasma exchange and intravenous immunoglobulin for obsessive–compulsive disorder and tic disorders in childhood. *Lancet, 354*(9185), 1153–1158.

Preble, O. T., & Torrey, E. F. (1985). Serum interferon in patients with psychosis. *American Journal of Psychiatry, 142*(10), 1184–1186.

Rapaport, M. H., Guylai, L., & Whybrow, P. (1999). Immune parameters in rapid cycling bipolar patients before and after lithium treatment. *Journal of Psychiatric Research, 33*(4), 335–340.

Rapaport, M. H., McAllister, C. G., Pickar, D., Nelson, D. L., & Paul, S. M. (1989). Elevated levels of soluble interleukin 2 receptors in schizophrenia. *Archives of General Psychiatry, 46*(3), 291–292.

Rybakowski, J. K. (2000). Antiviral and immunomodulatory effect of lithium. *Pharmacopsychiatry, 33*(5), 159–164.

Saxena, A. (2000). Diagnosis of rheumatic fever: current status of Jones criteria and role of echocardiography. *Indian Journal of Pediatrics, 67*(Suppl. 3), S11–S14.

Schott, K., Batra, A., Richartz, E., Sarkar, R., Gunthner, A., Bartels, M., & Buchkremer, G. (1998). Antibrain antibodies in mental disorder: No evidence for antibodies against synaptic membranes. *Journal of Neural Transmission, 105*(4–5), 517–524.

Selling, L. (1929). The role of infection in the etiology of tics. *Archives of Neurological Psychiatry, 22*, 1163–1171.

Singer, H. S., Giuliano, J. D., Hansen, B. H., Hallett, J. J., Laurino, J. P., Benson, M., & Kiessling, L. S. (1998). Antibodies against human putamen in children with Tourette syndrome. *Neurology, 50*(6), 1618–1624.

Sirota, P., Schild, K., Elizur, A., Djaldetti, M., & Fishman, P. (1995). Increased interleukin-1 and interleukin-3 like activity in schizophrenic patients. *Progress in Neuro-psychopharmacology and Biological Psychiatry, 19*(1), 75–83.

Song, C., Lin, A., Kenis, G., Bosmans, E., & Maes, M. (2000). Immunosuppressive effects of clozapine and haloperidol: Enhanced production of the interleukin-1 receptor antagonist. *Schizophrenia Research, 42*(2), 157–164.

Sourlingas, T. G., Issidorides, M. R., Havaki, S., Trikkas, G., & Sekeri-Pataryas, K. E. (1998). Peripheral blood lymphocytes of bipolar affective patients have a histone synthetic profile indicative of an active cell state. *Progress in Neuro-psychopharmacology and Biological Psychiatry, 22*(1), 81–96.

Spivak, B., Radwan, M., Brandon, J., Molcho, A., Ohring, R., Tyano, S., & Weizman, A. (1991). Cold agglutinin autoantibodies in psychiatric patients: Their relation to diagnosis and pharmacological treatment. *American Journal of Psychiatry, 148*(2), 244–247.

Stoll, A. L., Locke, C. A., Marangell, L. B., & Severus, W. E. (1999). Omega-3 fatty acids and bipolar disorder: A review. *Prostaglandins, Leukotrienes and Essential Fatty Acids, 60*(5–6), 329–337.

Stoll, A. L., Renshaw, P. F., Yurgelun-Todd, D. A., & Cohen, B. M. (2000). Neuroimaging in bipolar disorder: What have we learned? *Biological Psychiatry, 48*(6), 505–517.

Swedo, S. E. (1994). Sydenham's chorea: A model for childhood autoimmune neuropsychiatric disorders. *Journal of the American Medical Association, 272*(22), 1788–1791.

Swedo, S. E., Allen, A. J., Glod, C. A., Clark, C. H., Teicher, M. H., Richter, D., Hoffman, C., Hamburger, S. D., Dow, S., Brown, C., & Rosenthal, N. E. (1997). A controlled trial of light therapy for the treatment of pediatric seasonal affective disorder. *Journal of the American Academy of Child and Adolescent Psychiatry, 36*(6), 816–821.

Swedo, S. E., Leonard, H. L., Garvey, M., Mittleman, B., Allen, A. J., Perlmutter, S., Lougee, L., Dow, S., Zamkoff, J., & Dubbert, B. K. (1998). Pediatric autoimmune neuropsychiatric disorders associated with streptococcal infections: Clinical description of the first 50 cases. *American Journal of Psychiatry, 155*(2), 264–271.

Swedo, S. E., Leonard, H. L., Schapiro, M. B., Casey, B. J., Mannheim, G. B., Lenane, M. C., & Rettew, D. C. (1993). Sydenham's chorea: Physical and psychological symptoms of St. Vitus dance. *Pediatrics, 91*(4), 706–713.

Swedo, S. E., Pleeter, J. D., Richter, D. M., Hoffman, C. L., Allen, A. J., Hamburger, S. D., Turner, E. H., Yamada, E. M., & Rosenthal, N. E. (1995). Rates of seasonal affective disorder in children and adolescents. *American Journal of Psychiatry, 152*(7), 1016–1019.

Swedo, S. E., Rapoport, J. L., Cheslow, D. L., Leonard, H. L., Ayoub, E. M., Hosier, D. M., & Wald, E. R. (1989). High prevalence of obsessive–compulsive symptoms in patients with Sydenham's chorea. *American Journal of Psychiatry, 146*(2), 246–249.

Tsai, S. Y., Chen, K. P., Yang, Y. Y., Chen, C. C., Lee, J. C., Singh, V. K., & Leu, S. J. (1999). Activation of indices of cell-mediated immunity in bipolar mania. *Biological Psychiatry, 45*(8), 989–994.

Videbech, P. (1997). MRI findings in patients with affective disorder: A meta-analysis. *Acta Psychiatrica Scandinavica, 96*(3), 157–168.

Villemain, F., Magnin, M., Feuillet-Fieux, M. N., Zarifian, E., Loo, H., & Bach, J. F. (1988). Anti-histone antibodies in schizophrenia and affective disorders. *Psychiatry Research, 24*(1), 53–60.

Von Economo, C. (1931). *Encephalitis lethargica: Its sequelae and treatment.* London: Oxford University Press.

Weller, E. B., Weller, R. A., & Fristad, M. A. (1995). Bipolar disorder in children: Misdiagnosis, underdiagnosis, and future directions. *Journal of the American Academy of Child and Adolescent Psychiatry, 34*(6), 709–714.

Weller, R. A., Weller, E. B., Tucker, S. G., & Fristad, M. A. (1986). Mania in prepubertal children: Has it been underdiagnosed? *Journal of Affective Disorders, 11*(2), 151–154.

Wilcox, J. A. (1986). Perinatal distress and infectious disease as risk factors for catatonia. *Psychopathology, 19*(4), 196–199.

Wilcox, J. A., & Nasrallah, H. (1988). Sydenham's chorea and psychopathology. *Neuropsychobiology, 19*(1), 6–8.

Wozniak, J., Biederman, J., Kiely, K., Ablon, J. S., Faraone, S. V., Mundy, E., & Mennin, D. (1995). Mania-like symptoms suggestive of childhood-onset bipolar disorder in clinically referred children. *Journal of the American Academy of Child and Adolescent Psychiatry, 34*(7), 867–876.

Yolken, R. H., & Torrey, E. F. (1995). Viruses, schizophrenia, and bipolar disorder. *Clinical Microbiology Review, 8*(1), 131–145.

10

Sleep and Other Biological Rhythms

UMA RAO

From centuries of observation, it is apparent that mood changes in bipolar illness follow a rhythmic pattern, waxing and waning regularly in cycling patterns of euphoria, irritability, or sadness. Although these changes in clinical state appear to follow a seasonal pattern, research has shown that the fluctuations in mood are often accompanied by disturbances in innate biological rhythms, particularly those involving the circadian systems. In this chapter, the association between circadian dysregulation and bipolar disorder, and the hypothesized mechanisms of these disturbances, is described. Because the literature in child and adolescent populations in this area is almost nonexistent, extant data from adults will be reviewed along with all available information in youngsters. Based on these data, potentially fruitful areas for investigation in pediatric mood disorders will be outlined.

REGULATION OF CIRCADIAN RHYTHMS

Experimental studies indicate that external time cues, known as *zeitgebers*, synchronize circadian rhythms with the day–night cycle and also with one another. When entrained by zeitgebers, homeostatic mechanisms ensure that the various circadian rhythms keep distinct phase relationships to the environment and to one another. For instance, in humans, the temperature nadir almost always occurs during the last third of the night, just before dawn (Avery, Wilschiodz, & Rafaelsen,1982; Souêtre et al.,1988; Weitzman et al., 1974). Circadian rhythms that are normally synchronized with each other can dissociate when there is a disentrainment from the zeitgeber. The temperature rhythm of a night-shift worker, for example, might continue to be entrained to the day–night cycle but be dissociated from the sleep–wake cycle when the worker sleeps during the day. Such desynchronization suggests that the human circadian system is controlled by more than one oscillator. Although the nature and number of biological oscillators are subjects of controversy, the prevailing view is that human circadian rhythms are regulated by multiple self-sustained, coupled oscillators, which probably are organized hierarchically. However, many investigators believe in the existence of only one truly endogenous circadian oscillator (Czeisler, Kronauer, Mooney, Anderson, & Allan, 1987).

Experiments in animals and in humans have demonstrated that the suprachiasmatic nucleus (SCN), located in the anterior hypothalamus, serves as the primary endogenous oscillator (see Czeisler et al., 1987; Moore-Ede, Silzman, & Fuller, 1982; Reppert, Weaver, Rivkees, & Stopa, 1988). The SCN is almost impervious to environmental influences. The SCN, in turn, controls a much weaker circadian process that readily responds to environmental influences and regulates daily rhythms, such as rest–activity periods, the sleep–wake cycle, and sleep-dependent neuroendocrine activity (Moore-Ede et al., 1982). Proper functioning of the human circadian system depends on continuous sensory input from the environment. In addition to environmental influences, behavior regulates biological rhythms by subjecting a person to the entraining zeitgebers and serves a gating function. Principal environmental and behavioral events that are known to affect circadian organization include the light–dark cycle, temperature, humidity, food, and arousal state.

The timing of circadian rhythms relative to the day–night cycle, and to one another, is homeostatically controlled. Such a system may be altered by disease or by treatment interventions. Alterations can occur in the intrinsic periods of the oscillators, in the coupling between oscillators, or between the oscillators and the external day–night cycle. A better understanding of the circadian disturbances in manic–depressive illness potentially can be helpful in developing more effective treatment and preventive interventions for this disabling condition (Goodwin & Jamison, 1990).

RELATIONSHIP BETWEEN SLEEP AND MOOD DISORDERS

Among the various biological rhythms hypothesized to be involved in mood disorders, the sleep–wake cycle is believed to play an important role. For instance, sleep deprivation has significant, but transient, antidepressant effects in both unipolar and bipolar depressed subjects (Barbini et al., 1998; Leibenluft & Wehr, 1992; Wirz-Justice & Van den Hoofdakker, 1999). Clinical observations also suggest a close association between sleep loss and onset of manic episodes in patients with manic–depressive illness (Barbini, Bertelli, Colombo, & Smeraldi, 1996; Colombo, Benedetti,

Barbini, Campori, & Smeraldi, 1999; Wu & Bunney, 1990), specifically in those with rapid-cycling illness (Leibenluft, Albert, Rosenthal, & Wehr, 1996; Wehr, Goodwin, Wirz-Justice, Breitmaier, & Craig, 1982; Wehr, Sack, & Rosenthal, 1987). Other investigators have reported that treatment of patients with bipolar disorder with extended sleep may be helpful in preventing manic episodes and rapid cycling (Wehr et al., 1998; Wirz-Justice, Quinto, Cajochen, Werth, & Hock, 1999). Not only sleep duration, but also shifts in the timing of sleep can induce subsequent mood changes in patients with manic–depressive illness (Riemann et al., 1996; Sack, Nurnberger, Rosenthal, Ashburn, & Wehr, 1985; Wehr, Wirz-Justice, Goodwin, Duncan, & Gillin, 1979). Therefore, the timing and duration of sleep–wake cycles appear to be intrinsically related to the clinical state of bipolar disorder.

In addition to the connection between sleep–wake disturbances and the switch process in bipolar disorder, changes in sleep architecture have been reported. Electroencephalographic (EEG) sleep variables of adult patients with major depressive episode, including unipolar and bipolar depression, have been intensively studied (for a review, see Benca, Obermeyer, Thisted, & Gillin,1992; Kupfer & Thase, 1983). Furthermore, there are data to suggest that EEG sleep profiles may distinguish these two subtypes of depression (Duncan, Pettigrew, & Gillin, 1979; Feinberg, Gillin, Carroll, Greden, & Zis, 1982; Fossion et al., 1998; Giles, Rush, & Roffwarg, 1986; Jernajczyk, 1986; Jovanovic, 1977; Kupfer et al., 1972; Thase, Himmelhoch, Mallinger, Jarrett, & Kupfer, 1989).

The most consistent EEG sleep variables associated with major depressive disorder include sleep continuity disturbances, earlier onset of the first rapid eye movement (REM) sleep, higher phasic activity during REM sleep, altered temporal distribution of REM sleep (i.e., more REM sleep in the first half of the night), and diminished slow-wave (or delta) sleep (Benca et al., 1992). Approximately 50–75% of adult subjects, and up to 90% of geriatric patients, appear to manifest these sleep changes. Some data suggest that bipolar patients, specifically those with bipolar II subtype, may manifest hypersomnia (Feinberg et al., 1982; Fossion et al., 1998; Giles et al., 1986; Kupfer et al., 1972). Also, reduced REM latency may be less prevalent in bipolar depression (Giles et al., 1986; Jernajczyk, 1986; Jovanovic, 1977; Thase et al., 1989).

In contrast to the rich sources of data on EEG sleep profiles of individuals with unipolar and bipolar depression, systematic investigation of EEG sleep characteristics in subjects with bipolar disorder during manic or hypomanic state has been limited. Most of these data consist of case reports. Also, many of these patients were on psychotropic medication(s) at the time of these sleep studies, which potentially could influence the sleep variables (for a review, see Hudson, Lipinski, Frankenburg, Grochocinski, & Kupfer, 1988). In one of the better designed cross-sectional studies,

Hudson and colleagues (1988) found that, compared to age- and gender-matched controls, patients with mania exhibited significantly reduced sleep time, increased awake time, shortened REM latency, and increased phasic activity during REM sleep. In longitudinal studies of patients with rapid-cycling illness, changes in REM sleep variables and slow-wave sleep appear to be more accentuated during the depressive state than during the manic phase (Cairns, Waldron, MacLean, & Knowles, 1980; Post et al., 1977; Wehr, 1977; Wehr & Wirz-Justice, 1982).

In summary, these data indicate that sleep disturbances are common manifestations of unipolar and bipolar disorders. Also, dysregulation in the sleep–wake cycle may be associated with the switch process in bipolar disorder, suggesting that such disruptions may play an etiological role in these syndromes.

HYPOTHESIZED MECHANISMS OF SLEEP–WAKE DISTURBANCES IN MOOD DISORDERS

A number of theories have been proposed for the mechanisms underlying the sleep–wake disturbances observed in mood disorders. One of the first theories of disruption in biological rhythms associated with mood disorders was the hypothesis of *desynchrony*. This hypothesis proposes that the patient's own circadian rhythms are desynchronized either with one another (internal phase disorder) or with the entrainment to the day–night cycle (external phase disorder) (see Wehr et al., 1979). Other investigators have extended this model to explain the effects of sleep and sleep deprivation in mood disorders (see Table 10.1). Because more empirical data are available in patients with depression, and since depression is an integral part of bipolar illness, those data will be reviewed.

Process S Theory

Borbély and Wirz-Justice (1982) have hypothesized that the regulation of the sleep–wake cycle is determined by two factors: a circadian propensity for sleep (process C), and a sleepiness process (process S). According to this theoretical model, the level of sleep need depends on the duration of prior wakefulness and sleep: it increases exponentially with increasing duration of wakefulness and decreases during non-REM sleep. The hypothetical process S could play a signal role, providing information to the brain on how long it has been since the person has last slept. Sleep onset and sleep termination are determined by the accumulation of S and by a gating system consisting of two thresholds under control of the circadian process C. Therefore, the timing of non-REM sleep is dictated by sleep need and the circadian pacemaker. The regulation of REM sleep is more complex. In

TABLE 10.1. Theories of Sleep Regulation and Sleep Deprivation Effects in Mood Disorders

Theory	Proponents	Proposed pathophysiology in depression	Mechanism of action of sleep deprivation for antidepressant effect
Process S (antidepressant substance released during wakefulness)	Borbély & Wirz-Justice (1982)	Decreased secretion of process S factor(s)	Greater length of time available for S substance to accumulate and reach normal level.
Sleep-related depressogenic process (depressogenic substance released during sleep)	Wu & Bunney (1990)	Increased depressogenic substance released during sleep	Blockage of release of depressogenic substance by wakefulness; metabolism (or storage) of substance during wakefulness.
Internal coincidence (critical time period for production of depressogenic substance)	Wehr & Wirz-Justice (1981)	Phase advance of sleep-sensitive depression switch into sleep period	Prevention of the activation of depression switch by wakefulness during the critical period.

addition to a homeostatic component, REM sleep propensity and timing appear to be governed by an interaction between circadian and ultradian mechanisms, and by the reciprocal interaction of non-REM with REM sleep. It is hypothesized that there is a deficient buildup of process S, or sleep need, in depression, with process C remaining unaffected (Borbély & Wirz-Justice, 1982). Sleep deprivation is assumed to be therapeutic because the level of S is transiently elevated to normal, and relapse occurs after recovery sleep due to the return to low baseline levels (see Table 10.1).

Several investigators have considered potential endogenous compounds that might serve as sleep propensity (or S) factors. For instance, thyroid-stimulating hormone (TSH) is released with prolonged wakefulness, and alterations in TSH regulation have been reported in both unipolar and bipolar patients (Loosen & Prang, 1982; Sack, James, Rosenthal, & Wehr, 1988; Scanlon & Hall, 1989; Souêtre et al., 1988). TSH release appears to be mediated by two factors (Parker, Pekary, & Hershman, 1976). First, there is a circadian propensity for release of TSH beginning in the early evening. Then, sleep onset appears to curtail the release of TSH. Baumgartner and Meinhold (1986) observed higher levels of TSH release during sleep deprivation, and also noted an association between change in TSH levels and clinical improvement. Other neuroendocrine factors that are under circadian influence also may be involved in sleep regulation.

Sleep-Associated Depressogenic Process

In contrast to the process S theory (i.e., that a sleep regulatory mechanism occurring during wakefulness is related to the depressive phenomenon), Wu and Bunney (1990) have proposed that some process that takes place during sleep may be depressogenic (see Table 10.1). The strongest evidence that sleep is depressogenic comes from studies of relapse following the first night of sleep in those who show clinical improvement after sleep deprivation. Wu and Bunney reviewed 17 studies involving 158 subjects who responded to sleep deprivation, and found that 83% of patients who were not receiving any pharmacological treatment had a relapse after the first night of sleep. Some investigators reported that even a brief nap was sufficient to precipitate a relapse (Knowles et al., 1979; Kraft, Willner, Gillin, Janowsky, & Neborsky, 1984; Wiegand, Berger, Zulley, Lauer, & von Zerssen, 1987).

Wu and Bunney (1990) have suggested that some substance associated with depression may be released during sleep, and that the substance may be metabolized or stored during wakefulness, with a subsequent improvement in mood. Because profound changes in depressed mood can occur even after naps of 90-seconds duration (Kraft et al., 1984), the rapidity of this phenomenon suggests that sleep-related release of a depressogenic compound is more likely than the rapid metabolism during wakefulness. Instead of a depressogenic process, it is also possible to hypothesize that a euphorogenic substance is released during wakefulness and metabolized or stored during sleep. This theory is similar to the process S model (Borbély & Wirz-Justice, 1982).

A sleep-associated depressogenic process also could influence a regulatory mechanism or marker that measures the amount of sleep a person has had and determines when sleep should be terminated. If there is an excessive release or activity of this sleep-associated depressogenic process, the person's sleep might be interrupted even if he or she has not had sufficient sleep. This is akin to a faulty gas gauge that reads "full" even though the gas tank is empty. Wu and Bunney (1990) suggest that this could explain some of the sleep disturbances seen in patients with depression, such as frequent awakenings. As the patient improves, the excessive release or activity could be reduced to normal levels, thus preventing sleep interruption. This hypothesis also can account for the diurnal worsening of mood in the morning seen in some depressed patients, which becomes alleviated with wakefulness (Knowles et al., 1979).

Wu and Bunney (1990) suggest that one potential biological correlate of regulation of sleep length is increased REM density, which is frequently seen in subjects with depression. Aserinsky (1969) observed that in normal subjects who have had extended sleep, there is a tendency for the duration of successive REM periods to diminish, and there is also a high degree of phasic activity from one REM period to the next. Cortisol is an example of a potential substance released during sleep, with the greatest concentration occurring in the later half of the night when REM sleep is predominant (Rubin & Poland, 1982; Weitzman et al., 1971). Some studies have found that sleep deprivation may reduce cortisol secretion (Akerstedt, Palmblad, de la Torre, Marana, & Gillberg, 1980; Kant, Genser, Thorne, Pfalser, & Mougey, 1984), and that the reduction in cortisol secretion achieved by sleep deprivation may be associated with clinical improvement in depressed patients (Kasper, Moises, & Beckman, 1983; Kuhs, 1985; Nasarallah, Kuperman, & Coryell, 1980).

Internal Coincidence Theory

The internal coincidence hypothesis focuses on the timing of the sleep–wake schedule rather than on the duration of sleep (Wehr & Wirz-Justice, 1981). This is an extension of the phase advance hypothesis for depression (Wehr et al., 1979), and assumes that the phase angle between an advanced circadian pacemaker and the sleep–wake cycle is depressogenic (see Table 10.1). Similar to shift workers or transmeridian travelers, patients with depression sleep at the wrong biological clock time. It is postulated that sleep deprivation achieves its therapeutic effect by avoiding the coincidence of sleep with the critical phase.

Evidence for the critical phase angle comes from several studies. A 6-hour advance of sleep timing induced positive, sustained responses in a number of uncontrolled studies (see Van den Hoofdakker, 1997; Wehr et al., 1979). This suggests the possibility that it is the timing, not the duration, of sleep that determines the depressogenic character of sleep. Partial sleep deprivation during the second half of the night also was shown to be effective in inducing remission of depressive symptoms in some studies (Baxter et al., 1986; Philipp & Werner, 1979; Schilgen & Tolle, 1980), but not in others (Knowles et al., 1979). Also, a phase delay in sleep was shown to induce depressive symptoms (Surridge-David, MacLean, Coulter, & Knowles, 1987).

Because REM latency is reduced and most of the REM sleep occurs at an earlier time in individuals with depression, there may be an apparent phase advance of the timing of REM sleep. Other measures such as temperature and cortisol rhythms also may be phase-advanced in depression (Wehr & Sack, 1981). This phase advancement is consistent with the possibility of a vulnerable depression switch, which is moved into the sleep time during early morning.

REM Sleep Regulation

A related hypothesis suggests that abnormalities in the ultradian rhythm of REM sleep play a dominant role in depression, and that selective REM sleep deprivation would have an antidepressant effect (Vogel, Vogel,

McAbee, & Thurmond, 1980). There is also evidence to suggest that the occurrence of REM sleep during naps is specifically associated with onset of depression in some patients (Wiegand et al., 1987).

Slow-Wave Sleep Suppression

REM sleep deprivation experiments in healthy volunteers have led to gradual suppression of slow-wave activity (Beersma, Dijk, & Block, 1990; Brunner, Dijk, Tobler, & Borbély, 1990). Obviously, total sleep deprivation also is accompanied by acute suppression of slow-wave sleep. Because REM sleep deprivation in patients with depression leads to gradual improvement (Vogel et al., 1980), and total sleep deprivation results in acute improvement, it has been postulated that the suppression of slow-wave activity may play a more central role in the antidepressant effects of both REM sleep and total sleep deprivation (Beersma & Van den Hoofdakker, 1992).

Arousal–Cerebral Fatigue Theory

It is evident that sleep subserves restorative brain processes, and sleep loss, particularly loss of slow-wave sleep, causes "brain fatigue" (Horne, 1991). One paradoxical consequence of sleep loss in patients with depression is the subjective feeling of tiredness and sleepiness combined with improvement in mood and energy (Van den Burg, Beersma, Bouhuys, & Van den Hoofdakker, 1992). It is speculated that sleep-deprivation-induced cerebral fatigue might break the distressing state of hyperarousal in individuals with depression, resulting in simultaneous feelings of relief and tiredness.

Neurotransmitter Regulation of Sleep

In addition to being controlled by homeostatic and circadian processes, sleep regulation is controlled by neurochemical mechanisms (Cabeza, Zoltoski, & Gillin, 1994). For instance, McCarley and Hobson (1975) provided evidence for a sleep model based on the interaction of separate REM-enhancing and REM-inhibiting neuronal populations. This model postulates a balance between cholinergic and aminergic systems in the regulation of REM sleep. There is substantial evidence that cholinergic mechanisms are involved in generating REM sleep. There is also evidence, in both animals and humans, that aminergic neurotransmission is inhibitory to REM sleep (McCarley, Greene, Rainnie, & Portas, 1995). Wiegand and colleagues (1987) observed that the occurrence of REM sleep during naps precipitated depressive symptoms in patients who responded to sleep deprivation. These findings, together with data on REM sleep changes associated with depression, suggest that there may be enhanced cholinergic activity in depression (Hobson, Lydic, & Baghdoyan, 1986; Janowsky, Risch, & Gillin, 1983; Sitaram, Nurnberger, Gershon, & Gillin, 1982). There is also evidence to suggest that cholinergic activity may be reduced in the manic phase (Janowsky, el-Yousef, Davis, & Sekerke, 1972; Sokolski & DeMet, 2000).

Serotonin (5-HT) also is a major neurotransmitter candidate, being involved in both sleep and circadian rhythm regulation, as well as in the modulation of mood state (Maes & Meltzer, 1995; McCarley et al., 1995). There is evidence that 5-HT mechanisms, and in particular down-regulation of presynaptic 5-HT_{1A} receptors, may be involved in the antidepressant action of sleep deprivation (Prévot, Maudhuit, Le Poul, Hamon, & Adrien, 1996). Treatment with drugs affecting 5-HT systems have revealed interactions with sleep deprivation to potentiate antidepressant response or to prevent relapse (Benedetti et al., 1997; Kuhs, Farber, Borgstadt, Mrosek, & Tolle, 1996; Leibenluft & Wehr, 1992; Shelton & Loosen, 1993; Smeraldi, Benedetti, Barbini, Campori, & Colombo, 1999; Szuba et al., 1994). A recent study showed that a functional polymorphism within the promoter region of the 5-HT transporter gene, associated with good response to selective serotonin reuptake inhibitors (Smeraldi et al., 1998; Zanardi, Benedetti, Di Bella, Catalano, & Smeraldi, 1999), is also associated with better mood amelioration following sleep deprivation (Benedetti et al., 1999).

SLEEP STUDIES IN CHILDREN AND ADOLESCENTS WITH MOOD DISORDERS

As can be gleaned from the described data above, the literature on sleep deprivation and EEG sleep in adults with unipolar and bipolar disorders is extensive. But to the best of my knowledge, there are only three published reports on sleep deprivation effects in children and adolescents with depression, and none on children with bipolar disorder. King and colleagues (King, Baxter, Stuber, & Fish, 1987) studied the combined effects of partial sleep deprivation and medication in a 12-year-old child, and found mild beneficial effects with sleep deprivation. Detrinis and colleagues (1990) investigated the effects of partial sleep deprivation in adolescents, of whom four met criteria for major depressive disorder. All four subjects experienced improved mood and psychomotor activity. In contrast to the findings in adults, however, the beneficial effects lasted for up to 3–5 days after sleep deprivation.

Naylor and colleagues (1993) reported on 17 adolescent psychiatric patients who were deprived of sleep for 36 hours. There were four primary groups of patients: severely depressed, mildly depressed, partially remitted subjects, and nondepressed controls. Adolescents with severe depression showed a significant reduction in depressive symptoms after sleep deprivation, whereas remitted subjects and psychiatric controls had a worsening. Similar to the observations made by Detrinis and colleagues (1990), the effects of sleep deprivation persisted after one night of recovery sleep. The limited data in youngsters suggest a common pathophysiology between juvenile and adult depression, although there appear to be some developmental differences.

With regard to EEG sleep data, in contrast to the robust findings we see in studies of unipolar depression in adults, there is more variability in child and adolescent populations (see Table 10.2). Of four studies focusing on children with depression (Dahl et al., 1991; Emslie, Rush, Weinberg, Rintelmann, & Roffwarg, 1990; Puig-Antich et al., 1982; Young, Knowles, MacLean, Boag, & McConville, 1982), only one study, comprising an inpatient sample, reported prolonged sleep latency and reduced REM latency compared with controls (Emslie et al., 1990). Among 10 investigations conducted in adolescents, six reported sleep continuity disturbances, five showed shortened REM latency, and two studies found higher REM density (Appelboom-Fondu, Kerkhofs, & Mendlewicz, 1988; Dahl et al., 1990, 1996; Emslie, Rush, Weinberg, Rintelmann, & Roffwarg, 1994; Goetz et al., 1987, 1991; Khan & Todd, 1990; Kutcher, Williamson, Marton, & Szalai, 1992; Lahmeyer, Poznanski, & Bellur, 1983; Riemann, Kammerer, Löw, & Schmidt, 1995). None of these studies observed reduction in slow-wave sleep.

The discrepancy in EEG sleep findings between pediatric and adult populations should be placed in the context of comparable clinical profiles in the two groups. These data suggest that there may be maturational effects on sleep regulation that might have an influence on EEG sleep manifestations associated with depression. In addition to development, clinical course might play a role in the manifestation of polysomnographic changes. For instance, despite meeting adult criteria for major depressive disorder, depression prior to puberty does not show a strong temporal continuity with adult depression as compared to depression occurring after puberty (Harrington, Fudge, Rutter, Pickles, & Hill, 1990; Weissman, Wolk, Goldstein, et al., 1999; Weissman, Wolk, Wickramaratne, et al., 1999). It is possible that youngsters with depression who show high temporal stability in depressive episodes may manifest the most robust EEG sleep changes. Also, there is now clear evidence that early-onset depression is associated with a higher likelihood of conversion to bipolar disorder than the adult form of the illness (Geller, Fox, & Clark, 1994; Strober & Carlson, 1982; Strober, Lampert, Schmidt, & Morrell, 1993). As reviewed above, there are some distinctions between EEG sleep changes observed in unipolar and bipolar depression.

In a follow-up study initially reported by Dahl and colleagues (1990), we found that control subjects who subsequently developed depression

TABLE 10.2. Electroencephalographic Sleep Studies in Depressed
Children and Adolescents

Study	Sample	Sleep latency	Sleep efficiency	REM latency	REM density	Delta sleep
Studies in children						
Puig-Antich et al. (1982)	54 MDD; 11 NC	≅	≅	≅	≅	≅
Young et al. (1982)	12 MDD; 12 NC	≅	≅	≅	≅	≅
Emslie et al. (1990)	25 MDD; 25 NC	↑	≅	↓	≅	≅
Dahl et al. (1991)	36 MDD; 18 NC	≅	≅	≅	≅	≅
Studies in adolescents						
Lahmeyer et al. (1983)	13 MDD; 13 NC	≅	≅	↓	↑	≅
Goetz et al. (1987)	49 MDD; 40 NC	↑	↓	≅	≅	≅
Appelboom-Fondu et al. (1988)	9 MDD; 12 NC	≅	↓	≅	≅	≅
Dahl et al. (1990)	27 MDD; 30 NC	≅	≅	≅	≅	≅
Khan & Todd (1990)	10 MDD; 10 NC	≅	≅	≅	≅	≅
Goetz et al. (1991)	38 MDD; 37 NC	↑	≅	≅	≅	≅
Kutcher et al. (1992)	23 MDD; 28 NC	↑	≅	↓	≅	≅
Emslie et al. (1994)	31 MDD; 17 NC	↑	↓	↓	↑	≅
Riemann et al. (1995)	10MDD; 10 NC	≅	≅	↓	≅	≅
Dahl et al. (1996)	16 MDD; 21 NC	↑	≅	↓	≅	≅

Note. REM, rapid eye movement sleep; MDD, subjects with major depressive disorder; NC, normal control subjects; ≅, no difference between MDD and NC subjects; ↑, increased in MDD subjects compared with NC subjects; ↓, decreased in MDD subjects compared with NC subjects.

showed evidence of reduced REM latency and higher REM density long before the onset of depression, whereas youngsters with depression who switched to bipolar disorder had REM sleep measures that were consistent with normal controls (Rao et al., 1996, 2002). When the clinical course was taken into consideration, the unipolar group demonstrated the same EEG sleep pattern seen in adult depression, with the exception that there were no slow-wave sleep changes (see Table 10.3). In contrast to the unipolar group, initially depressed subjects who subsequently manifested bipolar illness showed a tendency for more stage 1 sleep and less slow-wave sleep (see Table 10.3). These findings highlight the importance of careful selection of experimental subjects and controls for the identification of biological markers for unipolar and bipolar disorders in youngsters. The results also suggest that the pathophysiological underpinnings of unipolar depression and manic–depressive illness may be different.

To my knowledge, there are no published data on EEG sleep manifestations of bipolar disorder in children and adolescents. We had collected sleep polysomnography measures in five adolescent subjects who were either in a manic, a hypomanic, or a mixed state. On clinical follow-up in early adult life, only two subjects showed evidence of bipolar disorder (Rao et al., unpublished data). We observed substantial variability in EEG sleep variables among these subjects, and the results are confounded by modest sample size and variability in clinical status. The experimental group did not differ from the controls on any of the major EEG sleep measures. However, the two subjects who showed evidence of bipolar illness on clinical follow-up had much less slow-wave sleep compared to the remaining three initially bipolar patients and normal controls.

HYPOTHESIZED MECHANISMS FOR EEG SLEEP CHANGES IN UNIPOLAR AND BIPOLAR DISORDERS

Kupfer and Ehlers (1989) have proposed that there may be two distinct pathways to reduced REM latency. In one model, there is increased REM pressure, resulting in REM sleep advancement at the expense of non-REM sleep. In the second model, the primary deficit is in slow-wave sleep, and shortened REM latency occurs secondary to reduction in non-REM sleep. Based on our pilot data in adolescents and based on data in adult subjects with bipolar illness, it is speculated that unipolar and bipolar mood disorders have distinct pathophysiological origins. Unipolar depression is characterized by increased REM sleep pressure. In the initial stages of illness, slow-wave sleep is preserved. This capacity may be reduced as the disease progresses and/or the individual matures, resulting in reduced slow-wave sleep in addition to the changes in REM sleep. In contrast to unipolar depression, bipolar illness is primarily associated with deficiency in slow-wave sleep. In younger subjects, this deficit is compensated by increased stage 1 and stage 2 sleep, thereby maintaining the temporal distribution of REM sleep. There may be an interaction between development and clinical course, however, leading to secondary changes in REM sleep in a subset of patients.

Developmental data in normal adolescent and adult volunteers suggest that cholinergic systems involved in REM sleep regulation may be relatively more active in adolescents compared with adults (Rao, Lutch-

TABLE 10.3. Selected EEG Sleep Variables (Mean ± *SD*) in Adolescents Based on Clinical Outcome in Adult Life

	Controls with no lifetime psychiatric disorder at follow-up (n = 20)	Initial controls who developed MDD at follow-up (n = 5)	Subjects with unipolar MDD at baseline and at follow-up (n = 19)	MDD subjects who converted to bipolar disorder at follow-up (n = 5)	p
Sleep architecture					
Stage 1 sleep (%)	3.4 ± 2.1	3.9 ± 3.3	3.0 ± 1.7	5.5 ± 2.3	NS
Stage 2 sleep (%)	50.4 ± 7.9	48.8 ± 5.9	48.3 ± 6.2	55.7 ± 3.4	NS
Stage 3 sleep (%)	6.4 ± 2.6	7.0 ± 2.1	7.8 ± 4.8	6.7 ± 3.5	NS
Stage 4 sleep (%)	18.2 ± 6.0	14.4 ± 5.9	17.1 ± 6.7	11.9 ± 1.3	NS
REM sleep (%)	$21.6 \pm 3.8_a$	$26.0 \pm 2.3_b$	$23.8 \pm 4.2_{a,b}$	$20.2 \pm 2.0_a$	.04
Sleep continuity					
Sleep latency (min)[a]	17.2 ± 10.4	21.6 ± 14.5	21.2 ± 12.2	14.1 ± 7.2	NS
Awake time (min)[a]	9.3 ± 5.6	14.3 ± 7.4	10.4 ± 8.1	16.7 ± 13.1	NS
Total sleep time (min)	460.0 ± 28.3	465.8 ± 13.2	466.2 ± 31.2	446.1 ± 30.0	NS
REM sleep					
REM latency (min)[a]	$104.1 \pm 48.2_a$	$67.3 \pm 20.2_b$	$78.2 \pm 35.0_b$	$136.6 \pm 54.4_a$	.02
REM density (units/ min)	$1.1 \pm 0.3_a$	$1.5 \pm 0.3_b$	$1.4 \pm 0.2_b$	$0.9 \pm 0.3_a$	.0001
REM duration (min)	$99.6 \pm 19.8_{a,c}$	$121.1 \pm 13.6_b$	$110.8 \pm 20.8_{a,b}$	$90.2 \pm 9.6_c$	.03
REM sleep in 1st sleep cycle (%)[a]	$12.4 \pm 5.9_a$	$17.5 \pm 0.3_b$	$18.3 \pm 7.5_b$	$9.2 \pm 2.8_a$	.003
1st REM sleep/2nd REM sleep[a]	$0.6 \pm 0.3_a$	$0.9 \pm 0.2_b$	$1.0 \pm 0.6_b$	$0.4 \pm 0.2_a$	.001

Note. MDD, major depressive disorder; NS, not significant.

[a]Analyses were performed on the logarithm; subscripts denote significant differences among groups.

mansingh, & Poland, 1999), whereas 5-HT activity is comparatively less in younger subjects (Rao, Lutchmansingh, & Poland, 2000). Therefore, developmental differences in EEG sleep changes observed in individuals with unipolar and bipolar disorders may occur within the context of maturational variations in the neuroregulatory systems controlling sleep. The up-regulated cholinergic systems in youngsters may be more sensitive to the effects of depression, thus fostering REM sleep. If 5-HT input, which is inhibitory to REM sleep, is reduced in youngsters as a consequence of depression, the enhanced cholinergic effects on REM sleep might not be counterbalanced. This could explain the observed REM sleep changes in adolescents with unipolar depression.

5-HT systems also are involved in the regulation of slow-wave sleep. There is evidence that 5-HT_2 receptors, specifically 5-HT_{2A} and 5-HT_{2C} receptor subtypes, are inhibitory to slow-wave sleep (Dugovic & Wauquier, 1987; Sharpley, Elliott, Attenburrow, & Cowen, 1994). 5-HT_{1A} receptors also have an influence on slow-wave sleep, but their effects are dose-dependent. Low doses of 5-HT$_{1A}$ agonists enhance slow-wave sleep (Bjørkum, Bjorvatn, Neckelmann, & Ursin, 1995; Monti & Jantos, 1992; Seifritz et al., 1996), whereas high doses may have the opposite effect (Tissier, Lainey, Fattaccini, Hamon, & Adrien, 1993). Slow-wave sleep may be maintained initially in unipolar depression because of the relatively low 5-HT$_{1A}$ receptor activity. As the illness progresses, it is possible that other changes occur in 5-HT systems, such as increased postsynaptic 5-HT$_2$ receptor sensitivity (Maes & Meltzer, 1995), that might contribute to slow-wave sleep deficits.

Previous neuroendocrine studies with 5-HT agonists have suggested similarities in 5-HT abnormalities in patients with unipolar and bipolar disorders (Coccaro et al., 1989; Nurnberger, Berretini, Simmons-Alling, Lawrence, & Brittain, 1990), as well as similarities between manic and depressive phases of bipolar illness (Meltzer et al., 1984). Recent investigations have found increased postsynaptic 5-HT$_{1A}$ receptor sensitivity in mania, which may be secondary to reduced 5-HT availability in central 5-HT synapses (Maes, Calabrese, Jayathilake, & Meltzer, 1997; Yatham, Shiah, Lam Tam, & Zis, 1999). However, in contrast to the observed changes in depression, presynaptic 5-HT$_{1A}$ receptor sensitivity may be relatively normal in bipolar disorder (Yatham et al., 1999). If it is true that postsynaptic 5-HT$_{1A}$ receptors are highly sensitive in bipolar disorder, this would explain the reduction in slow-wave sleep. Increased 5-HT$_{1A}$ receptor activity also would explain the possible suppression of REM sleep through its input on the pontine cholinergic neurons in a subset of patients (McCarley et al., 1995).

It is important to note that the above discussion on EEG sleep differences between unipolar and bipolar disorders is only speculative, based primarily on data in adult populations. In order to clarify the pathophysiological distinctions between unipolar and bipolar disorders, and also to assess the interactions between the development and the clinical course of these disorders, it is important to conduct controlled longitudinal EEG sleep studies of youth with unipolar and bipolar disorders.

ASSOCIATION OF OTHER BIOLOGICAL RHYTHMS WITH BIPOLAR DISORDER

In addition to sleep changes, alterations in temperature rhythm and in sleep-related neuroendocrine and neuropeptide activity have been reported in adult patients with bipolar illness. Depression is linked to higher mean daily body temperature compared with normal states, with most robust differences occurring during nighttime (Avery et al., 1982; Pflug, Johnsson, & Ekse, 1981; Smallwood, Avery, Paascualy, & Prinz, 1983; Souêtre et al.,

1988; Wehr, 1990). In a longitudinal study of patients with bipolar disorder, Pflug and colleagues (1981) observed higher temperature during the manic phase than during the depressed phase. The temperature rhythm disturbances returned to normal during recovery (Pflug et al., 1981; Souêtre et al., 1988). It is hypothesized that increased REM sleep in the second half of the night could overheat the brain, and this excess brain heat occurring at a critical circadian period might be associated with affective symptoms (Wehr, 1990). Consistent with this hypothesis, sleep phase advancement and sleep deprivation were associated with temperature reduction in subjects with depression (Souêtre et al., 1987; Wehr & Sack, 1981).

Among neuroendocrine measures, the hypothalamic–pituitary–adrenal (HPA) and thyroid axes have been best studied in bipolar disorder. HPA alterations associated with unipolar and bipolar mood disorders include elevated plasma cortisol, increased nocturnal secretion, early timing of cortisol rise, and insensitivity to feedback suppression with dexamethasone administration (Cassidy, Ritchie, & Carroll, 1998; Cookson, Silverstone, Williams, & Besser, 1985; Joyce, Donald, & Elder, 1987; Kiriike et al., 1988; Linkowski et al., 1994; Rybakowski & Twardowska, 1999; Stokes et al., 1984; Thase et al., 1989). Some reports suggest that HPA changes may be less robust in bipolar disorder than in unipolar illness (Christie et al., 1986; Schatzberg et al., 1983; Thase et al., 1989), whereas others have indicated that HPA alterations are, in fact, more marked in patients with bipolar disorder (Rybakowski & Twardowska, 1999). Some investigators have reported that HPA activity correlates more with depression than with mania in patients switching between mania and depression (Cookson, 1985; Joyce et al., 1987; Kennedy, Tighe, McVey, & Brown, 1989).

HPA activity might be related to hyperarousal or to aberrant stress responses (Depue, Kleiman, Davis, Hutchinson, & Krauss, 1985), or may have a nonspecific state-dependent relationship to bipolar disorder (Swann et al., 1990). The clinical significance of increased HPA activity is not clear, but data suggest that patients with depression with elevated cortisol levels do not adequately benefit from psychosocial interventions and may respond better to pharmacotherapy (Barden, Reul, & Holsboer, 1995; Robbins, Alessi, & Colfer, 1989; Thase et al., 1996).

Depression and mania can accompany both hypothyroid and hyperthyroid states (for reviews, see Goodwin & Jamison, 1990; Wehr, Sack, Rosenthal, & Cowdry, 1988). Following its circadian rhythm, plasma levels of TSH are highest at night, although the nocturnal increase is masked by sleep (Parker et al., 1976). One relatively consistent finding is that the nocturnal surge in TSH is blunted or absent during the depressive state in bipolar illness (Sack et al., 1988; Souêtre et al., 1988), which may be secondary to elevated nocturnal temperature. In patients with depression, sleep deprivation produces an increase in nocturnal TSH (Baumgartner & Meinhold, 1986), an effect that may reflect both release from inhibition by sleep and an interruption of REM, with the attendant decrease in brain warming (Sack et al., 1988). In addition to diminished nocturnal TSH levels, blunted TSH response to thyrotropin-releasing hormone has been reported in depressed patients (Loosen & Prange, 1982).

In contrast to the low TSH levels seen in depression, increased plasma TSH has been reported in relation to mania (Haggerty, Sinmon, Evans, & Nemeroff, 1987; Wehr et al., 1988). Thyroid hormones reportedly alter the clinical course of bipolar disorder (Bauer & Whybrow, 1988), potentiate the action of some antidepressant drugs (Goodwin, Prange, Post, Muscettola, & Lipton, 1982), and precipitate mania in some patients (Josephson & MacKenzie, 1980; Wehr & Goodwin, 1987). However, there is also evidence to suggest that thyroid hormones may be helpful in the treatment of manic–depressive illness, particularly in those having rapid-cycling episodes (Cowdry, Wehr, Zis, & Goodwin, 1983).

Among the neuropeptides influenced by circadian systems, melatonin has been investigated well in bipolar disorder. Melatonin synthesis is stimulated through a β-adrenergic receptor located on the pinealocyte membrane, and the secretion is highest at night (Moore & Klein, 1974). Bright light, which activates the retinohypothalamic tract, profoundly inhibits nighttime melatonin secretion (Lewy, Wehr, Goodwin, Newsome, & Markey, 1980). Patients with bipolar disorder were found to be relatively more sensitive to light (Lewy, Wehr, Goodwin, Newsome, & Rosenthal, 1981). Some patients with manic–depressive illness have had manic switches during phototherapy, suggesting a trait or vulnerability marker (Lewy et al., 1985; Schwitzer, Neudorfer, Blecha, & Fleischhacker, 1990).

Research has shown that patients with bipolar disorder or seasonal affective disorder have low baseline plasma melatonin levels and decreased nocturnal suppression compared with patients with unipolar disorder and healthy controls (Lam et al., 1990; Rosenthal et al., 1986; Thompson, Franey, Arendt, & Checkley, 1988). Nocturnal melatonin was found to be lower during the depressed phase and higher during the manic phase in rapidly cycling patients (Kennedy et al., 1989; Lewy et al., 1980). These data are consistent with a relative increase in pineal β-receptor activity in mania and a relative decrease in bipolar depression.

A few neuroendocrine investigations have been performed in child and adolescent subjects with unipolar depression (see Ryan & Dahl, 1993). Basal cortisol and thyroid studies performed in children and adolescents with unipolar depression are provided in Table 10.4 and in Table 10.5, respectively. Only changes in nighttime cortisol secretion have been reported in association with early-onset depression, whereas findings with respect to thyroid studies are variable. To the best of my knowledge, aside from the cited sleep data, no other circadian rhythms have been studied in patients with bipolar disorder.

TABLE 10.4. Baseline Cortisol Studies in Depressed Children and Adolescents

Study	Sample	Age range	Method and time of collection	Nighttime cortisol	Total cortisol
Puig-Antich et al. (1989)	45 MDD; 8 NC	6–12	24-hr plasma samples obtained at 20-min intervals	≅	≅
Dahl et al. (1989)	48 MDD; 40 NC	12–18	24-hr plasma samples obtained at 20-min intervals	≅	≅
Dahl et al. (1991)	27 MDD; 32 NC	12–18	24-hr plasma samples obtained at 20-min intervals	↑	≅
Kutcher et al. (1991)	12 MDD; 12 NC	16–19	Plasma samples obtained at 1, 2, 3, 4, 6, 22, and 24 hrs	↑	≅
Birmaher et al. (1992)	23 MDD; 9 NC	6–12	24-hr plasma samples obtained at 20-min intervals	≅	≅
Goodyer et al. (1996)	82 MDD; 40 NC	8–16	Salivary samples obtained at 8, 12, and 20 hours daily over a 48-hr period	↑	≅

Note. MDD, subjects with major depressive disorder; NC, normal control subjects; ≅, no difference between MDD and NC subjects; ↑, increased in MDD subjects compared with NC subjects.

POTENTIAL AREAS OF INVESTIGATION IN PEDIATRIC BIPOLAR DISORDERS

From the reviewed data in adults, it is apparent that circadian rhythm disturbances are intricately linked to manic–depressive illness. These results suggest that some circadian disturbances are common to both unipolar and bipolar disorders, but important differences also exist. Variations also are present between the depressed and the manic phases of bipolar disorder. From the limited data in youngsters, there is an indication that some developmental differences also may exist. Moreover, certain measures, including EEG sleep variables and hypersensitivity to light, may serve as vulnerability markers.

In attempts to clarify the distinctions between unipolar and bipolar disorder, and to better understand the interrelationships between biological markers and clinical course, we may be better served by studying the pediatric population. The vast majority of child and adolescent subjects with high vulnerability to bipolar disorder can be recruited prior to the onset of illness, or in their first episode, prior to developing other complications. Hence, this group of subjects potentially can be helpful in advancing our knowledge on the pathophysiology of manic–depressive illness, as well as in the assessment of interactions between neurobiological processes and clinical course. A better understanding of such interactions has the potential for developing more effective treatment and preventive strategies for

TABLE 10.5. Baseline Thyroid Studies in Depressed Children and Adolescents

Study	Sample	Age range	Method and time of collection	T4	T3	TSH
Kutcher et al. (1991)	12 MDD; 12 NC	16–19	Plasma samples at 1, 2, 3, 4, 6, 22, and 24 hrs	—	-	≅/↑[a]
Sokolov, Kutcher, & Joffe (1994)	14 MDD; 13 NC	14–20	Plasma samples obtained between 7:00 and 11:00 A.M.	↑	≅	≅
Dorn et al. (1996)	21 MDD; 20 NC	12–16	Plasma samples obtained at 7:30 A.M. and 7:30 P.M.	≅	≅	≅
Dorn et al. (1997)	45 MDD; 56 NC	7–13	Plasma samples obtained at various times of the day, primarily in the afternoon	≅/↓[b]	↓	≅/↓[b]

Note. MDD, subjects with major depressive disorder; NC, normal control subjects; T4, thyroxin; T3, triiodothyroinine; TSH, thyroid stimulating hormone; ≅, no difference between MDD and NC subjects; ↑, increased in MDD subjects compared with NC subjects; ↓, decreased in MDD subjects compared with NC subjects.

[a]No group differences in total or peak TSH secretion; MDD subjects secreted more secretion than NC subjects at 1:00 A.M.

[b]Only MDD boys had significantly less secretion than the controls.

this disorder in youth, and in adults as well. It is also important to note that, by studying the younger population, information prior to illness onset and changes due to clinical course can be obtained within a reasonably short time frame and in a cost-effective manner.

In addition to recruiting youngsters with manifest bipolar illness, it would be fruitful to include patients with unipolar depression when considering investigations of biological rhythms. In addition to facilitating the comparison of these two categories of mood disorders, there is a potential for detecting vulnerability markers for bipolar illness. Up to 20–30% of child and adolescent subjects with depression switch to bipolar disorder (Geller et al., 1994; Strober et al., 1993). Although this presents a challenge with respect to diagnosis and treatment, it can also provide a unique opportunity for gaining knowledge on the etiology and pathophysiology of manic–depressive illness.

In considering the potential areas for investigation, based on data in adults and also based on the available information in youth, sleep appears to be one logical choice. Sleep complaints are common symptoms of both depression and mania. Developmental influence(s) on rates of mood disorders and maturational changes in sleep regulation also imply a close connection between affective disorders and sleep regulation. Mood disorders are relatively rare prior to puberty, but increase dramatically during adolescence (Angold & Rutter, 1992; Giaconia et al., 1994). There is evidence that sleep regulation at younger ages is relatively "protected" against disruptions (Busby & Pivik, 1985; Carskadon, Orav, & Dement, 1983;

Feinberg, 1974; Williams, Karachan, & Hursch,1974). By mid- to late puberty, however, profound changes occur in sleep regulation, with a decrease in the threshold of arousal to disrupt sleep as well as a shift in circadian pattern (Busby, Mercier, & Pivik, 1994; Carskadon et al., 1983; Coble, Kupfer, Taska, & Kane, 1994; Coble, Reynolds, Kupfer, & Houck, 1987; Dahl et al., 1990). EEG sleep changes typically associated with adult depression are rarely seen in prepubertal depression, gradually emerge after puberty, and appear as consistent biological findings in later adolescence (Ryan & Dahl, 1993).

Increased risk for mood disorders during adolescence, vulnerability to perturbation of the sleep system after puberty, and relatively more robust EEG sleep changes in older adolescents suggest a link between sleep dysregulation and increased liability to mood disorders. Data also suggest that the sleep patterns in youth have changed significantly in recent decades as a result of social and occupational demands, resulting in irregular schedules and sleep debt (Wolfson & Carskadon, 1998). There is evidence that disruption of sleep–wake schedules has an adverse effect on functioning in emotional, behavioral, and cognitive domains (Wolfson & Carskadon, 1998). There is also evidence for a secular increase in mood disorders (Klerman et al., 1985; Kovacs & Gatsonis, 1994; Lasch, Weissman, Wickramaratne, & Bruce, 1990; Ryan et al., 1992). All of these factors point to connections among development, sleep regulation, and mood disorders. Hence, longitudinal investigations of sleep–wake rhythms in bipolar disorder potentially can be very fruitful.

In order to better understand the association between sleep regulation and pediatric mood disorders, clinicians and researchers might want to consider whether irregular sleep schedules increase the risk for depressive and/or manic episodes in youngsters with high vulnerability for these disorders. Within patient populations, an important question to consider is whether sleep–wake disturbances precipitate recurrent affective episodes and rapid cycling, and whether such episodes in turn trigger or worsen sleep–wake disruptions. Also, more studies are needed on the therapeutic effects of regular sleep–wake schedules as adjunctive interventions with pharmacological and/ or psychosocial treatments, as well as their effects on clinical course.

The role of extended bed rest and sleep deprivation in unipolar and bipolar disorders, and during manic, depressive, and mixed states, should be assessed systematically. In adult patients, sleep deprivation, prior to or in conjunction with antidepressant treatment, was found to be helpful. This is clinically very relevant for the pediatric group because a substantial minority of youngsters with depression do not respond to traditional antidepressant treatments, and those who do respond initially do not appear to show sustained remission. For investigating the underlying mechanisms of such interventions, laboratory behavioral, sleep, and neuroendocrine studies, as well as the use of pharmacological probes, might be considered.

In conclusion, numerous investigations in adults have shown that sleep–wake cycles and other circadian rhythms are associated with unipolar and bipolar mood disorders. Very limited data in children and adolescents also suggest such relationships. Although there are similarities between unipolar and bipolar disorders, important differences also exist. Also, some maturational effects have been observed. Systematic longitudinal studies of circadian systems in youth with unipolar and bipolar disorders potentially might be helpful in gaining knowledge on the pathophysiology of these disorders and the interactions between clinical course and neurobiological processes. Such knowledge has the potential for developing more effective treatment and preventive strategies for these disorders not only in youngsters, but also in adult patients.

ACKNOWLEDGMENTS

Support for this work was provided by Scientist Development Award No. MH01419 from the National Institute of Mental Health.

REFERENCES

Akerstedt, T., Palmblad, J., de la Torre, B., Marana, R., & Gillberg, M. (1980). Adrenocortical and gonadal steroids during sleep deprivation. *Sleep, 3*(1), 23–30.

Angold, A., & Rutter, M. (1992). Effects of age and pubertal status on depression in a large clinical sample. *Developmental Psychopathology, 4*, 5–28.

Appelboom-Fondu, J., Kerkhofs, M., & Mendlewicz, J. (1988). Depression in adolescents and young adults: Polysomnographic and neuroendocrine aspects. *Journal of Affective Disorders, 14*, 35–40.

Aserinski, E. (1969). The maximum capacity for sleep: Rapid eye motion density as an index of sleep satiety. *Biological Psychiatry, 1*, 147–159.

Avery, D. H., Wilschiodz, G., & Rafaelsen, O. J. (1982). Nocturnal temperature in affective disorder. *Journal of Affective Disorders, 4*, 61–71.

Barbini, B., Bertelli, S., Colombo, C., & Smeraldi, E. (1996). Sleep loss, a possible factor in augmenting manic episode. *Psychiatry Research, 65*, 121–125.

Barbini, B., Colombo, C., Benedetti, F., Campori, E., Bellodi, L., & Smeraldi, E. (1998). The unipolar–bipolar dichotomy and the response to sleep deprivation. *Psychiatry Research, 79*, 43–50.

Barden, N., Reul, J. M. H. M., & Holsboer, F. (1995). Do antidepressants stabilize mood through actions on the hypothalamic–pituitary–adrenocortical system? *Trends in Neurosciences, 18*, 6–11.

Bauer, M. S., & Whybrow, P. C. (1988). Thyroid hormones and the central nervous system in affective illness: Interactions that may have clinical significance. *Integrative Psychiatry, 6*, 75–100.

Baumgartner, A., & Meinhold, H. (1986). Sleep deprivation and thyroid hormone concentrations. *Psychiatry Research, 19*, 241–242.

Baxter, L. R., Liston, E. H., Schwartz, J. M., Altshuler, L. L., Wilkins, J. N., Richeimer, S., & Guze, B. H. (1986). Prolongation of the antidepressant response to partial sleep deprivation by lithium. *Psychiatry Research, 19,* 17–23.

Beersma, D. G. M., Dijk, D. J., & Block, C. G. (1990). REM sleep deprivation during 5 hours leads to an immediate REM sleep rebound and to suppression of NREM sleep intensity. *Electroencephalography and Clinical Neurophysiology, 76,* 114–122.

Beersma, D. G. M., & Van den Hoofdakker, R. H. (1992). Can non-REM sleep be depressogenic? *Journal of Affective Disorders, 24,* 101–108.

Benca, R. M., Obermeyer, W. H., Thisted, R. A., & Gillin, J. C. (1992). Sleep and psychiatric disorders: A meta-analysis. *Archives of General Psychiatry, 49,* 651–668.

Benedetti, F., Barbini, B., Lucca, A., Campori, E., Colombo, C., & Smeraldi, E. (1997). Sleep deprivation hastens the antidepressant action of fluoxetine. *European Archives of Psychiatry and Clinical Neuroscience, 247,* 100–103.

Benedetti, F., Serretti, A., Colombo, C., Campori, E., Barbini, B., di Bella, D., & Smeraldi, E. (1999). Influence of a functional polymorphism within the promoter of the serotonin-transporter gene on the effects of total sleep deprivation in bipolar depression. *American Journal of Psychiatry, 156,* 1450–1452.

Birmaher, B., Ryan, N. D., Dahl, R., Rabinovich, H., Ambrosini, P., Williamson, D. E., Novacenko, H., Nelson, B., Lo, E. S., & Puig-Antich, P. (1992). Dexamethasone suppression test in children with major depressive disorder. *Journal of the American Academy of Child and Adolescent Psychiatry, 31,* 291–297.

Bjørkum, A. A., Bjorvatn, B., Neckelmann, D., & Ursin, R. (1995). Sleep effects following intrathecal administration of the 5–HT$_{1A}$ agonist 8–OH-DPAT and the NMDA antagonist AP-5 in rats. *Brain Research, 692,* 251–258.

Borbély, A. A., & Wirz-Justice, A. (1982). Sleep, sleep deprivation and depression: A hypothesis derived from a model of sleep regulation. *Human Neurobiology, 1*(3), 205–210.

Brunner, D. P., Dijk, D. J., Tobler, I., & Borbély, A. A. (1990). Effect of partial sleep deprivation on sleep stages and EEG power spectra: Evidence for nonREM and REM sleep homeostasis. *Electroencephalography and Clinical Neurophysiology, 75,* 492–499.

Busby, K. A., Mercier, L., & Pivik, R. T. (1994). Ontogenetic variations in auditory arousal threshold during sleep. *Psychophysiology, 31,* 182–188.

Busby, K. A., & Pivik, R. T. (1985). Auditory arousal thresholds during sleep in hyperkinetic children. *Sleep, 8,* 332–341.

Cabeza, R. D. J., Zoltoski, R. K., & Gillin, J. C. (1994). Biochemical pharmacology of sleep. In S. Chokroverty (Ed.), *Sleep disorders medicine* (pp. 37–56). Boston: Butterworth-Heinemann.

Cairns, J., Waldron, J., MacLean, A. W., & Knowles, J. B. (1980). Sleep and depression: A case study of EEG sleep prior to relapse. *Canadian Journal of Psychiatry, 25,* 259–263.

Carskadon, M. A. Orav, E. J., & Dement, W. C. (1983). Evolution of sleep and daytime sleepiness in adolescents. In C. Guilleminault & E. Lugaresi (Eds.), *Sleep/wake disorders: Natural history, epidemiology and long-term evolution* (pp. 201–216). New York: Raven Press.

Cassidy, F., Ritchie, J. C., & Carroll, B. J. (1998). Plasma dexamethasone concentration and cortisol response during manic episodes. *Biological Psychiatry, 43,* 747–754.

Christie, J. E., Whalley, L. J., Dick, H., Blackwood, D. H. R., Blackburn, I. M., & Fink, G. (1986). Raised plasma cortisol concentrations a feature of drug-free psychotics and not specific for depression. *British Journal of Psychiatry, 148,* 58–65.

Coble, P. A., Kupfer, D. J., Taska, L. S., & Kane, J. (1984). EEG sleep of normal healthy children: Part 1. Findings using standard measurement methods. *Sleep,* 7(4), 289–303.

Coble, P. A., Reynolds, C. F., Kupfer, D. J., & Houck, P. (1987). Electroencephalographic sleep of healthy children: Part 2. Findings using automated delta and REM sleep measurement methods. *Sleep, 10,* 551–562.

Cocarro, E. F., Siever, L. J., Klar, H. M., Maurer, G., Cochrane, K., Cooper, T. B., Mohs, R. C., & Davis, K. L. (1989). Serotonergic studies in patients with affective and personality disorders. *Archives of General Psychiatry, 46,* 587–599.

Colombo, C., Benedetti, F., Barbini, B., Campori, E., & Smeraldi, E. (1999). Rate of switch from depression into mania after therapeutic sleep deprivation in bipolar depression. *Psychiatry Research, 86,* 267–270.

Cookson, J. C. (1985). The neuroendocrinology of mania. *Journal of Affective Disorders, 8,* 233–241.

Cookson, J. C., Silverstone, T., Williams, S., & Besser, G. M. (1985). Plasma cortisol levels in mania: Associated clinical ratings and changes during treatment with haloperidol. *British Journal of Psychiatry, 146,* 498–502.

Cowdry, R. W., Wehr, T. A., Zis, A. P., & Goodwin, F. K. (1983). Thyroid abnormalities associated with rapid-cycling bipolar illness. *Archives of General Psychiatry, 40,* 414–420.

Czeisler, C. A., Kronauer, R. E., Mooney, J. J., Anderson, J. L., & Allan, J. S. (1987). Biologic rhythm disorders, depression, and phototheraphy: A new hypothesis. *Psychiatric Clinics of North America, 10,* 687–709.

Dahl, R. E., Puig-Antich, J., Ryan, N. D., Nelson, B., Dachille, S., Cunningham, S. L., Trubnick, L., & Klepper, T. P. (1990). EEG sleep in adolescents with major depression: The role of suicidality and inpatient status. *Journal of Affective Disorders, 19,* 63–75.

Dahl, R. E., Puig-Antich, J., Ryan, N. D., Nelson, B., Novacenko, H., Twomey, J., Williamson, D., Goetz, R., & Ambrosini, P. J. (1989). Cortisol secretion in adolescents with major depressive disorder. *Acta Psychiatrica Scandinavica, 80,* 18–26.

Dahl, R. E., Ryan, N. D., Birmaher, B., Al-Shabbout, M., Williamson, D. E., Neidig, M., Nelson, B., & Puig-Antich, J. (1991). Electroencephalographic sleep measures in prepubertal depression. *Psychiatry Research, 38,* 201–214.

Dahl, R. E., Ryan, N. D., Matty, M. K., Birmaher, B., Al-Shabbout, M., Williamson, D. E., & Kupfer, D. J. (1996). Sleep onset abnormalities in depressed adolescents. *Biological Psychiatry, 39,* 400–410.

Dahl, R. E., Ryan, N. D., Puig-Antich, J., Nguyen, N. G. A., al-Shabbout, M., Meyer, V. A., & Perel, J. (1991). 24-hour cortisol measures in adolescents with major depression: A controlled study. *Biological Psychiatry, 30,* 25–36.

Depue, R. A., Kleiman, R. M., Davis, P., Hutchinson, M., & Krauss, S. P. (1985). The behavioral high-risk paradigm and bipolar affective disorder: Part 8. Serum free cortisol in nonpatient cyclothymic subjects selected by the General Behavioral Inventory. *American Journal of Psychiatry, 142,* 175–181.

Detrinis, R., Harris, J., Allen, R., et al. (1990). Effects of partial sleep deprivation in children with major depression and attention deficit hyperactivity disorder (ADHD). *Sleep Research, 19,* 322.

Dorn, L. D., Burgess, E. S., Dichek, H. L., Putnam, F. W., Chrousos, G. P., & Gold, P. W. (1996). Thyroid hormone concentrations in depressed and nondepressed adolescents: Group differences and behavioral relations. *Journal of the American Academy of Child and Adolescent Psychiatry, 35,* 299–306.

Dorn, L. D., Dahl, R. E., Birmaher, B., Williamson, D. E., Kaufman, J., Frisch, L., Perel, J. M., & Ryan, N. D. (1997). Baseline thyroid hormones in depressed and non-depressed pre- and early-pubertal boys and girls. *Journal of Psychiatric Research, 31,* 555–567.

Dugovic, C., & Wauquier, A. (1987). 5-HT$_2$ receptors could be primarily involved in the regulation of slow-wave sleep in the rat. *European Journal of Pharmacology, 137,* 145–146.

Duncan, W. C., Pettigrew, K. D., & Gillin, J. C. (1979). REM architecture changes in bipolar and unipolar depression. *American Journal of Psychiatry, 11,* 1424–1427.

Emslie, G. J., Rush, A. J., Weinberg, W. A., Rintelmann, J. W., & Roffwarg, H. P. (1990). Children with major depression show reduced rapid eye movement latencies. *Archives of General Psychiatry, 47,* 119–124.

Emslie, G. J., Rush, A. J., Weinberg, W. A., Rintelmann, J. W., & Roffwarg, H. P. (1994). Sleep EEG features of adolescents with major depression. *Biological Psychiatry, 36,* 573–581.

Feinberg, I. (1974). Changes in sleep cycle patterns with age. *Journal of Psychiatric Research, 10,* 283–306.

Feinberg, M., Gillin, J. C., Carroll, B. J., Greden, J. F., & Zis, A. P. (1982). EEG studies of sleep in the diagnosis of depression. *Biological Psychiatry, 17,* 305–316.

Fossion, P., Staner, L., Dramaix, M., Kempenaers, C., Kerkhofs, M., Hubain, P., Verbanck, P., Mendlewicz, J., & Linkowski, P. (1998). Does sleep EEG data distinguish between UP, BPI or BPII major depressions?: An age and gender controlled study. *Journal of Affective Disorders, 49,* 189–187.

Geller, B., Fox, L. W., & Clark, K. A. (1994). Rate and predictors of prepubertal bipolarity during follow-up of 6- to 12-year-old depressed children. *Journal of the American Academy of Child and Adolescent Psychiatry, 33*(4), 461–468.

Giaconia, R. M., Reinherz, H. Z., Silverman, A. B., Pakis, B., Frost, A. K., & Cohen, E. (1994). Ages of onset of psychiatric disorders in a community population of older adolescents. *Journal of the American Academy of Child and Adolescent Psychiatry, 33*(5), 706–717.

Giles, D. E., Rush, A. J., & Roffwarg, H. P. (1986). Sleep parameters in bipolar I, bipolar II, and unipolar depressions. *Biological Psychiatry, 21,* 1340–1343.

Goetz, R. R., Puig-Antich, J., Dahl, R. E., Ryan, N. D., Asnis, G. M., Rabinovich, H., & Nelson, B. (1991). EEG sleep of young adults with major depression: A controlled study. *Journal of Affective Disorders, 22,* 91–100.

Goetz, R. R., Puig-Antich, J., Ryan, N., Rabinovich, H., Ambrosini, P. J., Nelson, B., & Krawiec, V. (1987). Electroencephalographic sleep of adolescents with major depression and normal controls. *Archives of General Psychiatry, 44,* 61–68.

Goodwin, F. K., & Jamison, K. R. (1990). *Manic–depressive illness.* New York: Oxford University Press.

Goodwin, F. K., Prange, A. J., Jr., Post, R. M., Muscettola, G., & Lipton, M. A. (1982). Potentiation of antidepressant effects by L-triiodothyronine in tricyclic nonresponders. *American Journal of Psychiatry, 139,* 34–38.

Goodyer, I. M., Herbert, J., Altham, P. M., Pearson, J., Secher, S. M., & Shiers, H. M (1996). Adrenal secretion during major depression in 8- to 16-year-olds. I. Altered diurnal rhythms in salivary cortisol and dehydroepiandrosterone (DHEA) at presentation. *Psychological Medicine, 26,* 245–256.

Haggerty, J. J., Sinmon, J. S., Evans, D. L., & Nemeroff, C. B. (1987). Relationship of serum TSH concentration and antithyroid antibodies to diagnosis and DST response in psychiatric inpatients. *American Journal of Psychiatry, 144,* 1491–1493.

Harrington, R., Fudge, H., Rutter, M., Pickles, A., & Hill, J. (1990). Adult outcomes of childhood and adolescent depression. *Archives of General Psychiatry, 47,* 465–473.

Hobson, J. A., Lydic, R., & Baghdoyan, H. A. (1986). Evolving concepts of sleep cycle generation: From brain centers to neuronal populations. *Behavior and Brain Sciences, 9,* 371–448.

Horne, J. (1991). Dimensions to sleepiness: In T. H. Monk (Ed.), *Sleep, sleepiness and performance* (pp. 169–196). Chichester, UK: Wiley.

Hudson, J. I., Lipinski, J. F., Frankenburg, F. R., Grochocinski, V. J., & Kupfer, D. J. (1988). Electroencephalographic sleep in mania. *Archives of General Psychiatry, 45,* 267–273.

Janowsky, D. S., el-Yousef, M. D., Davis, J. M., & Sekerke, H. J. (1992). A cholinergic–adrenergic hypothesis of mania and depression. *Lancet, 2,* 632–635.

Janowsky, D. S., Risch, S. C., & Gillin, J. C. (1983). Adrenergic–cholinergic balance and the treatment of affective disorders. *Progress in Neuro-Psychopharmacology and Biological Psychiatry, 7,* 297–307.

Jernajczyk, W. (1986). Latency of eye movement and other REM sleep parameters in bipolar depression. *Biological Psychiatry, 21,* 465–472.

Josephson, A. M., & MacKenzie, T. B. (1980). Thyroxine-induced mania in hypothyroid patients. *British Journal of Psychiatry, 137,* 222–228.

Jovanovic, U. J. (1977). The sleep profile in manic–depressive patients in the depressive phase. *Waking and Sleeping, 1,* 199–210.

Joyce, P. R., Donald, R. A., & Elder, P. A. (1987). Individual differences in plasma cortisol changes during mania and depression. *Journal of Affective Disorders, 12,* 1–5.

Kant, G. J., Genser, S. G., Thorne, D. R., Pfalser, J. L., & Mougey, E. H. (1984). Effects of 72 hour sleep deprivation on urinary cortisol and indices of metabolism. *Sleep, 7(2),* 142–146.

Kasper, S., Moises, H. W., & Beckmann, H. (1983). Dexamethasone suppression test combined with total sleep deprivation in depressed patients. *Psychitrica Clinica, 16(1),* 17–25.

Kennedy, S. H., Tighe, S., McVey, G., & Brown, G. M. (1989). Melatonin and cortisol "switches" during mania, depression, and euthymia in a drug-free bipolar patient. *Journal of Nervous and Mental Disease, 177(5),* 300–303.

Khan, A. M., & Todd, S. (1990). Polysomnographic findings in adolescents with major depression. *Psychiatry Research, 33,* 313–320.

King, B. H., Baxter, L. R., Jr., Stuber, M., & Fish, B. (1987). Therapeutic sleep deprivation for depression in children. *Journal of the American Academy of Child and Adolescent Psychiatry, 26*(6), 928–931.

Kiriike, N., Izumiya, Y., Nishiwaki, S., Maeda, Y., Nagata, T., & Kawakita, Y. (1988). TRH test and DST in schizoaffective mania, mania, and schizophrenia. *Biological Psychiatry, 24,* 415–422.

Klerman, G. L., Lavori, P. W., Rice, J., Reich, T., Endicott, J., Andreasen, N. C., Keller, M. B., & Hirschfield, R. M. (1985). Birth cohort trends in rates of major depressive disorder among relatives of patients with affective disorder. *Archives of General Psychiatry, 42,* 689–693.

Knowles, J. B., Southmayd, S. E., Delva, N., MacLean, A. W., Cairns, J., & Letemendia, F. J. (1979). Five variations of sleep deprivation in a depressed woman. *British Journal of Psychiatry, 135,* 403–410.

Kovacs, M., & Gatsonis, C. (1994). Secular trends in age at onset of major depressive disorder in a clinical sample of children. *Journal of Psychiatric Research, 28,* 319–328.

Kraft, A. M., Willner, P., Gillin, C. G., Janowsky, D., & Neborsky, R. (1984). Changes in thought content following sleep deprivation in depression. *Comprehensive Psychiatry, 25*(3), 283–289.

Kuhs, H. (1985). Dexamethasone suppression test and sleep deprivation in endogenous depression. *Journal of Affective Disorders, 9,* 121–126.

Kuhs, H., Farber, D., Borgstadt, S., Mrosek, S., & Tolle, R. (1996). Amitriptyline in combination with repeated late sleep deprivation versus amitriptyline alone in major depression: A randomized study. *Journal of Affective Disorders, 37,* 31–41.

Kupfer, D. J., & Ehlers, C. L. (1989). Two roads to rapid eye movement latency. *Archives of General Psychiatry, 46,* 945–948.

Kupfer, D. J., Himmelhoch, J. M., Swartzburg, M., Anderson, C., Byck, R., & Detre, T. P. (1972). Hypersomnia in manic-depressive diseases (a preliminary report). *Diseases of the Nervous System, 33*(11), 720–724.

Kupfer, D. J., & Thase, M. E. (1983). The use of the sleep laboratory in the diagnosis of affective disorders. *Psychiatric Clinics of North America, 6,* 3–25.

Kutcher, S., Malkin, D., Silverberg, J., Marton, P., Williamson, P., Malkin, A., Szalai, J., & Katic, M. (1991). Nocturnal cortisol, thyroid stimulating hormone, and growth hormone secretory profiles in depressed adolescents. *Journal of the American Academy of Child and Adolescent Psychiatry, 30,* 407 414.

Kutcher, S., Williamson, P., Marton, P., & Szalai, J. (1992). REM latency in endogenously depressed adolescents. *British Journal of Psychiatry, 161,* 399–402.

Lahmeyer, H. W., Poznanski, E. O., & Bellur, S. (1983). EEG sleep in depressed adolescents. *American Journal of Psychiatry, 140*(9), 1150–1153.

Lam, R. W., Berkowitz, A. L., Berga, S. L., Clark, C. M., Kripke, D. F., & Gillin, J. C. (1990). Melatonin suppression in bipolar and unipolar mood disorders. *Psychiatry Research, 33,* 129–134.

Lasch, K., Weissman, M., Wickramaratne, P., & Bruce, M. L. (1990). Birth-cohort changes in the rates of mania. *Psychiatry Research, 33,* 31–37.

Leibenluft, E., Albert, P. S., Rosenthal, N. E., & Wehr, T. A. (1996). Relationship between sleep and mood in patients with rapid-cycling bipolar disorder. *Psychiatry Research, 63,* 161–168.

Leibenluft, E., & Wehr, T. A. (1992). Is sleep deprivation useful in the treatment of depression? *American Journal of Psychiatry, 149,* 159–168.

Lewy, A. J., Nurnberger, J. I., Wehr, T. A., Pack, D., Becker, L. E., Powell, R.-L., & Newsome, D. A. (1985). Supersensitivity to light: Possible trait marker for manic–depressive illness. *American Journal of Psychiatry, 142,* 725–727.

Lewy, A. J., Wehr, T. A., Goodwin, F. K., Newsome, D. A., & Markey, S. P. (1980). Light suppresses melatonin secretion in humans. *Science, 210,* 1267–1269.

Lewy, A. J., Wehr, T. A., Goodwin, F. K., Newsome, D. A., & Rosenthal, N. E. (1981). Manic–depressive patients may be supersensitive to light [Letter]. *Lancet, 1,* 383–384.

Linkowski, P., Kerkhofs, M., Van Onderbergen, A., Hubain, P., Copinschi, G., L'Hermite-Balériaux, M., Leclercq, R., Brasseur, M., Mendlewicz, J., & Van Cauter, E. (1994). The 24–hour profiles of cortisol, prolactin, and growth hormone secretion in mania. *Archives of General Psychiatry, 51,* 616–624.

Loosen, P. T., & Prange, A. J., Jr. (1982). Serum thyrotopin response to thyrotropin-releasing hormone in psychiatric patients: A review. *American Journal of Psychiatry, 139,* 405–416.

Maes, M., Calabrese, J., Jayathilake, K., & Meltzer, H. Y. (1997). Effects of subchronic treatment with valproate on L-5–HTP-induced cortisol responses in mania: Evidence for increased central serotonergic neurotransmission. *Psychiatry Research, 71,* 67–76.

Maes, M., & Meltzer, H. Y. M. (1995). The serotonin hypothesis of major depression. In F. E. Bloom & D. J. Kupfer (Eds.), *Psychopharmacology, the fourth generation of progress* (pp. 933–944). New York: Raven Press.

McCarley, R. W., Greene, R. W., Rainnie, D., & Portas, C. M. (1995). Brainstem neuromodulation and REM sleep. *Neuroscience/Seminars in Neuroscience, 7,* 341–354.

McCarley, R. W., & Hobson, J. A. (1975). Discharge patterns of cat pontine brain stem neurons during desynchronized sleep. *Journal of Neurophysiology, 38*(4), 751–766.

Meltzer, H. Y., Umberkoman-Wiita, B., Robertson, A., Tricou, B. J., Lowy, M., & Perline, R. (1984). Effect of a 5–hydroxytrytophan on serum cortisol levels in major affective disorders: Part 1. Enhanced response in depression and mania. *Archives of General Psychiatry, 41,* 366–374.

Monti, J. M., & Jantos, H. (1992). Dose-dependent effects of the $5-HT_{1A}$ receptor against 8–OH-DPAT on sleep and wakefulness in the rat. *Journal of Sleep Research, 1,* 169–175.

Moore, R. Y., & Klein, D. C. (1974). Visual pathways and the central neural control of a circadian rhythm in pineal serotonin N-acetyltransferase activity. *Brain Research, 71,* 17–33.

Moore-Ede, M. E., Silzman, F. M., & Fuller, C. A. (1982). *The clocks that time us: Physiology of the circadian timing system.* Cambridge, MA: Harvard University Press.

Nasarallah, H. A., Kuperman, S., & Coryell, W. (1980). Reversal of dexamethasone nonsuppression with sleep deprivation in primary depression. *American Journal of Psychiatry, 137,* 1463–1464.

Naylor, M. W., King, C. A., Lindsay, K. A., Evans, T., Armelagos, J., Shain, B. N., & Greden, J. F. (1993). Sleep deprivation in depressed adolescents and psychiatric controls. *Journal of the American Academy of Child and Adolescent Psychiatry, 32*(4), 753–759.

Nurnberger, J. I., Jr., Berrettini, W. H., Simmons-Alling, S., Lawrence, D., & Brittain, H. (1990). Blunted ACTH and cortisol response to afternoon tryptophan infusion in euthymic bipolar patients. *Psychiatry Research, 31*, 57–67.

Parker, D. C., Pekary, A. E., & Hershman, J. M. (1976). Effect of normal and reversed sleep–wake cycles upon nocturnal rhythmicity of plasma thyrotropin: Evidence suggestive of an inhibitory influence in sleep. *Journal of Clinical Endocrinology and Metabolism, 43*, 318–329.

Pflug, B., Johnsson, A., & Ekse, A. T. (1981). Manic–depressive states and daily temperature: Some circadian studies. *Acta Psychiatrica Scandinavica, 63*(3), 277–289.

Philipp, M., & Werner, C. (1979). Prediction of lofepramine-response in depression based on response to partial sleep deprivation. *Pharmacopsychiatry, 12*, 346–348.

Post, R. M., Stoddard, F. J., Gillin, J. C., Buchsbaum, M. S., Runkle, D. C., Black, K. E., & Bunney, W. E., Jr. (1977). Alterations in motor activity, sleep, and biochemistry in a cycling manic-depressive patient. *Archives of General Psychiatry, 34*, 470–477.

Prévot, E., Maudhuit, C., Le Poul, E., Hamon, M., & Adrien, J. (1996). Sleep deprivation reduces the citalopram-induced inhibition of serotoninergic neuronal firing in the nucleus raphé dorsalis of the rat. *Journal of Sleep Research, 5*, 238–245.

Puig-Antich, J., Dahl, R., Ryan, N., Novacenko, H., Goetz, D., Goetz, R., & Klepper, T. (1989). Cortisol secretion in prepubertal children with major depressive disorder: Episode and recovery. *Archives of General Psychiatry, 46*, 801 809.

Puig-Antich, J., Goetz, R., Hanlon, C., Davies, M., Thompson, J., Chambers, W. J., Tabrizi, M. A., & Weitzman, E. D. (1982). Sleep architecture and REM sleep measures in prepubertal children with major depression: A controlled study. *Archives of General Psychiatry, 39*(8), 932–939.

Rao, U., Dahl, R. E., Ryan, N. D., Birmaher, B., Williamson, D. E., Giles, D. E., Rao, R., Kaufman, J., & Nelson, B. (1996). The relationship between longitudinal clinical course and sleep and cortisol changes in adolescent depression. *Biological Psychiatry, 40*, 474–484.

Rao, U., Dahl, R. E., Ryan, N. D., Birmaher, B., Williamson, D. E., Rao, R., & Kaufman, J. (2002). Heterogeneity in EEG sleep findings in adolescent depression: Unipolar versus bipolar clinical course. *Journal of Affective Disorders, 70*, 273–280.

Rao, U., Lutchmansingh, P., & Poland, R. E. (1999). Age-related effects of scopolamine on REM sleep regulation in normal control subjects: Relationship to sleep abnormalities in depression. *Neuropsychopharmacology, 21*(6), 723–730.

Rao, U., Lutchmansingh, P., & Poland, R. E. (2000). Contribution of development to buspirone effects on REM sleep: A preliminary report. *Neuropharmacology, 22*(4), 440–446.

Reppert, S. M., Weaver, D. R., Rivkees, S. A., & Stopa, E. G. (1988). Putative melatonin receptors in a human biological clock. *Science, 242*, 78–81.

Riemann, D., Hohagen, F., Konig, A., Schwarz, B., Gomille, J., & Voderholzer, U. (1996). Advanced vs. normal sleep timing: Effects of depressed mood after response to sleep deprivation in patients with a major depressive disorder. *Journal of Affective Disorders, 37,* 121–128.

Riemann, D., Kammerer, J., Löw, H., & Schmidt, M. H. (1995). Sleep in adolescents with primary major depression and schizophrenia: A pilot study. *Journal of Child Psychology and Psychiatry, 36,* 313–326.

Robbins, D. R., Alessi, N. E., & Colfer, M. V. (1989). Treatment of adolescents with major depression: Implications of the DST and the melancholic clinical subtype. *Journal of Affective Disorders 17,* 99–104.

Rosenthal, N. E., Sack, D. A., Jacobsen, F. M., James, S. P., Parry, B. L., Arendt, J., Tamarkin, L., & Wehr, T. A. (1986). Melatonin in seasonal affective disorder and phototherapy. *Journal of Neural Transmission, 21,* 257–267.

Rubin, R. T., & Poland, R. E. (1982). The chronoendocrinology of endogenous depression. In E. E. Müller & R. M. MacLeod (Eds.), *Neuroendocrine perspectives* (Vol. 1, pp. 305–337). New York: Elsevier Biomedical Press.

Ryan, N. D., & Dahl, R. E. (1993). The biology of depression in children and adolescents. In J. J. Mann & D. J. Kupfer (Eds.), *Biology of depressive disorders: Part B. Subtypes of depression and comorbid disorders* (pp. 37–58). New York: Plenum Press.

Ryan, N. D., Williamson, D. E., Iyengar, S., Orvaschel, H., Reich, T., Dahl, R. E., & Puig-Antich, J. (1992). A secular increase in child and adolescent onset affective disorder. *Journal of the American Academy of Child and Adolescent Psychiatry, 31*(4), 600–605.

Rybakowski, J. K., & Twardowska, K. (1999). The dexamethasone/corticotropin-releasing hormone test in depression in bipolar and unipolar affective illness. *Journal of Psychiatric Research, 33,* 363–370.

Sack, D. A, James, S. P., Rosenthal, N. E., & Wehr, T. A. (1988). Deficient nocturnal surge of TSH secretion during sleep and sleep deprivation in rapid-cycling bipolar illness. *Psychiatry Research, 23,* 179–191.

Sack, D. A., Nurnburger, J., Rosenthal, N. E., Ashburn, E., & Wehr, T. A. (1985). The potentiation of antidepressant medications by phase-advance of the sleep–wake cycle. *American Journal of Psychiatry, 142,* 606–608.

Scanlon, M. F., & Hall, R. (1989). Thyroid-stimulating hormone: Synthesis, control of release, and secretion. In L. J. DeGroot, G. M. Besser, G. F. Cahill, J. C. Marshall, D. H. Nelson, W. D. Odell, J. T. Potts, Jr., A. H. Rubenstein, & E. Steinberger (Eds.), *Endocrinology* (Vol. 1, pp. 377–383). Philadelphia: Saunders.

Schatzberg, A. F., Rothschild, A. J., Stahl, J. B., Bond, T. C., Rosenbaum, A. H., Lofgren, S. B., MacLaughlin, R. A., Sullivan, M. A., & Cole, J. O. (1983). The dexamethasone suppression test: Identification of subtypes of depression. *American Journal of Psychiatry, 140,* 88–91.

Schilgen, B., & Tolle, R. (1980). Partial sleep deprivation as therapy for depression. *Archives of General Psychiatry, 37,* 267–271.

Schwitzer, J., Neudorfer, C., Blecha, H. G., & Fleischhacker, W. W. (1990). Mania as a side effect of phototherapy. *Biological Psychiatry, 28,* 532–534.

Seifritz, E., Moore, P., Trachsel, L., Bhatti, T., Stahl, S. M., & Gillin, C. (1996). The 5–HT$_{1A}$ agonist ipsapirone enhances EEG slow-wave activity in human sleep and produces a power spectrum similar to $5-HT_2$ blockade. *Neuroscience Letters, 209,* 41–44.

Sharpley, A. L., Elliott, J. M., Attenburrow, M. J., & Cowen, P. J. (1994). Slow wave sleep in humans: Role of $5-HT_{2A}$ and $5-HT_{2C}$ receptors. *Neuropharmacology, 33,* 467–471.

Shelton, R. C., & Loosen, P. T. (1993). Sleep deprivation accelerates the response to nortriptyline. *Progress in Neuro-Psychopharmacology and Biological Psychiatry, 17(1),* 113–123.

Sitaram, N., Nurnberger, J. I., Jr., Gershon, E. S., & Gillin, J. C. (1982). Cholinergic regulation of mood and REM sleep: Potential model and marker of vulnerability to affective disorder. *American Journal of Psychiatry, 139(5),* 571–576.

Smallwood, R. G., Avery, D. H., Paascualy, R. A., & Prinz, P. N. (1983). Circadian temperature rhythms in primary depression. *Sleep Research, 12,* 215.

Smeraldi, E., Benedetti, F., Barbini, B., Campori, E., & Colombo, C. (1999). Sustained antidepressant effect of sleep deprivation combined with pindolol in bipolar depression. *Neuropsychopharmacology, 20(4),* 380–385.

Smeraldi, E., Zanardi, R., Benedetti, F., Di Bella, D., Perez, J., & Catalano, M. (1998). Polymorphism within the promoter of the serotonin transporter gene and antidepressant efficacy of fluvoxamine. *Molecular Psychiatry, 3(6),* 508–511.

Solokov, T. H. S, Kutcher, S. P., & Joffe, R. T. (1994). Basal thyroid indices in adolescent depression and bipolar disorder. *Journal of the American Academy of Child and Adolescent Psychiatry, 33,* 469–475.

Souêtre, E., Salvati, E., Pringuey, D., Plasse, Y., Savelli, M., & Darcourt G. (1987). Antidepressant effects of the sleep/wake cycle phase advance. *Journal of Affective Disorders, 12,* 41–46.

Souêtre, E., Salvati, E., Wehr, T. A., Sack, D. A., Krebs, B., & Darcourt, G. (1988). Twenty-four-hour profiles of body temperature and plasma TSH in bipolar patients during depression and during remission and in normal control subjects. *American Journal of Psychiatry, 145,* 1133–1137.

Sokolski, K. N., & DeMet, E. M. (2000). Cholinergic sensitivity predicts severity of mania. *Psychiatry Research, 95,* 195–200.

Stokes, P. E., Stroll, P. M., Koslow, S. H., Maas, J. W., Davis, J. M., Swann, A. C., & Robins, E. (1984). Pretreatment DST and hypothalamic–pituitary–adrenocortical function in depressed patients and comparison groups. *Archives of General Psychiatry, 41,* 257–267.

Strober, M., & Carlson, G. (1982). Bipolar illness in adolescents with major depression. *Archives of General Psychiatry, 39,* 549–555.

Strober, M., Lampert, C., Schmidt, S., & Morrell, W. (1993). The course of major depressive disorder in adolescents: Part 1. Recovery and risk of manic switching in a follow-up of psychotic and nonpsychotic subtypes. *Journal of the American Academy of Child and Adolescent Psychiatry, 32(1),* 34–42.

Surridge-David, M., MacLean, A., Coulter, M., & Knowles, J. B. (1987). Mood change following an acute delay of sleep. *Psychiatry Research, 22(2),* 149–158. (Published erratum appears in *Psychiatry Research, 24(1),* 121.)

Swann, A. C., Secunda, S. K., Stokes, P. E., Croughan, J., Davis, J. M., Koslow, S. H., & Maas, J. W. (1990). Stress, depression, and mania: Relationship between perceived role of stressful events and clinical and biochemical characteristics. *Acta Psychiatrica Scandinavica, 81*(4), 389–397.

Szuba, M. P., Baxter, L. R., Jr., Altshuler, L. L., Allen, E. M., Guze, B. H., Schartz, J. M., & Liston, E. H. (1994). Lithium sustains the acute antidepressant effects of sleep deprivation: Preliminary findings from a controlled study. *Psychiatry Research, 51*(3), 283–295.

Thase, M. E., Dubé, S., Bowler, K., Howland, R. H., Myers, J. E., Friedman, E., & Jarrett, B. B. (1996). Hypothalamic–pituitary–adrenocortical activity and response to cognitive behavior therapy in unmedicated hospitalized depressed patients. *American Journal of Psychiatry, 153*, 886–891.

Thase, M. E., Himmelhoch, J. M., Mallinger, A. G., Jarrett, D. B., & Kupfer, D. J. (1989). Sleep EEG and DST findings in anergic bipolar depression. *American Journal of Psychiatry, 146*, 329–333.

Thompson, C., Franey, C., Arendt, J., & Checkley, S. A. (1988). A comparison of melatonin secretion in depressed patients and normal subjects. *British Journal of Psychiatry, 152*, 260–265.

Tissier, M. H., Lainey, E., Fattaccini, C. M., Hamon, M., & Adrien, J. (1993). Effects of ipsapirone, a 5-HT$_{1A}$ agonist, on sleep wakefulness cycles: Probably post-synaptic action. *Journal of Sleep Research, 2*, 103–109.

Van den Burg, W., Beersma, D. G. M., Bouhuys, A. L., & Van den Hoofdakker, R. H. (1992). Self-rated arousal concurrent with the antidepressant response to total sleep deprivation of the patients with a major depressive disorder: A disinhibition hypothesis. *Journal of Sleep Research, 1*, 211–222.

Van den Hoofdakker, R. H. (1997). Total sleep deprivation: Clinical and theoretical aspects. In A. V. Honig & H. M. Praag (Eds.), *Depression: Neurobiological, psychopathological and therapeutic advances* (pp. 564–589) Chichester, UK: Wiley.

Vogel, G. W., Vogel, F., McAbee, R. S., & Thurmond, A. J. (1980). Improvement of depression by REM sleep deprivation: New findings and a theory. *Archives of General Psychiatry, 37*, 247–253.

Wehr, T. A. (1977). Phase and biorhythm studies of affective illness. *Annals of Internal Medicine, 87*, 319–335.

Wehr, T. A. (1990). Effects of wakefulness and sleep on depression and mania. In J. Montplaisir & R. Godbout (Eds.), *Sleep and biological rhythms* (pp. 42–86). New York: Oxford University Press.

Wehr, T. A., & Goodwin, F. K. (1987). Can antidepressants cause mania and worsen the course of affective illness? *American Journal of Psychiatry, 144*, 1402–1411.

Wehr, T. A., Goodwin, F. K., Wirz-Justice, A., Breitmaier, J., & Craig, C. (1982). Forty-eight-hour sleep–wake cycles in manic–depressive illness: Naturalistic observations and sleep deprivation experiments. *Archives of General Psychiatry, 39*, 559–565.

Wehr, T. A., & Sack, D. A. (1981). Neuroendocrine/thermoregulatory mechanisms of sleep deprivation therapy. In W. P. Koella (Ed.), *Proceedings of the 6th European Congress on Sleep Research, Amsterdam* (pp. 384–406). Basel, Switzerland: Karger.

Wehr, T. A., Sack, D. A., & Rosenthal, N. E. (1987). Sleep reduction as a final common pathway in the genesis of mania. *American Journal of Psychiatry, 144*, 201–204.

Wehr, T. A., Sack, D. A., Rosenthal, N. E., & Cowdry, R. W. (1988). Rapid cycling affective disorder: Contributing factors and treatment responses in 51 patients. *American Journal of Psychiatry, 145*, 179–184.

Wehr, T. A., Turner, E. H., Shimada, J. M., Lowe, C. H., Barker, C., & Leibenluft, E. (1998). Treatment of a rapidly cycling bipolar patient by using extended bed rest and darkness to stabilize the timing and duration of sleep. *Biological Psychiatry, 43*, 822–828.

Wehr, T. A., & Wirz-Justice, A. (1981). Internal coincidence model for sleep deprivation and depression. *Sleep, 80*, 26–33.

Wehr, T. A., & Wirz-Justice, A. (1982). Circadian rhythm mechanisms in affective illness and in antidepressant drug action. *Pharmacopsychiatry, 15*, 31–39.

Wehr, T. A., Wirz-Justice, A., Goodwin, F. K., Duncan, W., & Gillin, J. C. (1979). Phase-advance of the circadian sleep–wake cycle as an antidepressant. *Science, 206*, 710–713.

Weissman, M. M., Wolk, S., Goldstein, R. B., Moreau, D., Adams, P., Greenwald, S., Klier, C. M., Ryan, N. D., Dahl, R. E., & Wickramaratne, P. (1999). Depressed adolescents grown up. *Journal of the American Medical Association, 281*, 1707–1713.

Weissman, M., Wolk, S., Wickramaratne, P., Goldstein, R. B., Adams, P., Greenwald, S., Ryan, N. D., Dahl, R. E., & Steinberg, D. (1999). Children with prepubertal-onset major depressive disorder and anxiety grown up. *Archives of General Psychiatry, 56*, 794–801.

Weitzman, E. D., Nogeire, C., Perlow, M., Fukushima, D., Sassin, J., McGregor, P., Gallagher, T. F., & Hellman, L. (1974). Effects of a prolonged 3–hour sleep–wake cycle on sleep stages, plasma cortisol, growth hormone and body temperature in man. *Journal of Clinical Endocrinology and Metabolism, 38*, 1018–1030.

Weitzman, E. D., Pukushima, D., Nogeire, C., Roffwarg, H., Gallagher, T. F., & Hellman, L. (1971). Twenty-four hour pattern of the episodic secretion of cortisol in normal subjects. *Journal of Clinical Endocrinology and Metabolism, 33*(1), 14–22.

Wiegand, M., Berger, M., Zulley, J., Lauer, C., & von Zerssen, D. (1987). The influence of daytime naps on the therapeutic effect of sleep deprivation. *Biological Psychiatry, 22*, 386–389.

Williams, R. L., Karachan, I., & Hursch, C. J. (1974). *Electroencephalography (EEG) of human sleep: Clinical applications.* New York: Wiley.

Wirz-Justice, A., Quinto, C., Cajochen, C., Werth, E., & Hock, C. (1999). A rapid-cycling bipolar patient treated with long nights, bed rest, and light. *Biological Psychiatry, 45*, 1075–1077.

Wirz-Justice, A., & Van den Hoofdakker, R. H. (1999). Sleep deprivation in depression: What do we know, where do we go? *Biological Psychiatry, 46*, 445–453.

Wolfson, A. R., & Carskadon, M. A. (1998). Sleep schedules and daytime functioning in adolescents. *Child Development, 69*, 875–887.

Wu, J. C., & Bunney, W. E. (1990). The biological basis of an antidepressant response to sleep deprivation: Review and hypothesis. *American Journal of Psychiatry, 147*, 14–21.

Yatham, L. N., Shiah, I., Lam, R. W., Tam, E. M., & Zis, A. P. (1999). Hypothermic, ACTH, and cortisol responses to ipsapirone in patients with mania and healthy controls. *Journal of Affective Disorders, 54*, 295–301.

Young, W., Knowles, J. B., MacLean, A. W., Boag, L., & McConville, B. J. (1982). The sleep of childhood depressives: Comparison with age-matched controls. *Biological Psychiatry, 17*, 1163–1168.

Zanardi, R., Benedetti, F., Di Bella, D., Catalano, M., & Smeraldi, E. (1999). Efficacy of paroxetine in depression is influenced by a functional polymorphism within the promoter of the serotonin transporter gene. *Journal of Clinical Psychopharmacology, 20*(1), 105–107.

11

The Genetics of Bipolar Disorder

Judith A. Badner

The genetics of bipolar disorder has been studied for many years. Most of these studies involve adult-onset bipolar disorder, but in recent years childhood-onset bipolar disorder has also been studied. There are several different methods to study whether genetic factors are important to the development of a trait. *Family studies* can determine if there are familial factors that increase the rate of a trait in relatives of individuals with the trait, but they cannot determine whether these familial factors are genetic or part of the shared environment. *Twin and adoption studies* can help separate out genetic factors from shared environmental factors. *Segregation analysis* can test the fit of specific genetic models to the pattern of transmission of a trait within families.

FAMILY STUDIES

A family study is a case–control study of the proportion of individuals with the trait among relatives of cases as compared to the proportion among relatives of controls. If the proportion is significantly higher in relatives of cases, that suggests that the trait is at least partly genetic, although shared nongenetic factors cannot be ruled out. Family studies can also show if other traits occur more frequently in relatives of cases versus controls (e.g., depression in relatives of individuals with bipolar disorder). A positive finding suggests that the second trait may be caused by similar familial factors as the first trait.

Several studies have shown an increase of affective disorders in relatives of cases as compared with controls (Gershon et al., 1982; Tsuang, Faraone, & Fleming, 1985; Weissman et al., 1984). Studies indicate that bipolar disorder, schizoaffective disorder, and unipolar depression are increased in the relatives of bipolar probands, with unipolar depression having the highest prevalence among the relatives. Among the relatives of unipolar depressed probands, the prevalence of unipolar depression is increased. Bipolar disorder is also increased but not to the same degree found in relatives of bipolar probands. This suggests a partial overlap in genetic factors for bipolar disorder and unipolar depression.

The interaction between the age of onset in bipolar probands and the probability of affective disorder has been studied. Simpson, Folstein, Meyers, and DePaulo (1992) showed that in families selected for the presence of a bipolar I proband and at least one affectively ill sib, *bilineality*, the presence of affective illness in the nonoffspring relatives of both parents, was associated with a younger age of onset in the affected sibs and the affected sibs were more likely to have recurrent unipolar depression (rather than schizoaffective–manic, bipolar I, or bipolar II disorder) and to have significantly fewer symptoms in the most severe depressive episode. In this study, families with two affectively ill parents were not studied. McMahon et al. (1994) studied families with a bipolar I proband and at least two siblings with diagnoses of bipolar I, bipolar II, or recurrent unipolar depression. Age of onset for bipolar I and bipolar II ranged from 5 to 60 years and was significantly earlier than recurrent unipolar depression, for which the age of onset ranged from 10 to 60. Significant risks factors for earlier age of onset were bilineality, diagnosis, and gender.

Strober (1992) summarized several studies that looked at the probability of affective disorder in first-degree relatives by the age of onset of the proband. For bipolar probands, when the cutoff was 30, 40, or 50 years, 4/4, 2/3, and 1/1 studies, respectively, showed increased likelihood of affectively ill relatives in the families of probands with younger ages of onset. A similar pattern was found for unipolar depressed probands. Schürhoff and colleagues (2000) ascertained 210 probands, of which 58 had age of onset before 18 years (early onset) and 39 had age of onset after 40 years (late onset). The prevalence of bipolar disorder was greater in the relatives of the early-onset group and there was no difference in the rate of unipolar depression in the early-onset group versus the late-onset group. The early-onset group also had more psychotic symptoms, had more mixed episodes, were more likely to have panic disorder, and were less likely to respond to lithium as compared with the late-onset group.

There have been many studies of families of probands with childhood onset of affective disorders. Most of these studies compare the rate of affective illness in the relatives with the rate of affective illness in relatives of children without psychiatric illness or with a different psychiatric illness. Puig-Antich and colleagues (1989) studied families of probands with prepubertal unipolar depression and families of nonill controls. They found an increase in the rate of unipolar depression, depressive spectrum disorders, and "other psychiatric" disorders in the first- and second-degree relatives of ill probands. Second-degree relatives also had an increase in alcoholism. There was no increase of mania or substance abuse in relatives of cases versus controls. Todd, Neuman, Geller, Fox, and Hickok (1993) studied 76 unipolar depressed probands for 2 to 5 years, during which time eight developed bipolar I disorder and 14 developed bipolar II disorder. Family history information was collected on first- and second-degree relatives and first cousins (of at least 15 years of age) of probands and unaffected controls with no affective illness in parents. Unipolar depression was increased in relatives of bipolar and unipolar depressed probands versus controls. Bipolar disorder was increased in first cousins of bipolar and unipolar depressed probands versus controls. There was no difference in the prevalence of bipolar disorder and unipolar depression in the relatives of bipolar probands versus unipolar depressed probands. In the same sample, Todd and colleagues (1996) also found an increased rate of alcoholism in relatives of bipolar and unipolar depressed probands as compared with controls. Wozniak, Biederman, Mundy, Mennin, and Faraone (1995) studied the families of probands with bipolar disorder (age no older than 12 years), probands with attention-deficit/hyperactivity disorder and no bipolar disorder, and unaffected controls. Of the 16 probands with bipolar disorder, 15 also met criteria for attention-deficit/hyperactivity disorder. There was an increased rate of bipolar disorder, attention-deficit/hyperactivity disorder, and unipolar depression in relatives of bipolar probands as compared with controls. There was an increased rate of attention-deficit/ hyperactivity disorder and unipolar depression in relatives of attention-deficit/hyperactivity disorder probands as compared with controls. Bipolar disorder was increased in relatives of bipolar probands as compared with relatives of attention-deficit/hyperactivity disorder probands.

Chang, Steiner, and Ketter (2000) looked at the children of families in which either one or both parents had bipolar disorder. The children had an average age of 11.1 years at the time of the study. There was a nonsignificant trend for bipolar disorder in the offspring to be associated with earlier age of onset in the parents as compared with nonill offspring but not with offspring with other illnesses. Bipolar disorder in the offspring was not associated with an increased rate of affective illness in relatives nor with lineality. Parents with bipolar disorder and a childhood history of attention-deficit/hyperactivity disorder were more likely to have a child with bipolar disorder but not a child with attention-deficit/hyperactivity disorder.

Neuman, Geller, Rice, and Todd (1997) compared the rate of affective illness in first-degree relatives of probands with prepubertal-onset bipolar disorder or unipolar depression versus probands with adult onset of these mood disorders. Family history information was obtained on first-degree relatives in both groups. Relatives of probands with prepubertal bipolar disorder were more likely to develop bipolar disorder or unipolar depression than relatives of probands with adult-onset bipolar disorder. Similarly, bipolar disorder and unipolar depression were increased in the relatives of probands with childhood-onset unipolar depression as compared with adult-onset unipolar depressed probands or adult-onset bipolar probands. This was true even when the birth cohort of the relatives was controlled for.

TWIN STUDIES

If family studies show an increase in the prevalence of a trait in relatives of cases as compared with relatives of controls, this may be due to the effects of susceptibility genes and/or familial nongenetic factors (such as shared environment). Identifying cases who are also part of a twinship and comparing the concordance of a trait among the monozygotic (i.e., identical) twins with the concordance among dizygotic (i.e., nonidentical) twins is a way of separating out the influence of genetics versus shared family environment. If the concordance is significantly higher among monozygotic twins, this suggests that genetic factors contribute to the development of the trait. *Heritability*, the percentage of phenotypic variation due to genetic variation, which can be estimated from twin studies, is a measure of the importance of genetic factors.

For affective illness, several studies have shown increased concordance among monozygotic twins as compared with dizygotic twins (Allen, 1976; Bertelsen, Harvald, & Hauge, 1977; Cardno et al., 1999; Kendler, Pedersen, Johnson, Neale, & Mathe, 1993). When one twin has bipolar disorder, the concordance rate, using narrow diagnostic criteria, ranges from 50% to 67% for monozygotic twins and from 17% to 24% for dizygotic twins. When broad diagnostic criteria are used for the second twin, the concordance range is 70–87% and 35–37% for monozygotic and dizygotic twins, respectively.

Estimates of heritability from twin studies for bipolar disorder range from 64% to 85% (Cardno et al., 1999; Kendler, Pedersen, Neale, & Mathe, 1995). Concordance for monozygotic twins is higher when one twin has bipolar disorder than when one twin has unipolar depression. Some twins are concordant for polarity (both bipolar or both unipolar) and some twins are discordant for polarity (one bipolar and one unipolar). This finding suggests that there are genetic factors in common for bipolar disorder and unipolar depression and that there are other factors unique to each disorder. The fact that the monozygotic concordance rate is not 100% suggests that genetic factors are not the only important factors in the development of bipolar disorder.

ADOPTION STUDIES

Another way of separating genetic and shared environmental influences is to look at adoption data. This can be done by comparing the frequency of the trait at issue in biological relatives of adoptees with the frequency of the trait in adoptive relatives of the adoptee. However, this method may be subject to biases when looking for psychiatric or medical disorders because the careful screening of adoptive parents in adoption placements would lead to a lower rate of these disorders in adoptive parents as compared with parents in the general population (Clerget-Darpoux, Goldin, & Gershon, 1986). However, comparing the incidence of illness in biological relatives of proband adoptees with the incidence of illness in biological relatives of control adoptees would not be subject to such biases.

Mendlewicz and Rainer (1977) observed affective disorder in a significantly higher proportion of biological parents than of adoptive parents of bipolar adoptee probands and in the biological and adoptive parents of control probands. Wender and colleagues (1986) observed an increase in suicide of biological relatives of probands with affective disorder as compared with adoptive relatives of these probands and biological and adoptive relatives of control adoptees. However, a significant increase of affective illness in biological relatives of affectively ill probands was not observed in this study, a finding that may be due to the exclusive reliance on medical records for diagnosis rather than also using direct interview and family history.

SEGREGATION ANALYSIS

Segregation analysis is a means of studying the pattern of transmission of a disease or trait within families and determining the mode of inheritance. It can be used to determine if a single locus is involved and whether the mode of inheritance of this single locus is dominant, recessive, or additive.

Segregation analysis has been applied to affective disorders (Goldin, Gershon, Targum, Sparkes, & McGinniss, 1983; Sham, Morton, & Rice, 1992; Tsuang, Bucher, Fleming, & Faraone, 1985) and to early-onset affective disorders (Todd et al., 1993). No clear evidence of a single major locus causing these disorders has been found through these analyses. It appears likely that these disorders are inherited by complex inheritance with one or more genes of small effect and environmental influences contributing to the development of the disorder. Segregation analysis has low power to distinguish between *oligogenic models*, models with few genes acting together with nongenetic factors, and *polygenic models*, models with many genes acting together with nongenetic factors. Also, even when clear evidence of a major locus is found, segregation analysis cannot distinguish between the same susceptibility locus being transmitted in all families (*genetic homogeneity*) or different susceptibility loci being transmitted in different families (*genetic heterogeneity*). However, modern molecular and statistical genetic methods make it possible to identify genes for oligogenic traits that do not show Mendelian transmission but that do show evidence of substantial heritability through family, twin, and/or adoption studies.

CONCLUSION

There is strong evidence of genes being important to the development of affective disorders, particularly bipolar disorder. The studies suggest that childhood-onset affective disorders share familial factors in common with adult-onset affective disorders and does not represent an etiologically distinct group. The studies that analyze bilineality suggest that younger ages of onset may occur when there are a greater number of familial factors present than in families with older ages of onset. Some have suggested that it would be better to try to identify genes for bipolar disorder in childhood-onset families rather than in adult-onset families because the former appear to have more genetic loading (Strober, 1992; Todd et al., 1993). However, this would only be true if the susceptibility alleles of genes for bipolar disorder are not common. If the susceptibility alleles are common, than families with childhood-onset bipolar disorder may be more likely to be homozygous for bipolar susceptibility genes which would lead to lower power in genetic linkage studies (Badner, Gershon, & Goldin, 1998). But this is something that will not be known until the genetic linkage studies are done in childhood bipolar disorder.

REFERENCES

Allen, M. G. (1976). Twin studies of affective illness. *Archives of General Psychiatry, 33*(12), 1476–1478.

Badner, J. A., Gershon, E. S., & Goldin, L. R. (1998). Optimal ascertainment strategies to detect linkage to common disease alleles. *American Journal of Human Genetics, 63*(3), 880–888.

Bertelsen, A., Harvald, B., & Hauge, M. (1977). A Danish twin study of manic–depressive disorders. *British Journal of Psychiatry, 130*(4), 330–351.

Cardno, A. G., Marshall, E. J., Coid, B., Macdonald, A. M., Ribchester, T. R., Davies, N. J., Venturi, P., Jones, L. A., Lewis, S. W., Sham, P. C., Gottesman, I. I., Farmer, A. E., McGuffin, P., Reveley, A. M., & Murray, R. M. (1999). Heritability estimates for psychotic disorders: The Maudsley twin psychosis series. *Archives of General Psychiatry, 56*(2), 162–168.

Chang, K. D., Steiner, H., & Ketter, T. A. (2000). Psychiatric phenomenology of child and adolescent bipolar offspring. *Journal of the American Academy of Child and Adolescent Psychiatry, 39*(4), 453–460.

Clerget-Darpoux, F., Goldin, L. R., & Gershon, E. S. (1986). Clinical methods in psychiatric genetics: Part 3. Environmental stratification may simulate a genetic effect in adoption studies. *Acta Psychiatrica Scandinavica, 74*(4), 305–311.

Gershon, E. S., Hamovit, J., Guroff, J. J., Dibble, E., Leckman, J. F., Sceery, W., Targum, S. D., Nurnberger, J. I., Jr., Goldin, L. R., & Bunney, W. E., Jr. (1982). A family study of schizoaffective, bipolar I, bipolar II, unipolar, and normal control probands. *Archives of General Psychiatry, 39*(10), 1157–1167.

Goldin, L. R., Gershon, E. S., Targum, S. D., Sparkes, R. S., & McGinniss, M. (1983). Segregation and linkage analyses in families of patients with bipolar, unipolar, and schizoaffective mood disorders. *American Journal of Human Genetics, 35*(2), 274–287.

Kendler, K. S., Pedersen, N., Johnson, L., Neale, M. C., & Mathe, A. A. (1993). A pilot Swedish twin study of affective illness, including hospital- and population-ascertained subsamples. *Archives of General Psychiatry, 50*(9), 699–700.

McMahon, F. J., Stine, O. C., Chase, G. A., Meyers, D. A., Simpson, S. G., & DePaulo, J. R. (1994). Influence of clinical subtype, sex, and lineality on age at onset of major affective disorder in a family sample. *American Journal of Psychiatry, 151*(2), 210–215.

Mendlewicz, J., & Rainer, J. D. (1977). Adoption study supporting genetic transmission in manic–depressive illness. *Nature, 268*(5618), 327–329.

Neuman, R. J., Geller, B., Rice, J. P., & Todd, R. D. (1997). Increased prevalence and earlier onset of mood disorders among relatives of prepubertal versus adult probands. *Journal of the American Academy of Child and Adolescent Psychiatry, 36*(4), 466–473.

Puig-Antich, J., Goetz, D., Davies, M., Kaplan, T., Davies, S., Ostrow, L., Asnis, L., Twomey, J., Iyengar, S., & Ryan, N. D. (1989). A controlled family history study of prepubertal major depressive disorder. *Archives of General Psychiatry, 46*(5), 406–418.

Schürhoff, F., Bellivier, F., Jouvent, R., Mouren-Simeoni, M. C., Bouvard, M., Allilaire, J. F., & Leboyer, M. (2000). Early and late onset bipolar disorders: Two different forms of manic–depressive illness? *Journal of Affective Disorders, 58*(3), 215–221.

Sham, P. C., Morton, N. E., & Rice, J. P. (1992). Segregation analysis of the NIMH Collaborative Study: Family data on bipolar disorder. *Psychiatric Genetics, 2*(3), 175–184.

Simpson, S. G., Folstein, S. E., Meyers, D. A., & DePaulo, J. R. (1992). Assessment of lineality in bipolar I linkage studies. *American Journal of Psychiatry, 149*(12), 1660–1665.

Strober, M. (1992). Relevance of early age-of-onset in genetic studies of bipolar affective disorder. *Journal of the American Academy of Child and Adolescent Psychiatry, 31*(4), 606–610.

Todd, R. D., Geller, B., Neuman, R., Fox, L. W., & Hickok, J. (1996). Increased prevalence of alcoholism in relatives of depressed and bipolar children. *Journal of the American Academy of Child and Adolescent Psychiatry, 35*(6), 716–724.

Todd, R. D., Neuman, R., Geller, B., Fox, L. W., & Hickok, J. (1993). Genetic studies of affective disorders: Should we be starting with childhood onset probands? *Journal of the American Academy of Child and Adolescent Psychiatry, 32*(6), 1164–1171.

Tsuang, M. T., Bucher, K. D., Fleming, J. A., & Faraone, S. V. (1985). Transmission of affective disorders: An application of segregation analysis to blind family study data. *Journal of Psychiatric Research, 19*(1), 23–29.

Tsuang, M. T., Faraone, S. V., & Fleming, J. A. (1985). Familial transmission of major affective disorders: Is there evidence supporting the distinction between unipolar and bipolar disorders? *British Journal of Psychiatry, 146*(3), 268–271.

Weissman, M. M., Gershon, E. S., Kidd, K. K., Prusoff, B. A., Leckman, J. F., Dibble, E., Hamovit, J., Thompson, W. D., Pauls, D. L., & Guroff, J. J. (1984). Psychiatric disorders in the relatives of probands with affective disorders: The Yale University–National Institute of Mental Health Collaborative Study. *Archives of General Psychiatry, 41*(1), 13–21.

Wender, P. H., Kety, S. S., Rosenthal, D., Schulsinger, F., Ortmann, J., & Lunde, I. (1986). Psychiatric disorders in the biological and adoptive families of adopted individuals with affective disorders. *Archives of General Psychiatry, 43*(10), 923–929.

Wozniak, J., Biederman, J., Mundy, E., Mennin, D., & Faraone, S. V. (1995). A pilot family study of childhood-onset mania. *Journal of the American Academy of Child and Adolescent Psychiatry, 34*(12), 1577–1583.

12

The Pharmacological Treatment of Child and Adolescent Bipolar Disorder

NEAL D. RYAN

There are several overlapping goals in our quest to understand the pharmacological treatment of child and adolescent bipolar disorder. The overarching goal of our quest for understanding is to learn how to better treat our patients. Bipolar disorder leads to considerable psychosocial dysfunction, morbidity, and mortality in children as well as in adults (Brent et al., 1994; Craney & Geller, in press; Geller et al., 2000a, 2001, 2002; Strober, Morrell, Lampert, & Burroughs, 1990; Strober et al., 1995). Therefore, we need to know how to treat acute episodes of both mania and depression and how to prevent recurrences—or, more realistically, to decrease the frequency of recurrences.

However, an almost equally important goal is to use "pharmacological dissection" to understand issues of continuities/discontinuities in bipolar disorder through development. While there are many similarities in the presentation of bipolar disorder in childhood and adolescence with its presentation in adulthood (Carlson, Davenport, & Jamison, 1977; Welner, Welner, & Fishman, 1979; Welner, Welner, & Leonard, 1977), nevertheless the clinical syndrome of bipolar disorder shows considerable developmental, age-specific features (Craney & Geller, in press). We have hypothesized that the development of the neural substrate involved in the control of mood may explain the seeming lack of efficacy of tricyclic antidepressants (TCAs; which are relatively noradrenergic) in the treatment of unipolar depression in youth while selective serotonin reuptake inhibitors (SSRIs) appear to be effective (Ryan & Varma, 1998). Alternatively, similar to other medical illnesses, childhood-onset depression may be a more severe illness (Childs & Scriver, 1986; Geller, Todd, Luby, & Botteron, 1996) and thus treatment-resistant to TCAs on this basis

Therefore, if we should find that adult-type treatment works for child and adolescent bipolar disorder we will be left with questions of safety, tolerability, kinetics, combination with psychotherapy, and a raft of other clinical questions about how to optimally treat this population. On the other hand, if we should find that some or many adult-type treatments are ineffective in child and/or adolescent bipolar disorder, this may lead to interesting hypotheses about the development of neural circuitry involved in affect as well as a considerable therapeutic conundrum as to what to try next for these severely impaired children. As of yet, there is surprisingly little data as to which of these two dramatically different alternatives are correct.

Finally, we will examine whether or not younger children and adolescents with bipolar disorder have like or unlike response to treatment. Evidence for differences by age comes from the work of Strober and colleagues (1988), who reported lithium resistance in adolescent mania that had a prepubertal onset. By contrast, older teenagers in several studies (Geller, Cooper, Sun, et al., 1998a; Strober et al., 1988) did well on drugs used for adult-onset mania. As described elsewhere in this book, there are differences through childhood in the presentation of this syndrome. In unipolar disorder, there is a clear maturational increase in depression and a shift in the sex ratio to a female excess that happens during the early teenage years and appears to be more associated with pubertal development than with age per se (Angold, Costello, & Worthman, 1998; Weissman, 2002). Thus, there is considerable precedent for the importance of maturational effects across youth in affective disorders.

LITHIUM

Historically, lithium has been the mainstay of treatment of bipolar disorder throughout the lifespan, with many studies demonstrating its efficacy in adulthood (Schou, 1997). Recent data suggest that lithium alone of antimanic agents may decrease suicide (Schou, 1998). Lithium has been the most used mood stabilizers in children (Youngerman & Canino, 1978), though there is, as yet, relatively modest evidence of its efficacy—as we will see.

Lithium appears relatively well tolerated in children and adolescents and its use has been reported in preschool children (Hagino, Weller, & Weller, 1995). Lithium kinetics have been studied in youth (Vitiello et al., 1988); one can use salivary levels to achieve rapid titration with this kinetic understanding (Malone et al., 1995; Vitiello, Behar, Ryan, Malone, & Delaney, 1987; Weller, Weller, & Fristad, 1986; Weller, Weller, Fristad,

Cantwell, & Tucker, 1987). Lithium side effects in children are much like those seen in adults (Rosenberg, Holttum, & Gershon, 1994; Silva et al., 1992). However, there is a suggestion that preschool children may experience more central nervous system effects (Hagino et al., 1995). In addition, several authors (Geller, Cooper, Zimerman, et al., 1998; Silva et al., 1992) have reported an uncommon, marked cognitive impairment at nontoxic lithium levels.

Open clinical experience and relatively small pilot studies with lithium has suggested efficacy in both children and adolescents (Brumback & Weinberg, 1977; DeLong & Aldershof, 1987; DeLong & Nieman, 1983; Kafantaris, 1995; McKnew et al., 1981; Varanka, Weller, Weller, & Fristad, 1988; Youngerman & Canino, 1978), though the relative scarcity of data makes comparison with adult efficacy difficult (Faedda et al., 1995). Lithium is frequently used as a first-line treatment for children and adolescents with bipolar disorder. In addition, in some (Campbell et al., 1984, 1995; Malone, Delaney, Luebbert, Cater, & Campbell, 2000), but not all (Rifkin et al., 1997; Silva, Gonzalez, Kafantaris, & Campbell, 1991), studies, lithium appears to have an antiaggressive effect in children and adolescents with conduct disorder.

In a randomized controlled acute treatment study, Geller, Cooper, Sun, and colleagues (1998) compared lithium to placebo in the treatment of adolescents (median age = 16.3; SD = 1.2) who had comorbid bipolar disorder and secondary substance dependence. This study consisted of a 2-week single-blind placebo washout phase followed immediately by a 10-week two-arm double-blind randomized trial of either lithium or placebo. Twenty-five subjects were enrolled. Those randomly assigned to lithium did significantly better both in terms of their bipolar disorder and in terms of their substance abuse than did those randomized to placebo. This is the first randomized controlled trial to demonstrate the efficacy of a mood stabilizer (and the only one to demonstrate the efficacy of lithium).

In another study by the same lead author, prepubertal children (median age = 10.7; SD = 1.2) with major depression (a group at high risk for future bipolarity) did not have a better antidepressant response to lithium than placebo in a randomized controlled trial of 30 children (Geller, Cooper, Zimerman, et al., 1998).

Kafantaris and colleagues (2001) took adolescents age 12 to 18 who had a manic or mixed bipolar I disorder and treated them openly with lithium for 4 weeks (or up to 8 weeks in those who initially required a neuroleptic in addition to the lithium). Those who responded were randomized to a double-blind discontinuation study. Forty adolescents entered the randomized discontinuation phase: 30 had been treated with lithium alone and 10 had received an adjunctive neuroleptic. Of those randomized to placebo, 62% showed an exacerbation, while 53% of those randomized to lithium continuation showed exacerbation (not a significant difference).

Strober and colleagues (1988) have reported that prepubertal children may be less responsive than adolescents to the mood-stabilizing effects of lithium. In an interesting open study, they found that patients who discontinued (against advice) their effective lithium treatment had a much shorter interval to next episode than those who continued their lithium treatment (Strober et al., 1990). It did not appear that the discontinuation of lithium was secondary to an occult relapse. Nevertheless, the discontinuation was obviously not at random, so those who discontinued may have been different in their hazard for relapse than those who followed advice and continued on medication.

Kowatch and colleagues (2000) randomly assigned 42 outpatient children and adolescents with bipolar disorder (mean age = 11.4 years) to 6 weeks of open treatment with either lithium, divalproex, or carbamazepine, thereby gathering data on the absolute and relative response rates for these agents in youth with bipolar disorder. Using a 50% or greater change on Young's Main Rating Scale (Y-MRS) scale to define response, the response rates on the three agents were 38% for lithium, 53% for divalproex, and 38% for carbamazepine. The rates were not significantly different. According to the Clinical Global Improvement (CGI) change score analyses, the relative rates were 46%, 40%, and 31%, respectively, so this study does not necessarily give a "signal" that divalproex is likely to be ultimately more effective than lithium. Nevertheless, by using modern diagnosis and serial assessment methods in a well-characterized sample, it appears that these agents are probably effective in a reasonable fraction (though possibly a minority) of children when given alone.

VALPROATE

Valproate and divalproex are widely used throughout childhood as an anticonvulsant, so its kinetics and side effects have been well studied (Battino, Estienne, & Avanzini, 1995; Botha, Gray, & Miller, 1995; Brouwer et al., 1992; Cloyd, Fischer, Kriel, & Kraus, 1993; Cloyd et al., 1992; Kriel, Fischer, Cloyd, Green, & Fraser, 1986; Sugimoto, Muro, Woo, Nishida, & Murakami, 1996)

Valproate side effects in childhood are, in general, much like those seen in adulthood (Rosenberg et al., 1994). In addition, there are two issues that deserve special attention. First, potentially lethal hepatic toxicity can occur with this compound in very young children, especially those under 2 years of age (Bryant & Dreifuss, 1996; Silberstein & Wilmore, 1996).

Second, in teenage women treated for epilepsy, there is an increased rate of polycystic ovaries (up to 80%) and hyperandrogenism (Isojarvi,

Laatikainen, Pakarinen, Juntunen, & Myllya, 1993; Rattya et al., 2001; Vainionpaa et al., 1999). While it has been suggested that this may be secondary to the weight gain seen with this compound (Jallon & Picard, 2001), with hyperinsulinemia and low levels of ILGF binding protein (Isojarvi et al., 1996), more recent data suggests that polycystic ovaries may occur as frequently in lean women on this agent (Isojarvi et al., 2001). The same authors in a study of three women with epilepsy found switching from valproate to lamotrigine resulted in decreased serum testosterone, reversal of weight gain (in the two women with weight gain), resumption of menstruation, and reversal of polycystic changes to ovaries (Isojarvi & Tapanainen, 2000). More recently, elevated testosterone levels have been reported in both male and female adolescents on valproate. The frequency of and risk for reproductive disorders in women with seizures is greater than that found in women without seizure disorder, so it is possible that the hazard of reproductive changes with valproate in adolescent girls with bipolar disorder without seizure disorder is lower than the very high rate seen in the studies in which valproate is used as an anticonvulsant (Morrell, 1999), but we simply do not yet know. In short, the final answer is not yet available on this very important question for teenagers with bipolar disorder. The adolescent girl on valproate should at least be carefully monitored for weight gain and amenorrhea; adolescents of both sexes should be monitored for testosterone levels.

In adults, divalproex sodium (or valproate) and lithium are the two first-line treatments for bipolar disorder with some indication that valproate may be superior to lithium alone in adults with mixed mania (Bowden, 1995; Calabrese, Fatemi, Kujawa, & Woyshville, 1996; Swann et al., 1997) or comorbid neurological conditions (Stoll et al., 1994).

There is limited case report and small series data concerning valproate use in children and adolescents (Deltito, Levitan, Damore, Hajal, & Zambenedetti, 1998; Donovan et al., 1997; Kastner, Friedman, Plummer, Ruiz, & Henning, 1990; Papatheodorou & Kutcher, 1993; Papatheodorou, Kutcher, Katic, & Szalai, 1995; West et al., 1994; Whittier, West, Galli, & Raute, 1995). One study compared a series of adolescents treated clinically with valproate to a historical series of similar adolescents treated with lithium (Strober, 1997). In that study, valproate was not superior to lithium for bipolar disorder except in the mixed mania group, where it performed better.

CARBAMAZEPINE

Carbamazepine is well studied in children as an anticonvulsant (Camfield et al., 1992; Cornaggia et al., 1993; Eeg-Olofsson et al., 1990; Liu &

Delgado, 1994). Like all available agents currently used to treat bipolar disorder, carbamazepine has significant potential side effects that include aplastic anemia and agranulocytosis (Olcay, Pekcan, Yalnizoglu, Buyuk-pamukcu, & Yalaz, 1995; Pellock, 1987; Rawson, Harding, Malcolm, & Lueck, 1998). In adults, while carbamazepine clearly has mood-stabilizing effects, it is generally felt to be less effective than either lithium or valproate in classical bipolar disorder. However, data from some (Cala-brese et al., 1996), but not all (Okuma, 1993), studies suggest that it may be superior to lithium alone in adults with mixed or rapid-cycling bipolar disorder and that lithium plus carbamazepine may be more effective than lithium alone in adult-onset mania (Solomon, Keitner, Ryan, & Miller, 1996).

There are a number of small studies examining carbamazepine in the treatment of children with attention-deficit/hyperactivity disorder-like be-havioral disturbance, frequently with concomitant electroencephalogram (EEG) abnormalities which in aggregate suggest superiority to placebo (see the meta-analysis in Silva, Munoz, & Alpert, 1996). The data in aggressive children without EEG abnormalities is mixed, but one randomized con-trolled study failed to find efficacy (Cueva et al., 1996).

The open randomized trial of Kowatch and colleagues (2000), in which they compared lithium, divalproex, and carbamazepine, did not find carbamazepine to be statistically significantly worse in outcome than the other two treatments, though it did not fare as well numerically.

ATYPICAL NEUROLEPTICS

Several groups have published data on their open series of trials for youth with bipolar disorder suggesting antimanic effects of the atypical neuro-leptics, including olanzapine (Chang & Ketter, 2000; Frazier et al., 2001; Soutullo, Casuto, & Keck, 1999) and risperidone (Frazier et al., 1999). These open data are consistently suggestive of a clinical effect for this class of compounds in treating juvenile bipolar disorder

DelBello, Schweiers, Rosenberg, and Strakowski (2001) have reported the only controlled trial of atypical neuroleptics. They treated 30 adoles-cents with bipolar I with divalproex and randomized half to adjunctive quetiapine and the other half to adjunctive placebo. Overall, both cells had significant improvement from baseline. In the reported completer analysis (of 22 subjects), those on divalproex plus quetiapine improved signifi-cantly more than those on divalproex plus placebo. It is also worth noting that the response rate seen in the divalproex plus placebo group (53%) matched that seen in the Kowatch and colleagues (2000) randomized open-treatment study in those subjects randomized to divalproex.

ANTIDEPRESSANTS

The question of whether or not antidepressants effectively treat bipolar depression (the depressive phase of the disorder) and whether or not they increase the risk for future episodes of mania or the risk for rapid cycling is very important. Several case reports suggest induction of mania by the use of SSRIs in youth (Achamallah & Decker, 1991; Christensen, 1995; Oldroyd, 1997). The Biederman group (Biederman, Mick, Spencer, Wilens, & Faraone, 2000) used a systematic chart review methodology to examine SSRI treatment of depressed bipolar youth. They found that SSRI treatment was associated both with greater improvement in bipolar depression and with greater probability of relapse of manic symptoms! Nevertheless, we await larger data sets and additional controlled data to provide a more definitive answer to this important question.

There is also data to suggest that antidepressants may not worsen the course of prepubertal mania. In a prospective longitudinal follow-up of 93 subjects with prepubertal and early adolescent mania, treatment was provided by the subjects' own practitioners (Geller et al., 2002). In this study, Geller and colleagues (2002) reported that antidepressants did not significantly effect rates of recovery or relapse.

OTHER AGENTS

To date, there are only a few case reports of the use of other potential mood stabilizers in juvenile bipolar disorder, including gabapentin (Soutullo et al., 1998), lamotrigine (Kusumakar & Yatham, 1997), and topiramate (Davanzo et al., 2001). The data is simply insufficient at present to hazard a meaningful guess as to whether some or all of these compounds will ultimately be shown to be effective in this population.

ONGOING STUDIES

Several ongoing studies have the potential to shed light in this still murky region. A randomized study by Ryan, Birmaher, Strober, and Keller should finish this year and its blind broken. In that study, adolescents with bipolar disorder were stabilized on a single mood stabilizer or a combination of mood stabilizers for 6 months and then were randomized to either a tapered discontinuation of medications (replaced by placebo) or were randomized to continue on medication.

In a recently initiated study, Kowatch, Findling, and Scheffer are conducting a randomized controlled trial of lithium versus divalproex versus placebo in children and adolescents with mania or mixed bipolar I disorder. The investigators plan a total sample of 150 subjects.

Several industry trials are being planned or are already underway for those mood stabilizers with remaining patent life. No data is yet available and it is unclear whether the recently proposed hiatus in the implementation of the U.S. Food and Drug Administration pediatric rule will slow down future industry study starts in youth.

CHILDREN AND ADOLESCENTS RESPOND DIFFERENTLY?

We now return to the third issue that we raised in the introduction to this chapter, whether or not current data suggest that youth through development have a similar response to mood stabilizers. Examination of single case reports gives a "signal" that compounds deserve more systematic study for efficacy but are not useful for understanding this question. Therefore, we examine larger naturalistic data sets and systematic open or randomized reports with examining response in multiple youth.

The large prospective naturalistic study by Geller and colleagues (Geller et al., in press; Geller, Zimerman, Williams, et al., 2000) examining prepubertal and early-onset bipolar disorder did not find that better course was associated with treatment provided by subjects' own practitioners with available mood stabilizers when grouped into categories of lithium, anticonvulsants, or neuroleptics or by a category of antimanic agents (lithium and/or anticonvulsants and/or neuroleptics). One exception found was that treatment with neuroleptic medications was associated with worse outcome. This "paradoxical" finding likely arises from the fact that in this naturalistic study medications were obviously not given randomly and neuroleptics are traditionally used only for treating children with the most severe illness.

Strober and colleagues (1998) compared adolescents with bipolar disorder treated with lithium who had a history of early childhood attention-deficit/hyperactivity disorder to those with bipolar disorder without a history of attention-deficit/hyperactivity disorder who were similarly treated. Those with a history of attention-deficit/hyperactivity disorder has less improvement overall and longer time to improvement. To the extent that the history of early childhood attention-deficit/hyperactivity disorder may have been early-onset bipolar disorder, this study may suggest that even as adolescents, the early-onset cases have worse prognosis. Strober (1992) also found that early age of onset of bipolar disorder predicted higher family genetic loading for the disorder, so one possible hypothesis is that early-onset bipolar disorder may be associated with higher genetic loading, and thereby to more difficult-to-treat forms of the disorder. Geller and colleagues (unpublished data) have also found far higher familial aggregation of bipolar disorders in prepubertal and early adolescent bipolar disorder compared to rates in studies of adult-onset mania.

The Kowatch and colleagues (2000) open randomized study had a mean age of 11.4 years, so it had both younger and older onset cases. In that study the overall reported response rates for the three agents were clinically important but overall across all three antimanic treatments the improvement response rate was less than 50%.

The mean age in the Kafantaris and colleagues (2001) study was 15.2 years. Of 108 subjects initially enrolled in the protocol, only 42% met response criteria when treated with lithium with neuroleptic augmentation as needed. This rate is very similar to the 38%–46% response rate (calculated in two different ways) in those subjects on lithium in the Kowatch and colleagues (2000) study who had a mean age almost 4 years younger. The range in the DelBello and colleagues (2001) augmentation study was 12–18 years of age and the response rate in that study in the divalproex-alone group exactly paralleled that in the Kowatch study on divalproex even though the subjects in the Kowatch study were younger on average.

Therefore, the evidence is mixed and ultimately inconclusive on the question of whether or not there are important differences in the response to mood stabilizers in younger and older children. The question, however, is of the essence in our understanding of this disorder. It will be imperative to directly study younger children with bipolar disorder in our treatment studies. There is certainly sufficient data to preclude mere extrapolation from adolescent studies down to make optimal clinical decisions regarding young children with bipolar disorder.

SUMMARY AND CONCLUSIONS

Most of our questions remain largely unanswered, including:

• Does acute mania and mixed or rapid-cycling bipolar disorder in children and adolescents respond to those mood stabilizers that have demonstrated efficacy in the adult forms of this disorder? There is evidence suggesting that they do—the majority of open clinical data and the controlled studies of Geller, Cooper, Sun, and colleagues (1998) with lithium and DelBello and colleagues (2001) examining quetiapine augmentation of divalproex, but the question still is substantially open.

• Do mood stabilizers prophylax against recurrence of bipolar disorder in youth? No randomized controlled data yet address this question. Open data of Strober and colleagues (1990) looking at those youth who, against advice, discontinued lithium compared to other youth who did not, suggest that lithium is effective in prophylaxis but this must be considered somewhat modest data since the medication discontinuation was obviously not even remotely at random.

• Are mood stabilizers or antidepressants effective in treating bipolar depression? The single randomized controlled trial of Geller, Cooper, Zimerman, and colleagues (1998) examining lithium in the treatment of depression in prepubertal children with a strong family history of bipolar disorder (a reasonable proxy for bipolar depression) did not find evidence that it is effective. A systematic chart review by Biederman and colleagues (2000) suggested that SSRIs may have efficacy. There is little other open clinical data addressing this point, which is therefore unresolved.

• Do mood stabilizers have the same effect in bipolar disorder throughout youth? Do they work the same in an 8-year-old child with mania as in a 16-year-old adolescent with mania? The data is insufficient to hazard a strong guess. It is not sufficient simply to extrapolate from adolescents to children without future studies in children because there are substantial age-related changes in bipolar disorder across this range.

Therefore, we are left with reasonable open data on how to use these agents in youth and somewhat reasonable data suggesting that they may well work. We desperately need more controlled studies to determine whether or not these preliminary data are leading us in the right direction and allowing us to take a more scientific approach to actually treating our patients with this serious disorder.

In designing future studies, a wide variety of clinical approaches, including placebo-controlled randomized trials, will be helpful in triangulating on the truth. One approach that may offer promise is that of equipoise stratification, suggested by Lavori (2001), which may allow us to get more information from more subjects in a more easily generalized approach. Almost all future treatment studies are likely to be multisite studies in order to enroll the minimum 100–300 subjects per study realistically needed to answer critical questions. Such studies are challenging and expensive, but this cost pales in comparison to the staggering cost of the disorder untreated or poorly treated in youth.

REFERENCES

Achamallah, N. S., & Decker, D. H. (1991). Mania induced by fluoxetine in an adolescent patient. *American Journal of Psychiatry 148*, 1404.

Angold, A., Costello, E. J., & Worthman, C. .M. (1998). Puberty and depression: The roles of age, pubertal status and pubertal timing. *Psychological Medicine, 28*, 51–61.

Battino, D., Estienne, M., & Avanzini, G. (1995). Clinical pharmacokinetics of antiepileptic drugs in paediatric patients: Part 1. Phenobarbital, primidone, valproic acid, ethosuximide and mesuximide. *Clinical Pharmacokinetics, 29,* 257–286.

Biederman, J., Mick, E., Spencer, T. J., Wilens, T. E., & Faraone, S. V. (2000). Therapeutic dilemmas in the pharmacotherapy of bipolar depression in the young. *Journal of Child and Adolescent Psychopharmacology, 10,* 185–192.

Botha, J. H., Gray, A. L., & Miller, R. (1995). A model for estimating individualized valproate clearance values in children. *Journal of Clinical Pharmacology, 35,* 1020–1024.

Bowden, C. L. (1995). Predictors of response to divalproex and lithium. *Journal of Clinical Psychiatry, 56*(Suppl. 3), 25–30.

Brent, D. A., Perper, J. A., Moritz, G., Baugher, M., Schweers, J., & Roth, C. (1994). Suicide in affectively ill adolescents: A case–control study. *Journal of Affective Disorders, 31,* 193–202.

Brouwer, O. F., Pieters, M. S., Edelbroek, P. M., Bakker, A. M., van Geel, A. A., Stijnen, T., Jennekens-Schinkel, A., Lanser, J. B., & Peters, A. C. (1992). Conventional and controlled release valproate in children with epilepsy: A crossover study comparing plasma levels and cognitive performances. *Epilepsy Research, 13,* 245–253.

Brumback, R. A., & Weinberg, W. A. (1977). Mania in childhood: Part 2. Therapeutic trial of lithium carbonate and further description of manic–depressive illness in children. *American Journal of Diseases of Children, 131,* 1122–1126.

Bryant, A. E., III, & Dreifuss, F. E. (1996). Valproic acid hepatic fatalities: Part 3. U.S. experience since 1986. *Neurology, 46,* 465–469.

Calabrese, J. R., Fatemi, S. H., Kujawa, M., & Woyshville, M. J. (1996). Predictors of response to mood stabilizers. *Journal of Clinical Psychopharmacology, 16*(Suppl. 1), 24S–31S.

Camfield, P., Hwang, P., Camfield, C., Fraser, A., Soldin, S., al-Quadah, A. K. (1992). The pharmacology of chewable versus regular carbamazepine in chronically treated children with epilepsy. *Canadian Journal of Neurological Sciences, 19,* 204–207.

Campbell, M., Adams, P. B., Small, A. M., Kafantaris, V., Silva, R. R., Shell, J., Perry, R., & Overall, J. E. (1995). Lithium in hospitalized aggressive children with conduct disorder: A double-blind and placebo-controlled study. *Journal of the American Academy of Child and Adolescent Psychiatry, 34,* 445–453. (Published erratum appears in Journal of the *American Academy of Child and Adolescent Psychiatry, 34*(5), 694)

Campbell, M., Small, A. M., Green, W. H., Jennings, S. J., Perry, R., Bennett, W. G., & Anderson, L. (1984). Behavioral efficacy of haloperidol and lithium carbonate: A comparison in hospitalized aggressive children with conduct disorder. *Archives of General Psychiatry, 41,* 650–656.

Carlson, G. A., Davenport, Y. B., & Jamison, K. (1977). A comparison of outcome in adolescent- and later-onset bipolar manic–depressive illness. *American Journal of Psychiatry, 134,* 919–922.

Chang, K. D., & Ketter, T. A. (2000). Mood stabilizer augmentation with olanzapine in acutely manic children. *Journal of Child and Adolescent Psychopharmacology, 10,* 45–49.

Childs, B., & Scriver, C. R. (1986). Age at onset and causes of disease. *Perspectives in Biological Medicine, 29,* 437–460.

Christensen, R. C. (1995). Paroxetine-induced psychotic mania. *American Journal of Psychiatry, 152,* 1399–1400.

Cloyd, J. C., Fischer, J. H., Kriel, R. L., & Kraus, D. M. (1993). Valproic acid pharmacokinetics in children: Part 4. Effects of age and antiepileptic drugs on protein binding and intrinsic clearance. *Clinical Pharmacology and Therapeutics, 53,* 22–29.

Cloyd, J. C., Kriel, R. L., Jones-Saete, C. M., Ong, B. Y., Jancik, J. T., & Remmel, R. P. (1992). Comparison of sprinkle versus syrup formulations of valproate for bioavailability, tolerance, and preference. *Journal of Pediatrics, 120,* 634–638.

Cornaggia, C., Gianetti, S., Battino, D., Granata, T., Romeo, A., Viani, F., & Limido, G. (1993). Comparative pharmacokinetic study of chewable and conventional carbamazepine in children. *Epilepsia, 34,* 158–160.

Craney, J. L., & Geller, B. (in press). Phenomenology and longitudinal course of children with a prepubertal and early adolescent bipolar disorder phenotype: A review. *Bipolar Disorder.*

Cueva, J. E., Overall, J. E., Small, A. M., Armenteros, J. L., Perry, R., & Campbell, M. (1996). Carbamazepine in aggressive children with conduct disorder: A double-blind and placebo-controlled study. *Journal of the American Academy of Child and Adolescent Psychiatry, 35,* 480–490.

Davanzo, P., Cantwell, E., Kleiner, J., Baltaxe, C., Najera, B., Crecelius, G., & McCracken, J. (2001). Cognitive changes during topiramate therapy. *Journal of the American Academy of Child and Adolescent Psychiatry, 40,* 262–263.

DelBello, M. P., Schweiers, M. L., Rosenberg, H. L., & Strakowski, S. M. (2001, December). *Quetiapine as adjunctive treatment for adolescent mania.* Paper presented at the annual meeting of American College of Neuropsychopharmacology, Waikoloa, HI.

DeLong, G. R., & Aldershof, A. L. (1987). Long-term experience with lithium treatment in childhood: Correlation with clinical diagnosis. *Journal of the American Academy of Child and Adolescent Psychiatry, 26,* 389–394.

DeLong, G. R., & Nieman, G. W. (1983). Lithium-induced behavior changes in children with symptoms suggesting manic–depressive illness. *Psychopharmacology Bulletin, 19,* 258–265.

Deltito, J. A., Levitan, J., Damore, J., Hajal, F., & Zambenedetti, M. (1998). Naturalistic experience with the use of divalproex sodium on an in-patient unit for adolescent psychiatric patients. *Acta Psychiatrica Scandinavica, 97,* 236–240.

Donovan, S. J., Susser, E. S., Nunes, E. V., Stewart, J. W., Quitkin, F. M., & Klein, D. F. (1997). Divalproex treatment of disruptive adolescents: A report of 10 cases. *Journal of Clinical Psychiatry, 58,* 12–25.

Eeg-Olofsson, O., Nilsson, H. L., Tonnby, B., Arvidsson, J., Grahn, P. A., Gylje, H., Larsson, C., & Noren, L. (1990). Diurnal variation of carbamazepine and carbamazepine-10,11-epoxide in plasma and saliva in children with epilepsy: A comparison between conventional and slow-release formulations. *Journal of Child Neurology, 5,* 159–165.

Faedda, G. L., Baldessarini, R. J., Suppes, T., Tondo, L., Becker, I., & Lipschitz, D. S. (1995). Pediatric-onset bipolar disorder: A neglected clinical and public health problem. *Harvard Review of Psychiatry, 3,* 171–195.

Frazier, J. A., Biederman, J., Tohen, M., Feldman, P. D., Jacobs, T. G., Toma, V., Rater, M. A., Tarazi, R. A., Kim, G. S., Garfield, S. B., Sohma, M., Gonzalez-Heydrich,

J., Risser, R. C., & Nowlin, Z. M. (2001). A prospective open-label treatment trial of olanzapine monotherapy in children and adolescents with bipolar disorder. *Journal of Child and Adolescent Psychopharmacology, 11,* 239–250.

Frazier, J. A., Meyer, M. C., Biederman, J., Wozniak, J., Wilens, T. E., Spencer, T. J., Kim, G. S., & Shapiro, S. (1999). Risperidone treatment for juvenile bipolar disorder: A retrospective chart review. *Journal of the American Academy of Child and Adolescent Psychiatry, 38,* 960–965.

Geller, B., Bolhofner, K., Craney, J. L., Williams, M., DelBello, M. P., & Gundersen, K. (2000). Psychosocial functioning in a prepubertal and early adolescent bipolar disorder phenotype. *Journal of the American Academy of Child and Adolescent Psychiatry, 39,* 1543–1548.

Geller, B., Cooper, T. B., Sun, K., Zimerman, B., Frazier, J., Williams, M., & Heath, J. (1998). Double-blind and placebo-controlled study of lithium for adolescent bipolar disorders with secondary substance dependency. *Journal of the American Academy of Child and Adolescent Psychiatry, 37,* 171–178.

Geller, B., Cooper, T. B., Zimerman, B., Frazier, J., Williams, M., Heath, J., & Warner, K. (1998). Lithium for prepubertal depressed children with family history predictors of future bipolarity: A double-blind, placebo-controlled study. *Journal of Affective Disorders, 51,* 165–175.

Geller, B., Craney, J. L., Bolhofner, K., DelBello, M. P., Williams, M., & Zimerman, B. (2001). One-year recovery and relapse rates of children with a prepubertal and early adolescent bipolar disorder phenotype. *American Journal of Psychiatry, 158,* 303–305.

Geller, B., Craney, J. L., Bolhofner, K., Nickelsburg, J., Williams, M., & Zimerman, B. (2002). Two year prospective follow-up of children with a prepubertal and early adolescent bipolar disorder phenotype. *American Journal of Psychiatry, 159,* 927–933.

Geller, B., Todd, R. D., Luby, J., & Botteron, K. N. (1996). Treatment-resistant depression in children and adolescents. *Psychiatric Clinics of North America, 19,* 253–267.

Geller, B., Zimerman, B., Williams, M., Bolhofner, K., Craney, J. L., DelBello, M. P., & Soutullo, C. A. (2000). Six-month stability and outcome of a prepubertal and early adolescent bipolar disorder phenotype. *Journal of Child and Adolescent Psychopharmacology, 10,* 165–173.

Hagino, O. R., Weller, E. B., Weller, R. A., Washing, D., Fristad, M. A., & Kontras, S. B. (1995). Untoward effects of lithium treatment in children aged four through six years. *Journal of the American Academy of Child and Adolescent Psychiatry, 34,* 1584–1590.

Isojarvi, J. I., Laatikainen, T. J., Knip, M., Pakarinen, A. J., Juntunen, K. T., & Myllyla, V. V. (1996). Obesity and endocrine disorders in women taking valproate for epilepsy. *Annals of Neurology, 39,* 579–584.

Isojarvi, J. I., Laatikainen, T. J., Pakarinen, A. J., Juntunen, K. T., & Myllyla, V. V. (1993). Polycystic ovaries and hyperandrogenism in women taking valproate for epilepsy. *New England Journal of Medicine, 329,* 1383–1388.

Isojarvi, J. I., & Tapanainen, J. S. (2000). Valproate, hyperandrogenism, and polycystic ovaries: A report of 3 cases. *Archives of Neurology, 57,* 1064–1068.

Isojarvi, J.I., Tauboll, E., Pakarinen, A. J., Van Parys, J., Rattya, J., Harbo, H. F., Dale, P. O., Fauser, B. C., Gjerstad, L., Koivunen, R., Knip, M., & Tapanainen, J. S.

(2001). Altered ovarian function and cardiovascular risk factors in valproate-treated women. *American Journal of Medicine, 111,* 290–296.

Jallon, P., & Picard, F. (2001). Bodyweight gain and anticonvulsants: A comparative review. *Drug Safety, 24,* 969–978.

Kafantaris, V. (1995). Treatment of bipolar disorder in children and adolescents. *Journal of the American Academy of Child and Adolescent Psychiatry, 34,* 732–741.

Kafantaris, V., Coletti, D. J., Dicker, R., Padula, G., Pleak, R., & Kane, J. M. (2001, December). *A double-blind placebo-controlled discontinuation study of lithium in the treatment of acute adolescent mania.* Paper presented at the annual meeting of American College of Neuropsychopharmacology, Waikoloa, HI.

Kastner, T., Friedman, D. L., Plummer, A. T., Ruiz, M. Q., & Henning, D. (1990). Valproic acid for the treatment of children with mental retardation and mood symptomatology. *Pediatrics, 86,* 467–472.

Kowatch, R. A., Suppes, T., Carmody, T. J., Bucci, J. P., Hume, J. H., Kromelis, M., Emslie, G. J., Weinberg, W. A., & Rush, A. J. (2000). Effect size of lithium, divalproex sodium, and carbamazepine in children and adolescents with bipolar disorder. *Journal of the American Academy of Child and Adolescent Psychiatry, 39,* 713–720.

Kriel, R. L., Fischer, J. H., Cloyd, J. C., Green, K. H., & Fraser, G. L. (1986). Valproic acid pharmacokinetics in children: Part 3. Very high dosage requirements. *Pediatric Neurology, 2,* 202–208.

Kusumakar, V., & Yatham, L. N. (1997). An open study of lamotrigine in refractory bipolar depression. *Psychiatry Research, 72,* 145–148.

Lavori, P. W., Rush, A. J., Wisniewski, S. R., Alpert, J., Fava, M., Kupfer, D. J., Nierenberg, A., Quitkin, F. M., Sackeim, H. A., Thase, M. E., & Trivedi, M. (2001). Strengthening clinical effectiveness trials: equipoise-stratified randomization. *Biological Psychiatry, 50,* 792–801.

Liu, H., & Delgado, M. R. (1994). Influence of sex, age, weight, and carbamazepine dose on serum concentrations, concentration ratios, and level/dose ratios of carbamazepine and its metabolites. *Therapeutic Drug Monitoring, 16,* 469–476.

Malone, R. P., Delaney, M. A., Luebbert, J. F., Cater, J., & Campbell, M. (2000). A double-blind placebo-controlled study of lithium in hospitalized aggressive children and adolescents with conduct disorder. *Archives of General Psychiatry, 57,* 649–654.

Malone, R. P., Delaney, M. A., Luebbert, J. F., White, M. A., Biesecker, K. A., & Cooper, T. B. (1995). The lithium test dose prediction method in aggressive children. *Psychopharmacology Bulletin, 31,* 379–382.

McKnew, D. H., Cytryn, L., Buchsbaum, M. S., Hamovit, J., Lamour, M., Rapoport, J. L., & Gershon, E. S. (1981). Lithium in children of lithium-responding parents. *Psychiatry Research, 4,* 171–180.

Morrell, M. J. (1999). Epilepsy in women: The science of why it is special. *Neurology, 53*(Suppl. 1), S42–S48.

Okuma, T. (1993). Effects of carbamazepine and lithium on affective disorders. *Neuropsychobiology, 27,* 138–145.

Olcay, L., Pekcan, S., Yalnizoglu, D., Buyukpamukcu, M., & Yalaz, K. (1995). Fatal agranulocytosis developed in the course of carbamazepine therapy: A case report and review of the literature. *Turkish Journal of Pediatrics, 37,* 73–77.

Oldroyd, J. (1997). Paroxetine-induced mania. *Journal of the American Academy of Child and Adolescent Psychiatry, 36,* 721–722.

Papatheodorou, G., & Kutcher, S. P. (1993). Divalproex sodium treatment in late adolescent and young adult acute mania. *Psychopharmacology Bulletin, 29,* 213–219.

Papatheodorou, G., Kutcher, S. P., Katic, M., & Szalai, J. P. (1995). The efficacy and safety of divalproex sodium in the treatment of acute mania in adolescents and young adults: An open clinical trial. *Journal of Clinical Psychopharmacology, 15,* 110–116.

Pellock, J. M. (1987). Carbamazepine side effects in children and adults. *Epilepsia, 28*(Suppl. 3), S64–S70.

Rattya, J., Pakarinen, A. J., Knip, M., Repo-Outakoski, M., Myllyla, V. V., & Isojarvi, J. I. (2001). Early hormonal changes during valproate or carbamazepine treatment: A 3-month study. *Neurology, 57,* 440–444.

Rawson, N. S., Harding, S. R., Malcolm, E., & Lueck, L. (1998). Hospitalizations for aplastic anemia and agranulocytosis in Saskatchewan: Incidence and associations with antecedent prescription drug use. *Journal of Clinical Epidemiology, 51,* 1343–1355.

Rifkin, A., Karajgi, B., Dicker, R., Perl, E., Boppana, V., Hasan, N., & Pollack, S. (1997). Lithium treatment of conduct disorders in adolescents. *American Journal of Psychiatry, 154,* 554–555.

Rosenberg, D. R., Holttum, J., & Gershon, S. (1994). *Textbook of pharmacotherapy for child and adolescent psychiatric disorders.* New York: Brunner/Mazel.

Ryan, N. D., & Varma, D. (1998). Child and adolescent mood disorders: Experience with serotonin-based therapies. *Biological Psychiatry, 44,* 336–340.

Schou, M. (1997). Forty years of lithium treatment. *Archives of General Psychiatry, 54,* 9–13; discussion, 14–15.

Schou, M. (1998). The effect of prophylactic lithium treatment on mortality and suicidal behavior: A review for clinicians. *Journal of Affective Disorders, 50,* 253–259.

Silberstein, S. D., & Wilmore, L. J. (1996). Divalproex sodium: Migraine treatment and monitoring. *Headache, 36,* 239–242.

Silva, R. R., Campbell, M., Golden, R. R., Small, A. M., Pataki, C. S., & Rosenberg, C. R. (1992). Side effects associated with lithium and placebo administration in aggressive children. *Psychopharmacology Bulletin, 28,* 319–326.

Silva, R. R., Gonzalez, N., Kafantaris, V., & Campbell, M. (1991). *Long-term use of lithium in aggressive conduct disorder children.* Paper presented at the annual meeting of the American Academy of Child and Adolescent Psychiatry, San Francisco.

Silva, R. R., Munoz, D. M., & Alpert, M. (1996). Carbamazepine use in children and adolescents with features of attention-deficit hyperactivity disorder: A meta-analysis. *Journal of the American Academy of Child and Adolescent Psychiatry, 35,* 352–358.

Solomon, D. A., Keitner, G. I., Ryan, C. E., & Miller, I. W. (1996). Polypharmacy in bipolar I disorder. *Psychopharmacology Bulletin, 32,* 579–587.

Soutullo, C. A., Casuto, L. S., & Keck, P. E., Jr. (1998). Gabapentin in the treatment of adolescent mania: A case report. *Journal of Child and Adolescent Psychopharmacology, 8,* 81–85.

Soutullo, C. A., Sorter, M. T., Foster, K. D., McElroy, S. L., & Keck, P. E. (1999). Olanzapine in the treatment of adolescent acute mania: A report of seven cases. *Journal of Affective Disorders, 53*, 279–283.

Stoll, A. L., Banov, M., Kolbrener, M., Mayer, P. V., Tohen, M., Strakowski, S. M., Castillo, J., Suppes, T., & Cohen, B. M. (1994). Neurologic factors predict a favorable valproate response in bipolar and schizoaffective disorders. *Journal of Clinical Psychopharmacology, 14*, 311–313.

Strober, M. (1992). Relevance of early age-of-onset in genetic studies of bipolar affective disorder. *Journal of the American Academy of Child and Adolescent Psychiatry, 31*, 606–610.

Strober, M. (1997). *The naturalistic prospective course of juvenile bipolar illness.* Paper presented at the meeting of the Second International Conference on Bipolar Disorder, Pittsburgh, PA.

Strober, M., DeAntonio, M., Schmidt-Lackner, S., Freeman, R., Lampert, C., & Diamond, J. (1998). Early childhood attention deficit hyperactivity disorder predicts poorer response to acute lithium therapy in adolescent mania. *Journal of Affective Disorders, 51*, 145–151.

Strober, M., Morrell, W., Burroughs, J., Lampert, C., Danforth, H., & Freeman, R. (1988). A family study of bipolar I disorder in adolescence: Early onset of symptoms linked to increased familial loading and lithium resistance. *Journal of Affective Disorders, 15*, 255–268.

Strober, M., Morrell, W., Lampert, .C, & Burroughs, J. (1990). Relapse following discontinuation of lithium maintenance therapy in adolescents with bipolar I illness: A naturalistic study. *American Journal of Psychiatry, 147*, 457–461.

Strober, M., Schmidt-Lackner, S., Freeman, R., Bower, S., Lampert, C., & DeAntonio, M. (1995). Recovery and relapse in adolescents with bipolar affective illness: A five-year naturalistic, prospective follow-up. *Journal of the American Academy of Child and Adolescent Psychiatry, 34*, 724–731.

Sugimoto, T., Muro, H., Woo, M., Nishida, N., & Murakami, K. (1996). Valproate metabolites in high-dose valproate plus phenytoin therapy. *Epilepsia, 37*, 1200–1203.

Swann, A. C., Bowden, C. L., Morris, D., Calabrese, J. R., Petty, F., Small, J., Dilsaver, S. C., & Davis, J. M. (1997). Depression during mania: Treatment response to lithium or divalproex. *Archives of General Psychiatry, 54*, 37–42.

Vainionpaa, L. K., Rattya, J., Knip, M., Tapanainen, J. S., Pakarinen, A. J., Lanning, P., Tekay, A., Myllyla, V. V., & Isojarvi, J. I. (1999). Valproate-induced hyperandrogenism during pubertal maturation in girls with epilepsy. *Annals of Neurology, 45*, 444–450.

Varanka, T. M., Weller, R. A., Weller, E. B., & Fristad, M. A. (1988). Lithium treatment of manic episodes with psychotic features in prepubertal children. *American Journal of Psychiatry, 145*, 1557–1559.

Vitiello, B., Behar, D., Malone, R., Delaney, M. A., Ryan, P. J., & Simpson, G. M. (1988). Pharmacokinetics of lithium carbonate in children. *Journal of Clinical Psychopharmacology, 8*, 355–359.

Vitiello, B., Behar, D., Ryan, P., Malone, R., & Delaney, M. A. (1987). Saliva lithium monitoring. *Journal of the American Academy of Child and Adolescent Psychiatry, 26*, 812–813.

Weissman, M. M. (2002). Juvenile-onset major depression includes childhood- and adolescent-onset depression and may be heterogeneous. *Archives of General Psychiatry, 59*, 223–234.

Weller, E. B., Weller, R. A., & Fristad, M. A. (1986). Lithium dosage guide for prepubertal children: A preliminary report. *Journal of the American Academy of Child Psychiatry, 25*, 92–95.

Weller, E. B., Weller, R. A., Fristad, M. A., Cantwell, M., & Tucker, S. (1987). Saliva lithium monitoring in prepubertal children. *Journal of the American Academy of Child and Adolescent Psychiatry, 26*, 173–175.

Welner, A., Welner, Z., & Fishman, R. (1979). Psychiatric adolescent inpatients: Eight- to ten-year follow-up. *Archives of General Psychiatry, 36*, 698–700.

Welner, A., Welner, Z., & Leonard, M. A. (1977). Bipolar manic–depressive disorder: A reassessment of course and outcome. *Comprehensive Psychiatry, 18*, 327–332.

West, S. A., Keck, P. E., McElroy, S. L., Minnery, K. L., McConville, B. J., & Sorter, M. T. (1994). Open trial of valproate in the treatment of adolescent mania. *Journal of Child and Adolescent Psychopharmacology, 4*, 263–267.

Whittier, M. C., West, S. A., Galli, V. B., & Raute, N. J. (1995). Valproic acid for dysphoric mania in a mentally retarded adolescent. *Journal of Clinical Psychiatry, 56*, 590–591.

Youngerman, J., & Canino, I. A. (1978). Lithium carbonate use in children and adolescents: A survey of the literature. *Archives of General Psychiatry, 35*, 216–224.

13

Psychotherapy for Children with Bipolar Disorder

JILL S. GOLDBERG-ARNOLD and MARY A. FRISTAD

Early-onset bipolar disorder wreaks havoc on family life, school functioning, and peer relationships. Prompt and effective treatment is critical to protect and maintain as much as possible the child's developmental trajectory. In addition to the importance of pharmacological treatment (see Chapter 12), family-based intervention (see Chapter 14) and individual psychotherapy play an important role in maximizing functional outcome. The symptoms of early-onset bipolar disorder, along with those of frequently co-occurring disorders (e.g., oppositional defiant disorder, attention-deficit/hyperactivity disorder, generalized anxiety disorder), interfere with social and emotional development, causing problems with peer relationships as well as interference at home and in school. Therapy can help children learn to understand and better manage their symptoms and to negotiate the challenges that their illnesses present.

Despite the seeming importance of psychotherapy in the treatment of bipolar disorder in children and adolescents, there has been little research on interventions for this population. Kaslow and Thompson (1998) recently reviewed empirically validated psychosocial treatments for children and adolescents with depression. Only two met criteria for being "probably efficacious." Neither of these studies examined clinically depressed children (Kaslow & Thompson, 1998); rather, each examined and treated subsyndromal children in school settings (Stark, Brookman, & Frazier, 1990; Stark, Reynolds, & Kaslow, 1987). Our recent review (Fristad, Goldberg-Arnold, & Gavazzi, 2002b) indicated that there are no currently developed psychosocial treatments, empirically validated or otherwise, described in the scientific literature for children or adolescents with bipolar disorder.

This chapter reviews a child group therapy program developed as part of a larger multifamily psychoeducation program for families of preadolescent children (e.g., 8–11 years) with mood disorders. Multifamily psychoeducation groups (MFPGs) were developed to include children with bipolar and depressive spectrum illnesses and their parents. To date, a series of preliminary studies on the efficacy of the Family Psychoeducation Program have been conducted (Fristad, Gavazzi, Centolella, & Soldano, 1996; Fristad, Gavazzi, & Soldano, 1998; Fristad, Goldberg-Arnold, & Gavazzi, 2002a; Fristad et al., 2002b; Goldberg-Arnold, Fristad, & Gavazzi, 1999). The program was initially developed to include six weekly 1¼-hour sessions. Feedback from participants suggested the need for more and longer sessions. Thus, the program was recently revised to include eight weekly 1½-hour sessions. This format was piloted in a clinical setting; a full-scale randomized study is underway to further establish the efficacy of the program. As outcome data from the preliminary studies have been described and discussed elsewhere, the primary focus of this chapter is to describe the therapeutic techniques used in the children's groups and their applications to individual and family therapy settings. Developmental considerations for adapting therapeutic techniques for children of other age groups are discussed as well.

REVIEW OF PILOT STUDY FINDINGS

A pilot study of the 6-week protocol was recently completed with 35 children and their parents (47 parents participated). Families were randomly assigned to either immediate participation in MFPGs along with treatment as usual or to a 6-month waitlist control group along with treatment as usual. An MFPG consists of a group for parents (described in more detail in Chapter 14) and a group for children (described in detail below) that run concurrently. Families were recruited from a variety of sources, including our local National Alliance for the Mentally Ill (NAMI) chapter (1), via a newspaper article (11), from the university inpatient and outpatient units (8), and from local pediatricians (6), school psychologists (5), and mental health providers (4). Treatment histories ranged from no prior mental health contact to multiple inpatient hospitalizations along with intensive outpatient treatment and/or residential placement. Referral sources and treatment histories were equally distributed between the treatment groups.

At study entry, children's mood disorder diagnoses and their illness severity also spanned a wide spectrum (major depressive disorder, $n = 9$; dysthymic disorder, $n = 3$; dysthymic disorder/major depressive disorder, $n = 7$; bipolar I, $n = 4$; bipolar II, $n = 12$). The average Children's Global

Assessment Scale (C-GAS) score was 51 (range = 35–68; SD = 6.8) (Shaffer et al., 1983). Diagnoses were made using the Children's Inventory of Psychiatric Syndromes (ChIPS) child and parent versions (Rooney, Fristad, Weller, & Weller, 1999), the Child Depression Rating Scale—Revised (Poznanski et al., 1984), and the Mania Rating Scale (Young, Biggs, Ziegler, & Meyer, 1978). The mean number of additional comorbid diagnoses (behavior, anxiety, other) was 3.6 (range = 1–7). The children's mean age was 10.1 years (range = 7.7–11.8; SD = 1.2 years). Of the 35 children, 27 were boys (77%) and 29 (83%) were prescribed psychotropic medications. Further description of the participants can be found in Fristad and colleagues (2002a).

Assessments were conducted prior to study entry (T_1); 2 months after study entry, after the immediate treatment group completed MFPG (T_2); 6 months after study entry (4 months after MFPG completion for the immediate treatment group and just prior to MFPG for the waitlist group, T_3). Just the waitlist group was assessed again after completing MFPG (T_4). The Understanding Mood Disorders Questionnaire (UMDQ) was used to assess parental knowledge about mood disorder symptoms and treatments (Gavazzi, Fristad, & Law, 1997) and the Expressed Emotion Adjective Checklist (EEAC) was used to assess family environment (Friedmann & Goldstein, 1993). A detailed description of the assessment protocol is available in Fristad and colleagues (2002a).

For the purposes of this chapter, study results will be briefly summarized. There was no difference in baseline knowledge between the immediate and waitlist groups. However, both immediately after intervention and at the 6-month follow-up, parents in the immediate treatment group had greater knowledge about childhood mood disorders than did parents in the waitlist group. Parental ratings of the parent–child relationships improved for immediate treatment families and declined for the waitlist group from baseline to immediately and 4-months posttreatment. Children who participated in treatment reported a significant increase in perceived social support from parents and a trend toward increased perceived support from peers 4 months posttreatment. At 6-month follow-up, families who participated in treatment significantly improved their "consumer skills" (i.e., their ability to obtain appropriate services) compared to the waitlisted families (82% vs. 20%).

TREATMENT OVERVIEW

Bipolar disorder is an extremely difficult illness for children and adolescents. In both group and individual therapy, children and teens need to be given the message that they are not to *blame* for their symptoms and that they do not *cause* their symptoms. Rather, they share responsibility for *managing* their symptoms along with their parents and their treatment team. Therapy attempts to provide children and teens with as many tools as possible to assist them in taking increased responsibility for symptom management. To accomplish this, children and teens need to learn about bipolar disorder, accept the need for treatment, take medications as prescribed, learn coping strategies, and make healthy choices about thoughts and behaviors.

BEHAVIOR MANAGEMENT CAVEATS

Children with bipolar disorder can be a challenging population to treat. Group therapy is no exception. Many children with bipolar disorder have comorbid diagnoses (e.g., attention-deficit/hyperactivity disorder, oppositional defiant disorder), the symptoms of which present significant behavior management challenges of their own. In order for children to benefit from group sessions, it is necessary to create a positive atmosphere in which group members can have positive peer interactions and feel successful. Therefore, a positive discipline strategy is needed to provide structure, support, and sometimes extra motivation. A range of different point systems that vary in complexity can be used, based on the age of the participating children and the number of adults working with the children's group. For the group described below, points are given for completing group homework as well as for following group rules established during the initial session (e.g., only one person talks at a time, treat others respectfully, no "put-downs"). At the end of each session, group members and group leaders discuss and vote on points for each member. Points are tracked throughout the length of the group, then redeemed for small rewards during the final session.

Flexibility is critical to balance the needs of individual children with the goal of providing a positive experience for all group members. Working with a cotherapist allows the flexibility to provide breaks from the group for children who need it. For example, in a recent group, an 11-year-old boy with early-onset bipolar disorder and oppositional defiant disorder was experiencing a high level of agitation during most of the 2-month period in which group occurred. Provision of a break about 30 to 40 minutes into the 90-minute session allowed his continued participation in the group process. Without a planned break, he would escalate, refuse to take a break, and disrupt group for the other participants. With the cooperation of the cotherapist, it was arranged for this group member to leave with the lead therapist (also his individual therapist) to help with an errand related to the group. In this way, he was able to leave without being disruptive, without undue stigma, and then return successfully to the group a few minutes later.

GROUP THERAPY GOALS

Overall goals for the children's group are to (1) increase knowledge of mood disorder symptoms and treatments, (2) improve symptom management, (3) increase coping skills (e.g., anger management, anxiety management, communication, problem solving), and (4) improve peer and family relationships. While children are repeatedly given the message that they are not to *blame* for their mood symptoms, they are taught skills to more effectively and responsibly *manage* their symptoms and are encouraged to take responsibility for the choices they *can* make.

The content and goals for each of the eight group sessions are described in detail below. Although these groups are structured with goals, activities, and homework assignments predetermined for each session, the group therapist must maintain flexibility and change course as necessary and appropriate. For example, if a relevant but "out-of-sequence" topic arises based on input from the children, it can be discussed at that point rather than according to the preordained schedule. Also, groups vary in response to activities. Some are more receptive to discussion while others will work better with short discussions followed by more hands-on activities. Thus, the description below serves as a template rather than as a rigid schedule.

GENERAL PROGRAM DESCRIPTION

Each session begins with a brief meeting of parents and children together. Snacks are served at the beginning of each session to foster a congenial atmosphere and to provide an opportunity for casual conversation. Providing snacks is also a pragmatic consideration, as children are often quite hungry during the late afternoon or early evening, especially if "coming off" their stimulant dose. During the initial session, introductions are made and the format of the group is explained. Parents are given a booklet and children are given a folder containing information to be covered during group. The children's folders contain some basic materials initially; more is added during subsequent sessions. During the remaining sessions, the conjoint family time is used to review project assignments that parents and children have completed together during the previous week. The children then leave with their therapists. The two groups are conducted in adjacent rooms. Important features for the children's groups include a board to write on and a large area that can be used for *in vivo* practice (e.g., a gymnasium in the building).

The final 15–20 minutes of each 90-minute session is spent engaged in recreational activities, which serves as *in vivo* practice. Group games provide an opportunity to encourage and support appropriate social interactions and to develop friendships. Teamwork, rather than "winning," is emphasized, which is of particular importance for less athletically skilled children. Group leaders participate in the activities to model social skills, to facilitate teamwork, to ensure that teams are evenly matched, and to closely monitor social interactions. Children with early-onset bipolar disorder often find unstructured playtime (e.g., school recess) particularly challenging. Provision of close supervision during the *in vivo* practice time provides opportunities to reinforce positive behavior and to correct negative behavior. Group leaders have to be prepared to put on their sneakers and get involved with the activities! Each session ends with the children voting on their points and then rejoining the parent group, where they provide a report of their activities. During this time, upcoming family projects are explained. For a summary of all eight sessions, see Table 13.1.

Session 1

During the initial conjoint phase, group members introduce themselves and share some common information such as their name, age, grade, and name of their school. Following this discussion, children go to their own room with their group therapists. Once there, they reintroduce themselves and complete further "get-to-know-you" exercises (e.g., sharing names and types of pets, age and gender of siblings, favorite vacation site). After introductions, group rules are discussed, generated, and recorded as discussed previously. The point system is explained (e.g., each member can earn a maximum of 10 points for each session, including 2 points for bringing his or her completed homework). Group members are told that the points will be recorded at the end of each session and that they will be able to redeem their points for prizes during the eighth and final session.

The purpose of the group is then discussed and group members identify reasons for participating in the group (e.g., gaining knowledge about their diagnoses, learning ways to cope with resultant problems, and having an opportunity to meet others with similar problems). From the outset, group members frequently experience, and express, considerable relief at being able to look around the room and see that they are "not the only one." Most children with early-onset bipolar disorder are accustomed to having the most problems within their social setting. In group, all members have problems and almost everyone takes medication. Group members experience immediate social gains as a result of realizing that they are accepted within the group milieu. For children who have been uniformly rejected in their other social settings, this may provide their first opportunity to become leaders and to be "popular."

After reviewing the general group rules and the purpose of group, the discussion shifts to education about mood symptoms. Handouts included in the children's folders that describe depressive and manic symptoms are

TABLE 13.1. Summary of Session Goals, Activities, and Home Projects

Session	Goals	Activities	Home project
1	Introductions/orientation/learn about mood symptoms	"Get to know you" activities, group discussion, mood symptoms review	No child project (family project given through adjunct parent group)
2	Distinguish symptoms from self/learn about medications	"Naming the Enemy" exercise, medication review with association to symptoms	Naming the Enemy along with parents
3	Anger management	"Taking Charge of the Mad, Bad Feelings" exercise, "Building the Tool Kit" exercise	Anger management practice (record signals, triggers, and responses)
4	Responsibility/choices	"Thinking–Feeling–Doing" exercise	Use Thinking–Feeling–Doing worksheet to work through a negative mood state
5	Problem solving	"Stop–Think–Plan–Check" exercise is introduced, the group using the paradigm to discuss problems experienced by group members	Use Stop–Think–Plan–Check worksheet to evaluate a problem experienced during the week
6	Nonverbal communication	"Thoughts/Feelings Charades"	No words communication worksheet (practice nonverbal communication with parents)
7	Verbal communication	Human knot, empathic listening, or practicing giving clear instructions; discuss helpful versus unhelpful communication (including listening)	Discuss the Let's Talk worksheet with parents
8	Review/closure	Game to review content, sharing of phone numbers	Continue practicing and progressing!!

reviewed. The children discuss mood symptoms and other associated symptoms they have experienced. Alternate ways of labeling or describing symptoms are listed on the board (e.g., "everything gets on my nerves," "self-hatred," "being hyper"). Prior to rejoining the parents, children move to the play area and participate in a physical game (e.g., basketball, tag).

Session 2

From this session on, children participate in a brief check-in with parents, then move to "their" room to have a snack while briefly summarizing the previous session's content and reviewing their project of the week. The first "new" activity in this session is the "Naming the Enemy" exercise (see Figure 13.1; Fristad, Gavazzi, & Soldano, 1999). This exercise was developed initially for use with individual families (Fristad et al., 1999). We have successfully adapted it for use as a children's group exercise followed by completion at home with the parents as a family project. A large sheet of paper is taped to the board and used to record this exercise. A simple picture of a person is drawn at the top center of the paper, with two columns below it. Group members are asked to generate positive descriptions about themselves, which are written in the first column (e.g., respectful, good at basketball, takes care of animals, good at math, smart, funny). The group then generates a collective list of symptoms they have experienced. These are grouped into di-

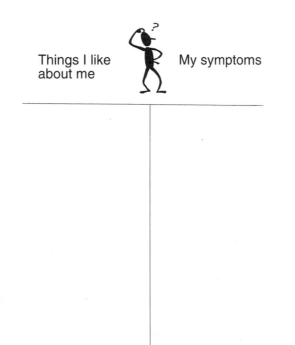

FIGURE 13.1. During Session 2, the "Naming the Enemy" exercise is used to help group members recognize how their strengths and positive characteristics can be masked by mood symptoms.

My Medicine

Name	Dose	Reason

FIGURE 13.2. In conjunction with a review of mood symptoms, each child is provided with information about his or her specific medications and then is asked to complete this chart, which is designed to help identify the reasons for each medication.

agnostic categories (e.g., depression, mania, anxiety) and written in the second column. Once symptoms have been generated, group leaders initiate a discussion of how symptoms can mask positive attributes and strengths. The paper is folded in half to graphically demonstrate how symptoms "mask" or "cover up" positive attributes and strengths.

Using the list of symptoms as a guide, group leaders then shift into a discussion about medications. Each child is given a set of information sheets corresponding to their currently prescribed medications. Target symptoms for each medication are reviewed. Children are then handed "child-friendly" forms on which they list their own medications (see Figure 13.2), then write the target symptoms they experience next to each relevant medication name. The group then pairs medications with symptoms listed on the board (e.g., Zoloft for depression, Depakote for mania). Children are then instructed about the coming week's family project: to complete the Naming the Enemy exercise along with their parents. These instructions are repeated at the closing phase of the session, when the children rejoin their parents.

Session 3

This session begins with a review of the Naming the Enemy exercise along with parents. Following this conjoint time, the children separate to their own room and the focus turns to developing coping skills. An integrated set of skills is taught sequentially in Sessions 3 through 7. Anger management is the first skill taught, using the "Taking Charge of the Mad, Bad Feelings" framework (see Figure 13.3). Anger is described as a normal and natural emotion that everyone experiences, but that must be managed to avoid hurtful outcomes. Anger triggers (i.e., what sets you off) and anger signals (i.e., signs of building anger) are identified and discussed for each child. The discussion then shifts to how signals (from the child or teen, or from the parent) can be used to facilitate a "stop before you react" game plan. Different strategies for managing anger are reviewed and practiced, including calming strategies that can be used in the moment (e.g., deep breaths, counting to 10, taking a break from the situation, and using "I messages").

The "Building the Tool Kit" exercise is introduced. Children are encouraged to assemble a wide range of "tools" to help them cope with difficult emotions and problem situations. For this discussion, four circles are drawn on the board (see Figure 13.4) and labeled "Physical" (e.g., running outside, punching a pillow), "Creative" (e.g., drawing, listening to music), "Social" (e.g., talking with a trusted person, playing with a friend, spend-

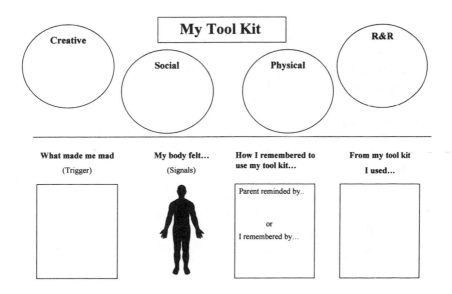

FIGURE 13.3. The "Taking Charge of the Mad, Bad Feelings" exercise is used during Session 3 to teach anger management.

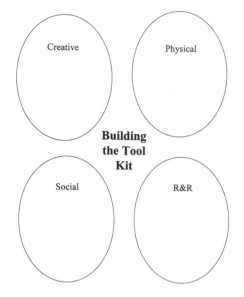

FIGURE 13.4. In conjunction with teaching anger management, the "Building the Tool Kit" exercise is used to help group members identify different realms of coping tools.

ing time with a pet), and "R&R" (e.g., restorative activities such as getting a drink or snack, going to a "private place" such as a bedroom or corner of the playground, taking a warm bath, taking a nap). Group members are asked to generate strategies to fit in each sphere. As strategies are suggested, they are listed in the appropriate circles on the board. Each child is asked to identify his or her favored strategies within the coping realms (i.e., physical, creative, social, or R&R). The need for a variety of strategies is emphasized. The session wraps up with a discussion of the importance of recognizing anger and taking responsibility for one's behavior when angry. Again, the separateness of feelings and behavior is emphasized. Children are reminded that they are *not to blame* for feeling angry but they *are responsible* for what they do when they are angry. Children are given an "Anger Management Worksheet" (Figure 13.3) to complete before the next session, on which children are asked to personalize their own tool kit, then describe an anger-provoking situation, record their anger signals, describe how they remembered to use their tool kit, and finally, explain how they handled the situation.

Session 4

After a brief check-in, snacks, and review of the Anger Management Worksheet, the session turns to extending the theme of responsibility and the power of choices. The "Thinking–Feeling–Doing" (T–F–D) exercise, a

simplified method of teaching cognitive-behavioral principles, is introduced to teach the relationship between thoughts, feelings, and behavior
(Fristad & Holderle, 2001). A picture is drawn on the board as well as
given to the children as a worksheet (see Figure 13.5). The picture depicts a
stick-figure person with a thought bubble, a heart, and a box. The heart
represents feelings and the box represents actions. Each shape (e.g.,
thought bubble, feelings heart, action box) is divided into top and bottom
parts. Beginning with the heart, the group is prompted for examples of unpleasant mood states (e.g., sad, angry, anxious), which are listed on the
bottom side of the heart. The group is then prompted for the preferred
mood states (e.g., happy, calm, relaxed), which are listed on the top side of
the heart. The group then shifts focus to the actions box. The top half of
the box is labeled "helpful" and the bottom is labeled "hurtful." The
group is asked for examples of how an individual might choose to act
when he or she is angry, sad, or anxious. Helpful choices (e.g., talking to
someone about how you are feeling) are listed in the top part of the box
and hurtful choices (e.g., hitting someone) are listed in the bottom part.
The group then shifts again to the thought bubble. The top half of the bubble is labeled "helpful" and the bottom half is labeled "hurtful." The
group then works together to identify examples of self-talk or thought processes that are either helpful (e.g., "I can work this out"; "I just made a

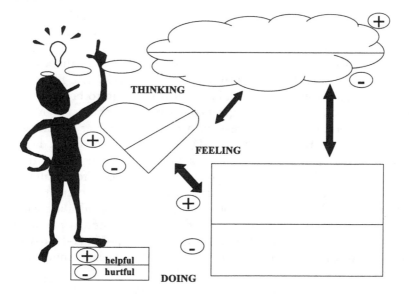

FIGURE 13.5. During Session 4, the focus turns to being responsible for making helpful choices. The "Thinking–Feeling–Doing" exercise is used to teach the connections between feelings, thoughts, and actions and to differentiate between helpful and hurtful
choices.

mistake but it will work out") or hurtful (e.g., "I wish I would die"; "Everybody hates me"), and then these are listed in the appropriate boxes. Once examples have been generated for each part of each shape, the group is prompted to consider the relationships between thinking, feeling, and doing. The idea that it is very difficult to "will yourself" out of a negative mood and into a better mood is emphasized. Instead, two-way arrows are drawn from thoughts to actions, thoughts to feelings, and actions to feelings. The individual's ability to change his or her actions and thoughts to bring about the desired mood change is emphasized. Group members are again reminded that they are not to blame for negative moods. Rather, they now can choose to act on helpful behaviors and focus on helpful thoughts—they have tools available to change their negative moods.

Once these general ideas have been taught, individual group members are encouraged to give examples of times they have experienced painful moods. The group works together to identify hurtful actions and thoughts and to generate helpful behavioral choices and thoughts. Each child is given an extra copy of the T–F–D worksheet and asked to use it during the upcoming week to work through a negative mood state. When the children rejoin their parents, this exercise is also explained to the parents so they can facilitate the process.

Session 5

After checking in with parents and reviewing the T–F–D worksheets completed during the previous week, focus shifts to problem solving. Session 5 content builds on awareness gained in Sessions 1 and 2 and skills taught in Sessions 3 and 4. Group members are taught to think of problem solving in several steps: "Stop–Think–Plan–Check" (see Figure 13.6). The first step, "Stop," involves calming down enough to be able to think (in other words, to use the anger management strategies taught during Session 3). Group members are then asked to volunteer problems they have experienced recently. The T–F–D figure is drawn on the board so that the group can explore helpful actions and thoughts to try (the "Think" step). The group votes on the best strategies for dealing with the problem (the "Plan" step). Examples of problems articulated by recent group members include negotiating sibling conflict, dealing with suicidal thoughts, and coping with an unreliable noncustodial parent. Each group member is given another copy of the "Stop–Think–Plan–Check" worksheet to explore solutions to a problem during the coming week as a family project.

Session 6

This session begins with a review of the "Stop–Think–Plan–Check" worksheet done at home. Group members share problems they experi-

The Problem:_____

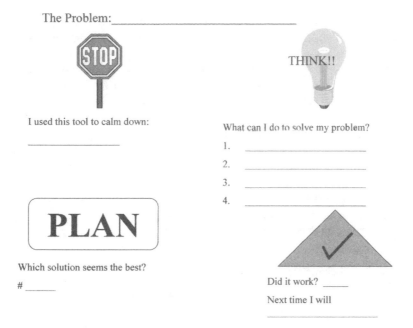

FIGURE 13.6. During Session 5, impulse control strategies are taught using the "Stop–Think–Plan–Check" exercise.

enced and how they resolved them. Group members' actions are discussed using the "Stop–Think–Plan–Check" paradigm to reinforce the use of these four steps in solving problems. The focus then shifts to communication skills, specifically, nonverbal communication. Observations of children with mood disorders suggests that they often demonstrate poor social skills due to current symptoms as well as to developmental interruptions caused by episodes of mania and depression. This can be exacerbated by right-hemisphere weaknesses that contribute to an impaired ability to interpret social cues, interpersonal distance, and humor. A specific area in which children with early-onset bipolar disorder often lag behind peers is their awareness of and sensitivity to their own and others' nonverbal communication (e.g., asking for things in an irritable tone of voice, not noticing that a comment has hurt a peer's feelings and then continuing to make hurtful comments).

In order to raise awareness and develop skills, a game of "Thoughts/Feelings Charades" is introduced. Prior to the game, group members are asked to generate examples of ways that people communicate (e.g., talking, tone of voice, body language, facial expression). Group members then take turns demonstrating a thought or feeling using only body language, with prompts ranging from simple (e.g., "I feel angry") to complex (e.g., "I feel guilty"). Group members attempt to guess the thought or feeling. After playing the game for several rounds, the group discusses the importance of reading others' body language and being aware of one's own body language. Members generate examples of how paying attention to nonverbal communication might help relationships. After working with body language and facial expressions, the group shifts to tone of voice. Group members practice different tones, including angry and whiny, then demonstrate more appropriate tones. The importance of making sure that vocal tone matches the situation is emphasized (e.g., using a polite tone instead of an angry tone when you want someone to do something for you). Each group member is given a worksheet to take home (see Figure 13.7). They are asked to practice nonverbal communication with their parents. On the form, they are asked to record whether their parents can correctly guess the emotion they are expressing, then if they can correctly guess the emotion their parent is demonstrating.

Session 7

After a review of the nonverbal communication assignment, the discussion turns to verbal communication and listening skills. A variety of different exercises can be used to teach and underscore different aspects of verbal communication, depending on the level of the group. A fun and active opening exercise is to have the group form a human knot. The group is then instructed to disentangle *without* speaking. The process of disentan-

Feeling	Child Practices-- Can Adult Guess? ☺ = yes ? = not sure	Adult Practices-- Can Child Guess? ☺ = yes ? = not sure
Happy		
Sad		
Scared		
Angry		
Bored		
Other:_____		

FIGURE 13.7. During Session 6, nonverbal communication is taught. The "No Words" exercise is sent home as a family project to provide additional practice.

gling is timed. Once the group is finished, they are asked what made the process easy and/or difficult. After a brief discussion, they are asked to form a knot a second time. They are then asked to disentangle using as much verbal communication as possible (i.e., no one moves without explaining what he or she plans to do). This process is also timed. The group compares their two "disentangling experiences" (e.g., no talking vs. talking through the process) and discusses the importance of communication in solving problems.

Different verbal communication activities can be used, depending on the composition of the group. For particularly verbal children, the focus might be placed on using empathic listening and communication strategies; less verbal children might benefit from a focus on more basic aspects of verbal communication. One exercise that can be used with less verbally skilled children demonstrates the importance of clear communication. For this exercise, each group member takes a turn at being the "instructor." As instructor, the child is given a geometric design and then is asked to describe the design such that the other group members can accurately draw it without seeing it. The "instructor" is coached, as needed, to give specific clear commands. Once instructions are completed, the "instructor" looks at the drawings to compare them to the model and to appraise his or her success at describing the design. After each member has had a turn as "instructor," the session turns from this nonthreatening topic to one that is more sensitive. The group works together to generate helpful and unhelpful ways in which family members listen and communicate with each other. This discussion gives the children an opportunity to evaluate their own communication strategies, including their listening skills. During a recent group, one boy with early-onset bipolar disorder and oppositional defiant disorder talked about how unhelpful it is when he argues with his mother about a simple request because he wants to watch TV instead. He noted that if he would do what she requested right away, he would be done in a few minutes and would still be able to watch his show rather than spending the whole show arguing with her. Group members are then instructed to record polite requests for improved communication with their parents on the top half of the "Let's Talk" Worksheet (see Figure 13.8). They share this with their parents (who have been instructed to listen and not comment) when they rejoin the parents' group. Parents are asked to complete the bottom half of the "Let's Talk" Worksheet at home, then discuss it with their children.

Session 8

The final session is dedicated to review and closure. A game-show format is used to review material presented in the seven previous groups. As a point system has been used throughout group, this last session includes an opportunity for group members to trade in their points for small rewards (e.g., inexpensive games and toys purchased at a party supply store). Trading of phone numbers is encouraged if group members initiate the idea (this usually occurs).

APPLICATIONS IN INDIVIDUAL THERAPY

Much of the session content described above readily transports to work with individual children and families. Advantages of the group (i.e., increased social support, peer feedback, *in vivo* practice, role plays, and discussions with same-age peers) are lost, but advantages of "individual family" work are gained. These advantages include ease in scheduling and the opportunity to individualize content to address the specific needs of the child and his or her family.

Naming the Enemy

This exercise is particularly useful early in treatment to help the child and his or her family establish a constructive framework for communicating in a noncritical manner about the child's symptoms (Fristad et al., 1999).

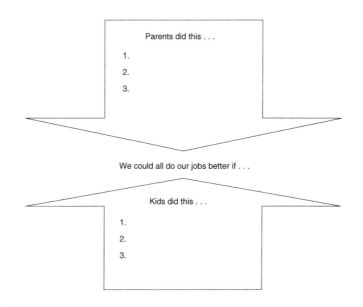

FIGURE 13.8. During Session 7, verbal communication is practiced. The "Let's Talk" exercise is started in the children's group, then sent home to complete as a family project.

When a first episode occurs during adulthood, self-identity is well established. When onset occurs during childhood, self-identity is in the process of emerging. The earlier the age of onset of mood symptoms, the more difficult it can become to disentangle symptoms from other characteristics of the child. The Naming the Enemy exercise can be conducted with a child and his or her parents toward the end of an initial evaluation or early in therapy to facilitate the disentanglement of symptoms from personality and to establish the mood disorder as the "common enemy" of the child and family. This also helps to decrease tension between family members, including the child, as they utilize a common nonblaming language to discuss problems associated with the child's illness. As in group, the family is initially asked to generate positive attributes and strengths of the child, which are listed in one column (see Figure 13.1). After the strengths are listed, the family is then asked to generate a list of symptoms. The symptoms are listed in the second column and grouped according to diagnoses. Once the two lists are completed, the paper is folded in half so that the symptoms physically cover up the strengths. This very concrete exercise is used to help remind the family of the child's positive characteristics and the tendency of mood symptoms to mask or cover up strengths. The mood disorder is established as "the enemy," while the parents, child, and treatment providers are "on the same team" fighting "against the enemy." In this framework, the goal of treatment can be to help the child's preexisting strengths to reemerge.

For example, Chris is an 8-year-old male diagnosed with early-onset bipolar disorder and attention-deficit/hyperactivity disorder. At the time of his initial evaluation, he had recently begun taking a mood stabilizer and his behavior had started to improve. He and his parents listed many strengths for him (e.g., good at sports, including soccer and football; good-looking; good at math; very loving; kind; thoughtful; interested in animals; inquisitive). When asked about the symptoms he had been experiencing, they listed a number of problems which were grouped under the headings "Bipolar" (e.g., really mad; hits people; grumpy; can't fall asleep; silly; hyper; talks fast, loud, and a lot; thoughts race) and "ADHD" (e.g., get in trouble a lot, can't sit still, hard to concentrate, not listening, bored easily). Once the two lists were generated, the paper was folded in half to graphically represent how symptoms cover up positive qualities. Chris experienced some relief at hearing his parents talk about his strengths. Chris's family all benefited by seeing his *symptoms* as the primary problem rather than seeing *him* as "bad."

Building the Tool Kit

An important goal of therapy for both children and adolescents with bipolar disorder is to build their coping resources. The Building the Tool Kit exercise can also be used with individual children and adolescents. When working with children, a more concrete approach can be used. For example, Ian is an 11-year-old with bipolar disorder. His moods cycle rapidly, with a predominance of mixed mood states. He becomes easily overwhelmed in group settings. In therapy, however, Ian is insightful and able to eloquently describe his mood states. He labels his mood as "overstimulated," which he defines as a combination of excitement, sadness, anger, happiness, anxiety, and worry. His mother reports significant opposition from him whenever she notices him becoming "overstimulated." She has tried to encourage him to remove himself from situations (e.g., playing with a group of peers) when this occurs. As part of therapy, Ian and his therapist discussed his need to take increasing responsibility for managing his mood. Along with referring him to a child psychiatrist to adjust his medications and help him achieve greater mood stability, he and his therapist began to develop a tool kit. Initially, Ian objected to being asked to remove himself from situations, as he perceived this as punishment. To help change his perceptions, Ian and his therapist developed plans for an actual tool kit that he would assemble at home with his mother's cooperation. Ian and his therapist talked about what things could be placed in his tool kit that he would enjoy using to help himself settle down. First, he identified some music, so several compact discs (CDs) and a portable CD player were included in his kit. Next, Ian named reading certain books and playing with army figures as favorite activities, and so these items were also placed in the tool kit. Emphasis was placed on Ian taking responsibility and utilizing his mother as an important resource in managing his moods.

Ian is at the older end of the continuum for using such a concrete approach. With teenagers, the tool kit can be assembled in both abstract and concrete ways. A decorated box can hold bath salts, a favorite CD, and "cue cards" with reminders of pleasurable, calming activities. Encouraging development of options from a range of categories (e.g., physical, creative, social, restorative) is important, as some activities may be more applicable to different situations. For example, a teenager struggling with depressive symptoms may find comfort in running, but, after dark, may need to choose another strategy such as calling a friend to improve her mood.

Thinking–Feeling–Doing

This exercise (see Figure 13.5) can also be used very successfully with children and teens in an individual or family setting. The cartoon format, although simple, is well received by children and adolescents. This exercise can be used on an ongoing basis to help children and teens work through challenging problems and to teach and reinforce the idea that moods are not chosen but do have to be managed.

For example, Brian, a 9-year-old Caucasian male, was having considerable difficulty managing frustration and anger. Following the onset of his mood disorder, the T–F–D exercise was used to help him develop his resources for coping with negative affect. Previously, Brian had worked on building his toolkit (see previous section) and had developed lists of his preferred coping strategies within the four spheres (e.g., creative activities included playing the piano, drawing, and building models; physical activities included riding his bike, kicking a ball, and hitting a tennis ball; social activities included playing video games with a friend, talking problems over with parents, and playing with the family dog; restorative activities included taking a bath, playing Gameboy, and laying on the bed). The T–F–D diagram was next used in therapy to help him make the connections between his affect, his thoughts, and his actions. Brian reported "mad" as the mood he most often needed to manage, with "happy" and "calm" as the preferred options. He easily grasped the idea that it is extremely difficult to just decide to stop being mad and to start being happy. His attention was then directed to the "Doing" boxes. Brian was asked to describe hurtful things that he sometimes does when he feels mad. He generated several examples, including shutting down and refusing to talk, screaming and yelling, and throwing things. He readily recognized that these actions result in negative consequences as well as a continuation of negative mood. Brian was then asked to generate some helpful actions. This was more difficult for him, but by referring to his toolkit, Brian was able to come up with some alternatives, including going to his room and playing with his dog. Attention was next shifted to his thoughts. Brian identified several examples of hurtful thoughts, including "nothing ever goes my way" and "everything is always ruined." He was then coached through developing more helpful thoughts, including "I'm just mad right now" and "Things will seem better when I'm calm."

Divide and Conquer

The overarching goal for both individual and group psychotherapy for children and young adolescents with bipolar disorder is to reduce the impact of mood symptoms on everyday functioning by increasing coping skills. Teaching the "Divide and Conquer" technique can be extremely helpful. During depressive episodes, children are often easily overwhelmed by tasks. The object of Divide and Conquer is for children to learn strategies to break tasks and situations down into manageable chunks. For example, during a particularly severe and nonremitting depressive episode, a 16-year-old girl would become overwhelmed and immobilized when faced with school assignments that she would have previously found to be simple. The focus of therapy became helping her to divide her assignments into smaller chunks so that she could "conquer" her academic tasks.

Putting on the Brakes

The opposite approach is used for children experiencing increased energy during manic or hypomanic episodes. This is an attempt to increase self-awareness, thereby helping the child to limit his or her activities, thus avoiding becoming overwhelmed or making damaging choices. For example, a child experiencing the beginnings of a manic episode can be coached to limit her activities and manage her sleep regimen to prevent an escalation of symptoms. For one 16-year-old male, "putting on the brakes" translated to staying home from school on days that he was not sure he could control his anger and interact appropriately in social situations. In this way, he was able to prevent himself from damaging his social support system.

DEVELOPMENTAL CONSIDERATIONS

For both group and individual settings, developmental status plays an important role in setting goals and planning therapy. For young children (e.g., preschool, early elementary school) many of the therapeutic activities previously described can be introduced in sessions along with parents, then carried out at home. For example, parents and children can build a tool kit together in therapy, then the parents can reinforce their child at home for turning to the tool kit when necessary. For young adolescents, gaining autonomy from family is an important developmental task. The therapist can play an important role in helping adolescents to appropriately accept the responsibility that comes with increased freedom, while supporting parents in the "letting-go" process. The content and process of group therapy varies greatly for different age ranges. Young children (e.g., 6–8) need an activity-based group with frequent opportunities for hands-on activities and practice of skills. Older children (e.g., 8–11) continue to need practice and activities but can absorb information about their illness and participate in more in-depth discussions. Adolescents may benefit from a different type of group with a much greater focus on discussion and peer support and less overt leadership from a therapist. Considerable negotiation around issues of separation and individuation are inherent to working with adolescents. Areas of predictable discussion are determining "who's in charge" in regard to medication adherence, therapy attendance, and school special services involvement, and addressing issues related to self-medication (i.e., substance use).

CONCLUSIONS

We have a great deal to learn about treating bipolar disorder in children and young adolescents. The techniques discussed in this chapter have been developed as part of an empirically supported but not yet empirically validated program. Additional research is needed to further develop, refine, and test psychosocial interventions for children and adolescents with bipolar disorder.

ACKNOWLEDGMENT

This work was supported in part by grants from the Ohio Department of Mental Health and the National Institute of Mental Health (R01 MH61512).

REFERENCES

Friedmann, M. S., & Goldstein, M. J. (1993). Relatives' awareness of their own expressed emotion as measured by a self-report adjective checklist." *Family Process, 32*, 459–471.

Fristad, M., Gavazzi, S. M., Centolella, D., & Soldano, K. (1996). Psychoeducation: An intervention strategy for families of children with mood disorders. *Contemporary Family Therapy, 18*, 371–383.

Fristad, M. A., Gavazzi, S. M., & Soldano, K. W. (1998). Multi-family psychoeducation groups for childhood mood disorders: A program description and preliminary efficacy data. *Contemporary Family Therapy, 20*(3), 385–402.

Fristad, M. A., Gavazzi, S. M., & Soldano, K. W. (1999). Naming the enemy: Learning to differentiate mood disorder "symptoms" from the "self" that experiences them. *Journal of Family Psychotherapy, 10*(1), 81–88.

Fristad, M. A., Goldberg-Arnold, J. S., & Gavazzi, S. M. (2002a). *The efficacy of multi-family psychoeducation as an adjunctive intervention for families of children with mood disorders.* Manuscript submitted for publication.

Fristad, M. A., Goldberg-Arnold, J. S., & Gavazzi, S. M. (2002b). Multifamily psychoeducation groups (MFPG) for families of children with bipolar disorder. *Bipolar Disorders, 4*, 254–262.

Fristad, M. A., & Holderle, K. E. (2001). *Thinking–Feeling–Doing: A practical approach to cognitive-behavioral therapy for children and adolescents.* Unpublished manuscript.

Gavazzi, S. M., Fristad, M. A., & Law, J. (1997). The Understanding Mood Disorders Questionnaire. *Psychological Reports, 81*, 172–174.

Goldberg-Arnold, J. S., Fristad, M. A., & Gavazzi, S. M. (1999). Family psychoeducation: Giving caregivers what they want and need. *Family Relations, 48*, 411–417.

Kaslow, N. J., & Thompson, M. P. (1998). Applying the criteria for empirically supported treatments to studies of psychosocial interventions for child and adolescent depression. *Journal of Clinical Child Psychology, 27*(2), 146–155.

Poznanski, E. O., Grossman, J. A., Buchsbaum, Y., Banegas, M., Freeman, L., & Gibbons, R. (1984). Preliminary studies of the reliability and validity of the Children's Depression Rating Scale. *Journal of the American Academy of Child Psychiatry, 23*, 191–197.

Rooney, M. T., Fristad, M. A., Weller, E. B., & Weller, R. A. (1999). *Children's Inter-

view for Psychiatric Syndromes: Administration manual. Washington, DC: American Psychiatric Press.

Shaffer, D., Gould, M. S., Brasic, J., Ambrosini, P., Fisher, P., Bird, H., & Aluwahlia, S. (1983). A children's global assessment scale (CGAS). *Archives of General Psychiatry, 40,* 1228–1231.

Stark, K. D., Brookman, C. S., & Frazier, R. (1990). A comprehensive school-based treatment program for depressed children. *School Psychology Quarterly, 5,* 111–140.

Stark, K. D., Reynolds, W. M., & Kaslow, N. J. (1987). A comparison of the relative efficacy of self-control therapy and a behavioral problem-solving therapy for depression in children. *Journal of Abnormal Child Psychology, 15,* 91–113.

Young, R. C., Biggs, J. T., Ziegler, V. E., & Meyer, D. A. (1978). A rating scale for mania: Reliability, validity and sensitivity. *British Journal of Psychiatry, 133,* 429–435.

14

Family Interventions for Early-Onset Bipolar Disorder

MARY A. FRISTAD and JILL S. GOLDBERG-ARNOLD

The clinical interventions described below have been developed based on our cumulative clinical and research experience in treating families in groups (Fristad, Arnett, & Gavazzi, 1998; Fristad, Gavazzi, Centolella, & Soldano, 1996; Fristad, Gavazzi, & Soldano, 1998) as well as individually (Fristad, Arnett, & Gavazzi, 1999) when a child within the family has an early-onset bipolar disorder. We value the openness and candidness of the families with whom we have had the opportunity to work and collaborate. Likewise, we greatly appreciate our local advocacy groups and national online support groups for giving us vital "insider" perspectives on what does and does not assist families in coping with early-onset bipolar disorder, which is, without doubt, a very difficult and trying illness.

CLINICAL CAVEATS

It is important for family members and clinicians to note that "one size does *not* fit all" when preparing a treatment plan. The label "bipolar disorder" describes one of probably an assortment of diagnoses experienced by the child, and does not in full define the child. To further complicate matters, children's symptoms will vary as they develop for at least three reasons: changes in the child, changes in the child's environment, and the vacillating nature of the illness. As a result, successful programming for a child with bipolar disorder requires tremendous flexibility. Thinking of the child's treatment and educational needs as "moving targets" provides the players in the system with a positive and productive mindset.

Likewise, it is helpful to "think globally, act locally." This phrase, borrowed from the world of social activism, is quite fitting here. First, parents of children with early-onset bipolar disorder often describe themselves as social activists working on behalf of their children. Second, "think globally, act locally" also refers to the need for the coordinating clinician to have a broad awareness of bipolar disorder and its changing manifestations in children and adolescents, and then to arrange for individual therapeutic components to address the various needs of the child and his or her family, as the specific situation demands.

To facilitate family-based treatment planning, we discuss common trouble spots for families contending with early-onset bipolar disorder. Then we describe therapeutic interventions to address these concerns.

PREDICTABLE PROBLEMS AND PROMISING POSSIBILITIES

The Child's Perspective

Children with bipolar disorder often have tremendous difficulties getting along with other family members, although these are the same individuals who ultimately can provide the greatest support and resources for the ill child. In large part, these difficulties can be attributed to their frequently occurring rages, which can be unpredictable and dangerous. Thus, it is essential that adults in the home are in agreement about the development and utilization of a safety plan. Frank discussions with family members, including siblings, regarding safety rules (e.g., clarifying the difference between "tattling" and getting reinforcements, when needed, for safety) can defuse some of the tension related to rages.

It is quite difficult for children with early-onset bipolar disorder *not* to become demoralized. As a result, children with early-onset bipolar disorder can begin to blame the illness for their behavior and then make no attempt to manage, or take responsibility for, their own symptoms (an unhealthy variation of "the devil made me do it!"). A key therapeutic goal is to help children internalize the message "It's not your fault, but it is your challenge." By this we mean that neither the child nor his or her parents are to blame for the illness. However, the child and his or her family ultimately will be most affected by the consequences of the illness, so the more they are able to communicate and problem-solve about symptom management, the better off they will be. More details about developing these skills in children with early-onset bipolar disorder appear in Chapter 13, on therapy for children with early-onset bipolar disorder.

The Sibling Perspective

Siblings quite likely experience one or more predictable struggles while growing up in a home with a brother or sister who has early-onset bipolar disorder. Many siblings resent the different sets of rules laid down by parents ("Why do *I* have to make my bed—you don't make *Jennifer* make hers!"). Whenever possible, it is useful to point out the uniformity of rules (e.g., *all* family members are expected not to hurt others with words or actions, consequences occur if they do), as well as rule modifications made for reasons other than the sibling's illness (e.g., younger children are assigned less demanding chores than older children). Beyond this, having candid discussions within the home about each family member's unique strengths and weaknesses can help the sibling to accept different expectations for different family members. Some siblings struggle with the fear that they, too, will become ill like their brother or sister. In many cases, parents can alleviate this concern by pointing out the differences in temperament that suggest the sibling will *not* follow in his brother or sister's footsteps. In some cases, however, more than one child in a family does develop a mood disorder. If this occurs, parents are urged to address each child's treatment needs separately, as the course of illness will not necessarily be the same for each child.

Another common problem is "getting lost in the shuffle." Parents often are made aware of this through the nonverbal actions of siblings (e.g., misbehaving to get attention, withdrawing). As much as parents can, they are encouraged to carve out one-to-one time to spend with nonaffected siblings. This gives nonaffected siblings the clear message that they can get positive attention without acting out. If not, brothers and sisters learn that negative actions result in attention, which inevitably leads to imitation of negative behaviors. Such imitative behavior occurs with great regularity in younger siblings, but can also occur with older siblings. Although parents of children with early-onset bipolar disorder may be intellectually aware of siblings' needs, it often takes specific focus in family therapy sessions to assist overwhelmed and exhausted parents to make realistic plans to address the needs of their other children. Doing so, however, can reap the reward of diminished copycat behavior in siblings. Finally, brothers and sisters need to understand clearly that imitating negative behavior is not considered acceptable within the family home.

A concern particularly relevant for older siblings is that they will "drift away," getting their emotional needs met (or not met) through other sources—whether healthy (e.g., a church youth group, a sports team) or unhealthy (e.g., drugs, sex, alcohol). While all teenagers increasingly turn toward peers and away from family as part of their normal development, parents should still be available as their "anchor." If teenagers who have siblings with early-onset bipolar disorder perceive their parents as emotionally unavailable, they will not benefit from the important grounding that their parents can provide.

Many siblings experience tremendous embarrassment, especially when their ill brother or sister has had a manic episode. This embarrassment can go hand in hand with tremendous loyalty toward and defensiveness on behalf of the ill child. Both parents and siblings benefit from the acknowledgment that such mixed feelings can occur, and, in fact, are predictable.

Finally, some siblings, particularly older/eldest siblings, often try to protect their brother or sister with early-onset bipolar disorder and/or take on the role of a "third" parent (or, for the many single parents raising a child with early-onset bipolar disorder, the "second" parent role). Siblings should be commended on their care and compassion, then given clearly defined guidelines regarding what assistance is appropriate (and not appropriate) for them to provide.

For all the issues described above—resentment, fear, imitation, loneliness, embarrassment, and pseudomaturity—the need for effective family communication is highlighted. Making clear plans to address the emotional (and sometimes practical physical needs) of siblings is very important. This may involve recruiting additional adults into the family's day-to-day life, such as a grandparent, aunt, or uncle. Siblings will benefit from having someone outside the home with whom they can candidly express their feelings. In addition to support coming from a loving adult friend or relative, support might also come from a sibling group run by a local mental health agency or consumer support group, a school guidance counselor, or a private therapist. To grow up psychologically healthy in a family of origin affected by early-onset bipolar disorder, siblings ultimately will need to be able to define and articulate their feelings, to not be ashamed of them, and to have well-defined coping strategies.

The Parent's Perspective

Perhaps most draining for parents can be the lack of concordance between the adults in caretaking roles. This can be as "simple" as two parents within a home disagreeing or as "complicated" as various coalitions of parents, stepparents, and extended relatives disagreeing over the most appropriate care for the ill child. The amount of disagreement between parents/caregivers on child-rearing matters has been linked to higher rates of child problem behaviors (Jouriles et al., 1991), poor marital quality (Lamb, Hwang, & Broberg, 1989), lower levels of family problem solving (Vuchinich, Vuchinich, & Wood, 1993) and overall parental effectiveness (Deal, Halverson, & Wampler, 1989). Cole and Rehm (1986) found that fathers provided significantly less positive reinforcement for their children during a challenging task than mothers, regardless of whether the child was depressed or nondepressed. This reinforces findings that mothers and fathers approach parenting tasks differently and suggests that fathers in particular may benefit from interventions designed to increase positive parent–child interactions.

In addition to the problem of concordance, there is the practical concern of sheer exhaustion for the parent of a child with early-onset bipolar disorder. Physical, mental, and emotional exhaustion can develop after a parent has spent hours in therapeutic holds until a child with early-onset bipolar disorder comes out of a rage, after restless or sleepless nights worrying about the nighttime wanderings and behaviors of a manic child, or after attending countless meetings with schools, police, therapists, physicians, social welfare agencies, and so forth in regard to the ill child. It is critical that parents adopt the mindset that they are running a marathon (i.e., they will be parenting their child for many years to come!) and not a sprint, and they will need to pace themselves accordingly. As difficult as it can be, it is essential that parents value taking care of themselves. Otherwise, they will find that they have nothing left to give their ill child and his or her siblings (not to mention their spouse or significant other, colleagues at work, etc.). This sometimes requires assisting families to reexamine "the big picture"—to determine what is a reasonable amount of stress and strain the family realistically can manage. This may result in the parents deciding to reduce their expenditures in order to live on one or one and a half incomes instead of two, for example, or to find other ways to simplify their lifestyle in an effort to "buy" more time and energy for the family's needs.

Parents commonly feel guilty about their child's difficulties. Education regarding the biological underpinnings of bipolar disorder can be useful to defuse this guilt. However, this frequently produces the unwanted consequence of spouses pointing fingers at each other's family of origin. It is critical that parents learn to accept the reality that "we don't get to choose the genes we get, or the ones we give." Blaming themselves or their spouses for "their family history" is damaging. Helping the family to refocus on accepting the present reality and moving forward to proactively manage symptoms is essential. When parents are successfully "deguiltified," they have much more emotional energy to turn toward the very difficult task of parenting a child with early-onset bipolar disorder.

Isolation is another common sequelae for families. Often, friends and/ or relatives do not understand or do not want to be bothered with the additional effort often required to have a child with early-onset bipolar disorder in their home. Likewise, parents may be too fearful or ashamed to bring their child to social gatherings. In single-parent homes in particular, the logistics of leaving the home can become difficult, as the child with early-onset bipolar disorder requires monitoring and may not be cooperative about attending siblings' events. Online support groups have been extremely useful in providing social support to parents who feel isolated (Sisson & Fristad, 2001). Another strategy is for parents to candidly explain their situation to family members or friends with whom they feel comfortable, and who can provide respite or support, as needed. Some parents have found that sharing educational materials (e.g., handouts summarizing key features of the illness) with friends and family helps build their credibility when attempting to convey the information that their child has a "real" disorder.

The Family's Perspective

It is very easy for the illness to "take over" family life. Doing so diverts attention from other family developmental issues (e.g., becoming involved as a family with outside groups such as churches, celebrating family milestones, planning family vacations). Family therapy can be used by parents to regain perspective and focus on "the big picture" when the family is not in a crisis stage.

Families can also experience tremendous financial strain from the cost of treatment, which is typically not covered adequately (or with parity to physical illnesses) by the family's insurance policy, the cost of added specialized childcare and medications, and reduced wage-earning potential on the part of one or more parent(s). Parents' roles as social activists are revisited here. Although parents of children and adolescents with early-onset bipolar disorder quite likely feel as if their time, energy, and resources are completely occupied by the demands of raising a child with early-onset bipolar disorder, they might wish to encourage others to participate in local lobbying and campaigning for insurance parity, increased availability of treatment resources, and other issues of importance. Local support group chapters (e.g., local National Alliance for the Mentally Ill or Mental Health Association chapters) often provide an organized resource for such individuals wishing to "do their part."

In addition to coping with the lack of insurance parity, dealing with insurance carriers can be a nightmare in and of itself. Horror stories of promised coverage that vanishes once charges are accrued are commonplace. Lengthy waits on hold, disconnects, contradictory information, and being assigned to providers unsophisticated in the assessment and treatment of early-onset bipolar disorder are frequently experienced. While there are no satisfactory answers to this dilemma, we encourage families to contact their state insurance commission to lodge formal complaints against any insurance carrier that does not appear to be maintaining its contractual agreement for timely and adequate service (within the confines of what the policy promises to deliver).

Finally, some predictable negative family cycles can ensue for families in which one (or more) member(s) is experiencing a serious mental illness (Holder & Anderson, 1990). The ill family member is often overly sensitive and preoccupied with him- or herself. Despite the parents' best intentions, reassurance does not help and the child's negative behavior can appear to be done "on purpose." When the parents' expectations are not met, the child continues to want to be in control even though he or she is failing with regular responsibilities. Families often describe themselves as "walking on eggshells" to avoid conflict. They try to help by coaxing, reassuring, and/or protecting the child, who does not respond positively to this approach. Family members then tend either to try harder or to withdraw. Often, one parent tries "Strategy A" (try harder) while the other parent tries "Strategy B" (withdraw). Next, the two parents begin quarreling with each other about how the other's strategy is not working. While this provides some initial relief to the child (parental attention is no longer focused on him or her), it accomplishes no productive goal, and, in fact, is destructive to the marital system. The child with early-onset bipolar disorder feels more alienated and the family feels rejected. Parents either withdraw, get angry, or both. Ultimately, the family feels guilty, goes back to coaxing, and so forth, while the child feels unworthy, hopeless, and infantilized. Families can burn out over time, with anger and guilt left over as residual effects. The end result of this negative cycle is alienation and/or overprotection.

STRATEGIES FOR FAMILIES

Holder and Anderson (1990) outline coping strategies for families. While originally developed for families of adult members with chronic, severe mental illness, these strategies also apply readily to families of children and adolescents with early-onset bipolar disorder.

Avoid Traps

Behaviors to avoid include:

- Rapidly reassuring the child—telling a child that "everything is fine" when the child does not feel "fine" does not ultimately reassure the child. Rather, this message can induce panic or demoralization (i.e., "If the current situation is 'fine,' what will things be like when my parents say it 'Isn't fine?' ").
- Taking comments literally—when children are at a "high" or a "low" in their mood swing, they may say things they would not say (or mean) at any other time. Parents do well to erase these hateful comments from their memory as soon as possible.
- Attempting to be constantly available and positive—parents need to understand that it is impossible to "cheer" their child out of a depressive phase, and that the price they will pay for trying to do so is exhaustion.
- Feeling guilty for not meeting the child's every "need"—this cannot, and should not, be done. Independent of the illness is a developing child. Satisfying any child's every whim will create a "monster"!

- Allowing the disorder to take over family life—the reality is that a child with early-onset bipolar disorder will have multiple crisis points (e.g., a hospitalization). During these times family life probably will revolve around the illness. Between crisis points, however, family life needs to revert back to a "new normal" to avoid "secondary damage" (e.g., ignored siblings turning to substance abuse, ignored spouses turning to divorce).
- Making big decisions (e.g., about custody, about divorce) during an episode—families will do best to postpone such major decision making until 3–6 months after the crisis has subsided. This will prevent rash decisions from being made in response to the crisis event.

Create a Balance

Three considerations are useful here. First, it is critical to distinguish the child from the disorder (Fristad, Gavazzi, & Soldano, 1999). The more the family learns how to join forces against "the enemy" (i.e., the illness), rather than exerting effort to oppose each others' efforts in symptom management, the better.

Second, family members need to learn to recognize multiple realities. When a child's mood is very high or very low, the child may truly perceive the world differently from those around him or her. Calmly conveying the message that "I understand you see the situation this way, but I see it that way" provides a reality check for the child or teenager in a nonconfrontational manner. This is particularly important for adolescents, who developmentally are attempting to differentiate themselves from their parents.

Finally, it is critical for parents to be supportive and patient, without taking on the role of "analyst." Communicating a willingness to talk and to listen is essential to improved family functioning. Children, and adolescents to an even greater extent, complain when their parents attempt to "analyze" why they are feeling down or moody.

Change Expectations

When the child is acutely ill, it is necessary to temporarily decrease expectations. Even during this phase, however, children can resent being "babied." Thus, it is critical to build good communication skills when the child is out of episode, so that clear negotiations regarding expectations can occur while the child is in episode.

While not "babying" their child, parents can provide realistic support and reinforcement, via opportunities for activity scheduling and providing appropriate structure in the child's life. Parents typically benefit from therapeutic input regarding how and when to modify expectations about activities, schoolwork, and so on, as their ill children wax in and out of more significant symptomatology. This becomes increasingly challenging as children grow older and expect to operate with more autonomy. Families who deal with early-onset bipolar disorder in prepubertal children can anticipate "renegotiating contracts" as their children age into each stage (early, middle, and late) of adolescence.

Finally, parental recognition of early-onset bipolar disorder as an illness, with episodes from which their child needs time and space to recover, is helpful. Throughout the recovery phase, it is important to remain hopeful—the scientific understanding of early-onset bipolar disorder has increased dramatically in the past 5–10 years. In the lifetime of children currently being treated with this condition, we can best anticipate a myriad of new, and increasingly effective, treatments. So, even if there is no single medicine or treatment now that addresses all the family's needs, there should always be at least "one more thing" to try in a methodical fashion. Maintaining hope for improvement is the best available "antidote" for demoralization of the child and family—and is essential for progress to occur.

Self-Preservation Skills

Three concepts are relevant here. First, parents require much encouragement and support (our society does not fully reinforce these notions) to take time away to rejuvenate themselves and to avoid "martyrdom" (e.g., it is highly recommended that parents go out on a date and thoroughly enjoy themselves, after arranging for adequate childcare for the ill child and siblings).

Second, it is critical for parents to accept their negative feelings about their child's illness. This is a necessary first step for acceptance, which precedes families' ability to proactively and effectively manage early-onset bipolar disorder. After all, not many people enjoy the kinds of treatment often "saved" by the ill child for those he or she loves most: being spat upon, hit, berated, insulted, and/or threatened. When parents are able to admit to hating the illness, their emotional energy is much more available to actively manage the illness.

Finally, it is important to minimize the impact the illness has on the self-esteem of parents. Rather than seeing how they are "worse" parents than others up or down the street, it is essential that parents learn to judge how well they are able to successfully negotiate through the land mines of parenting a child with early-onset bipolar disorder.

Improve Communication

Any meta-analysis of marital or family therapy indicates that the key to a successful intervention at the marital or family level will involve improving two critical skills: communication and problem solving. Families of children with early-onset bipolar disorder are no exception to that rule. De-veloping clear, direct communication, about both the illness and its man-agement, as well as family life in general, is a sine qua non of effective families who learn to successfully deal with early-onset bipolar disorder.

Skills for families to master include:

- Listen to, without correcting, each others' feelings and concerns.
- Ask the child if he or she wants suggestions before giving advice (we remind families that in the Charlie Brown TV cartoons, we never hear the adult voices, just a lot of "bwah, bwah, bwah"—that is how parental lectures come across to kids!).
- Talk directly with the family member involved about matters of concern.
- Choose your battles. Try to pick one or two target symptoms at a time to deal with—let the others go, if at all possible.
- Address issues when they are small instead of letting them build up—this avoids explosions of pent-up hostility.
- Keep rules simple and clear.
- Keep expectations reasonable (therapist input can be particularly useful for this, as appropriate levels of expectations can vary, based on the variable symptom presentation of the child).
- Give praise and positive feedback whenever it is legitimate—im-provement occurs gradually and cannot be measured by the same yardstick as used for siblings or same-aged peers!
- Deliver criticism in a calm voice.
- Word requests for change positively (e.g., When you do X, I feel Y: I would like you to do Z).
- Nonverbal communication (body language) can be even more im-portant than verbal communication (e.g., glaring while positively stating a request turns the communication into a negative inter-change).
- Do not use siblings as an outlet to vent frustrations, fears, or anger.

Improve Problem Solving

Discuss symptoms matter-of-factly as problems to be solved. Utilize stan-dard steps of problem solving to address matters of concern.

- Communicate the problem to the necessary people.
- Brainstorm possible solutions.
- Weigh the pros and cons of each possible solution.
- Decide upon a solution to try.
- Evaluate its effectiveness.
- Try another solution if the first one didn't work.

- Remain flexible.
- Continue to attempt solutions until you achieve success.

Specific Issues in Managing Manic Symptoms

Much of "good" parenting can be boiled down to three key ingredients: nurturance, discipline, and making developmental modifications as children grow and change. However, parenting a child with early-onset bipolar disorder takes special skills and education that are *not* taught in standard parenting books! It is critical for parents to become aware of their child's mood symptoms and the appropriate treatment for them. When parents become familiar with how their children cycle, they will be less likely to get carried away with a "high" mood (and also will be less likely to misinterpret a return from depression to euthymia as a flight into mania).

In addition to understanding the basic phenomenology of mania and depression, families also benefit from understanding the biopsychosocial triggers that can ignite a child's episode. For example, highly stimulating situations, sleep deprivation, or major transitions are frequently reported as triggers for new episodes.

Arguing with someone who is manic is counterproductive. Reminding the individual about the foolish or embarrassing behaviors that occurred during the manic episode after the mania has subsided is cruel, unless the child or adolescent refuses to acknowledge that he or she has a disorder that requires treatment.

Allow time for recovery. Then, as quickly as possible, the family should go back to business as usual!

Managing Suicidal and Other Emergency Behavior

Suicidal threats and gestures need to be taken seriously. All available methods for suicide (e.g., guns) that can be removed from the home should be. We routinely share the admonition, based on the classic study by Brent, Perper, and Allman (1987), that locking up guns in one part of the house and ammunition in another part of the house is insufficient. Guns simply cannot be justified in the home of a child with early-onset bipolar disorder. When children are acutely at risk, we work with parents to develop either a 1:1 monitoring system until the crisis passes, or strongly recommend hospitalization to keep the child safe. The family should develop a crisis plan with their therapist and review it with other members of the treatment team, so that parents know how to access their therapist, physician, police, and/or local community crisis center, as appropriate, at any time of day or night.

We emphasize that inpatient care (or the local community equivalent) should be accessed when a child is at risk to him- or herself, to others, or to property. Most hospitalizations in this current climate of managed care are very brief. Hospitalization should never be conceptualized or conveyed to a child as punishment or respite.

Multiple Family Members in Treatment

When a child is diagnosed with early-onset bipolar disorder, it is extremely likely that other immediate family members, siblings and/or parents, will also require mental health intervention. Often, we find that the "ticket in" for these family members is the effective treatment of the ill child. Especially for parents who remember ineffective treatment of their relatives of the previous generation, stereotypes of treatment "taking forever and not working" can be broken with the provision of modern, compassionate, and effective care.

Stress Management

While most families we work with would rather have learned these lessons the "easier" way, we also focus on the development of healthy lifestyles. We emphasize the importance of good sleep hygiene, eating healthfully, maintaining a balance between work and play, avoiding "overload" in demands on time and energy, developing stress reduction techniques (e.g., deep breathing exercises, imagery, muscle relaxation, physical activity), maintaining an active support network (e.g., friends, sports teams, church or temple, Scouts), developing a creative outlet to express feelings, and giving altruistically to others in need (e.g., one child with early-onset bipolar disorder volunteers during the school day with a physically handicapped child).

SCHOOL FUNCTIONING

Scope of the Problem

Children with "serious emotional disturbance" (SED; the educational label often assigned to children with early-onset bipolar disorder as well as with other emotional and behavioral disorders) are four times more likely to drop out of high school than their peers (21.4% vs. 85% high school completion rate) (U.S. Department of Education, 1999). Thus, not only are there issues related to the management of the child while he or she is *in* school, but the long-term vocational implications of this illness are profound.

Impact of Illness on Learning

There are a multitude of ways in which learning can be negatively impacted in children with early-onset bipolar disorder. First, the "primary" symptoms of mania and depression can interfere with classroom learning. A child who is agitated, lethargic, unfocused, or unmotivated is not an ideal student. Second, most children with early-onset bipolar disorder also have comorbid conditions. Impulsivity, hyperactivity, oppositionality, anxiety, and learning disabilities often accompany early-onset bipolar disorder, and each negatively affects school performance. Third, the "secondary" symptoms of early-onset bipolar disorder can interfere with learning. For example, children whose peer relations are not developing adequately tend to feel particularly vulnerable on the playground, in the lunchroom, and at the gym. Being the perennial "last pick" as a science project partner or baseball teammate does not induce peak performance in most of the children we know. Finally, medication side effects can result in poor handwriting, fatigue, and a "duller" class performance. Sometimes this can be managed by reducing the dosage or adjusting the administration time for medication doses. However, some side effects do not completely go away for some children, no matter how carefully medications are prescribed and monitored.

Understanding School Rules and Regulations

It is critical that both mental health clinicians and families understand some basic terminology, classifications, and programming mechanisms used by schools, so that effective programming can occur:

- IDEA: The Individuals with Disabilities Education Act—this is a federal funding statue whose purpose is to provide financial aid to states in their efforts to ensure adequate and appropriate services for children with disabilities.
- Section 504—this is a broad civil rights law that protects the right of individuals with disabilities in programs and activities that receive financial support from the U.S. Department of Education.

The similarities and differences between accessing school-based assistance for children via these two mechanisms are outlined in Table 14.1.

Build Bridges, Don't Burn Them

As the family clinician working with parents of children with early-onset bipolar disorder, it is important to help parents strategize for a long-term partnership with the school district. Even if the parents are, for example, currently working with an inflexible teacher or an unsympathetic principal, they need to carefully consider how they negotiate and make requests for their child, assuming they plan to interact with the same school district from school entry through high school graduation. This is important both for the child with early-onset bipolar disorder and for his or her siblings.

TABLE 14.1. Achieving a Free and Appropriate Education via IDEA versus Section 504

Mechanism	Individuals with Disabilities Education Act (IDEA)	Section 504
Eligibility	Must meet one of 13 qualifying categories.	Eligible if handicapping condition is present.
Requirements	A written individualized educational plan (IEP) is developed based on a multifactored evaluation (MFE).	An agreed-upon 504 plan.
Advantages	Provides additional federal money to the school district. Usually results in more extensive modifications.	Expedient. Often more flexible.
Disadvantages	Requires more paperwork, time to complete, testing.	No additional money to the school district. Sometimes not adhered to as strictly.

Parents should be coached to (1) demonstrate their knowledge about their child's illness; (2) educate the educators (e.g., by supplying a copy of a book or relevant up-to-date webpage printouts about bipolar disorder); (3) become an asset to the school (e.g., actively participate in fundraising efforts, volunteer in the library); and (4) work as a team member, assuming (and assertively requesting) good-faith effort on the part of the school.

While parents can often make significant headway in their efforts to build an effective team, some school districts simply don't have the financial (or other) resources to effectively program for a child with early-onset bipolar disorder. If that appears to be the case, the clinician might find it most expeditious to ask the question "Do you own or rent?" (i.e., Can the family manage to get into another school district presumed to be more responsive/have more resources to meet their needs?).

Assemble the Team

Assuming headway can be made, it is important to cultivate the mindset that it *does* "take a village" to raise and teach a child with early-onset bipolar disorder. Team members from the school might be selected from the principal, assistant principal, teacher(s), school psychologist, guidance counselor, special education faculty, enrichment teacher (bipolar disorder is the one psychiatric condition associated with above-average intelligence and a greater-than-chance likelihood of creative ability [DeLong & Aldershof, 1988; Richards, Kinney, Lunde, Benet, & Merzel, 1988]), speech/

language pathologist, learning disabilities tutor, school nurse, and—last but not least—secretarial and/or custodial staff. Some of these staff may address problems caused by comorbid conditions (e.g., an expressive language disorder, an arithmetic disorder). Secretarial/custodial staff can at times provide some alternative programming options (e.g., for a child who needs adults to "look after" him or her rather than face the gauntlet of going to recess after lunch).

The team from the "home front" should include the child (input is increasingly important as the child progresses to more advanced grades), parents, the prescribing physician (often via written documents), the therapist (typically through oral or written communication), and possibly an additional adult support (attending a school meeting at which one parent meets five or more school personnel can be very intimidating for most parents, who benefit from a spouse, relative, and/or friend accompanying her or him and taking notes for the primary caretaker).

At the end of the meeting, clear patterns of preferred communication should be established (i.e., it is often neither necessary nor desirable for a parent to be in separate communication with a half-dozen school personnel). One person, such as the special education coordinator, should be designated as the "point person" through whom all routine communication is channeled.

Free to Low-Cost Interventions

School personnel typically welcome suggestions for strategies that are inexpensive or that come without cost. Parents can ask, for example, that their child be provided with (1) preferential seating assignments (e.g., close to the teacher but not in the "center of attention"); (2) breaks, as needed, throughout the day, with a clearly identified "safe zone" where the child can retreat, as needed (e.g., the guidance counselor's office or antechamber if he or she is with another student); (3) use of a laptop computer in class (particularly for older students with significant medication-induced tremor or other graphomotor weaknesses); (4) an adjusted schedule (e.g., staying home for the first two periods, choir and study hall, thereby avoiding riding on a bus at 6:45 A.M.); (5) test accommodations (e.g., taking tests with extended time in the guidance counselor's office); (6) grade adjustments (e.g., not giving homework, grading based on work done during class and in a one-to-one tutorial); (7) peer mentoring (e.g., having a National Honor Society high school student coach a sixth-grader in math); (8) home schooling (this is not a frequent recommendation, as parents and children with early-onset bipolar disorder often prefer to have a break from one another, but it is an option to consider in some unique cases); (9) GED (if completion of a traditional or even a nontraditional high school curriculum ultimately becomes too challenging); and (10) a flexible attitude from school personnel. The latter is critical for any school plan. The former suggestions should be applied in a tailor-made fashion to meet the unique needs of the individual child and his or her family and school.

Moderate to High-Cost Interventions

At times, more expensive options are clearly in order. Moderate cost interventions include use of a resource room, in-school tutor, home-based instruction (partial or full, with the caveats as noted above for home schooling), specialized part- or full-time staff assisting the mainstreamed child, a self-contained special needs classroom, and/or an alternative school, if available within the district. As a last resort, high-cost interventions such as enrollment in a specialized day or residential treatment program can be considered. However, the reality is that these programs are scarce and expensive, making them an unrealistic alternative for many, if not most, families.

PEER RELATIONS

Who Needs Trophies, Anyway?

The sad reality for many children with early-onset bipolar disorder (and their parents) is that they don't "fit in" to standard group experiences of childhood. Soccer medals, piano recitals, and Scout outings simply may not happen for these families. This results in a need for the parents to remourn (or mourn, if they haven't done the work yet) the loss of their "ideal" child. Many children dealing with early-onset bipolar disorder either do not develop the skills that form the fabric of social interaction or they are delayed or distorted in their development. Specific skills that can be addressed in individual or group therapy are outlined in Chapter 13 in this volume. Several tips pertinent to the family, however, are in order. First, parents need to accept that they can "set the stage," but they cannot "direct the play." In other words, parents should be encouraged to make available a variety of recreational opportunities for their child with early-onset bipolar disorder. Then they need to sit back and let their child experience some autonomy in making choices about his or her comfort level with each activity.

Find the Right Fit

It is best if a variety of sports, music, social, and other creative outlets are considered. Some children with early-onset bipolar disorder will do better in individual activities (e.g., tae kwon do) rather than in group activities (e.g., baseball). As children grow, their interests and degree of success in various activities can change. For example, if team sports were not a realistic option for a child with early-onset bipolar disorder during grade school and middle school, that same child might develop interest in a new sport available only at the high school level (e.g., crew).

Persistence in finding a "good fit" can pay off if the child's skills lead to increased self-esteem based on excelling in a particular activity, or if relationship-building and social skills development occurs following success in a group activity. However, if the child is not successful, parents are encouraged to cut their losses relatively quickly. Forcing a child to "stick it out" to learn "commitment" is probably a less beneficial lesson if the child is failing miserably or acting out in public settings. Finally, if the child has an opportunity to participate in group therapy with other children experiencing similar difficulties, this might provide an opportunity for significant social benefits (Fristad, Goldberg-Arnold, & Gavazzi, 2002).

TIPS FOR THE THERAPIST/CASE MANAGER

The family clinician is encouraged to utilize psychoeducational principles in working with families of children with early-onset bipolar disorder. Many family therapists practicing today were trained in an era that emphasized labeling "family pathology." However, more recent influences from the consumer movement have resulted in the development of a more supportive, growth-oriented stance in working with families (Marsh, 1995). Specifically, clinicians are encouraged to:

- Teach family members about early-onset bipolar disorder and its treatment.
- Do not blame family members for symptoms.
- Rely on family members' strengths while focusing on skill building.
- Teach families special coping skills above and beyond those needed for "regular" family life.
- Encourage families to accept and tolerate those symptoms that do not change readily.
- Build a treatment team and an educational team that includes the family.
- Communicate regularly with team members.
- Develop a long-term, mutually respectful partnership with families.
- Work to increase social support:
  - for the child
  - for the family
  - for the treatment providers.

SUMMARY

Our knowledge of early-onset bipolar disorder—its phenomenology, course, and biopsychosocial treatment—is expanding rapidly. Families dealing with this illness today, however, need immediate and practical solutions. Central to family-based interventions for children with early-onset bipolar disorder is access to a clinician well versed in the manifestations of this illness. As early-onset bipolar disorder is a "moving target," the family clinician needs to be prepared to move along with it, helping the family to adopt a flexible treatment plan that can accommodate the vicissitudes of the illness.

Early-onset bipolar disorder produces a host of issues to be addressed in order to maximize the psychological health of all family members: the ill child him- or herself, siblings, and parents. We have outlined in this chapter both predictable problems as well as strategies to address them. The challenge of educating a child with early-onset bipolar disorder is also high. A proactive stance to help the family deal with these family-based and school issues is necessary.

While the guidelines provided in this chapter offer families of children with early-onset bipolar disorder and the clinicians working with them a frame of reference from which they can work, much more programmatic research is needed in the field to further develop, refine, and test effective biological, psychological, and social/environmental interventions for children struggling with early-onset bipolar disorder.

ACKNOWLEDGMENT

This work was supported in part by grants from the Ohio Department of Mental Health and the National Institute of Mental Health (R01 MH61512).

REFERENCES

Brent, D. A., Perper, J. A., & Allman, C. J. (1987). Alcohol, firearms, and suicide among youth: Temporal trends in Allegheny County, Pennsylvania, 1960–1983. *Journal of the American Medical Association, 257*, 3369–3372.

Cole, D. A. R., & Rehm, L. P. (1986). Family interaction patterns and childhood depression. *Journal of Abnormal Child Psychology, 14*, 297–314.

Deal, J. E., Halverson, C. F., & Wampler, K. S. (1989). Parental agreement on child-rearing orientations: Relations to parental, marital, family and child characteristics. *Child Development, 60*, 1025–1034.

DeLong, G. R., & Aldershof, A. L. (1988). An association of special abilities with juvenile manic–depressive illness. In L. K. Obler & D. Fein (Eds.), *The exceptional brain: Neuropsychology of talent and special abilities* (pp. 387–395). New York: Guilford Press.

Fristad, M. A., Arnett, M. M., & Gavazzi, S. M. (1998). The impact of psychoeducation workshops on families of mood disordered children. *Family Therapy, 25*(3), 151–159.

Fristad, M. A., Gavazzi, S. M., Centolella, D. M., & Soldano, K. W. (1996). Psychoeducation: A promising intervention strategy for families of children and adolescents with mood disorders. *Contemporary Family Therapy, 18*(3), 371–383.

Fristad, M. A., Gavazzi, S. M., & Soldano, K. W. (1998). Multi-family psychoeducation groups for childhood mood disorders: A program description and preliminary efficacy data. *Contemporary Family Therapy, 20*(3), 385–402.

Fristad, M. A., Gavazzi, S. M., & Soldano, K. W. (1999). Naming the enemy: Learning to differentiate mood disorder "symptoms" from the "self" that experiences them. *Journal of Family Psychotherapy, 10*(1), 81–88.

Fristad, M. A., Goldberg-Arnold, J. S., & Gavazzi, S. M. (2002). Multi-family psychoeducation groups (MFPG) for families of children with mood disorders. *Bipolar Disorders, 4*, 254–262.

Holder, D. A., & Anderson, B. M. (1990). Psychoeducational family intervention for depressed patients and their families. In B. I. Keitner (Ed.), *Depression and families: Impact and treatment* (pp. 157–184). Washington, DC: American Psychiatric Press.

Jouriles, E. N., Murphy, C. M., Farris, A., Smith, D. A., Richters, J. E., & Waters, E. (1991). Marital adjustment, parental disagreements about child rearing, and behavior problems in boys: Increasing the specificity of the marital assessment. *Child Development, 62*, 1424–1433.

Lamb, M. E., Hwang, C. P., & Broberg, A. (1989). Associations between parental agreement regarding child-rearing and the characteristics of families and children in Sweden. *International Journal of Behavioral Development, 12*(1), 115–129.

Marsh, D. T. (1995). *Serious mental illness and the family: The practitioner's guide.* New York: Wiley.

Richards, R., Kinney, D. K., Lunde, I., Benet, M., & Merzel, A. P. C. (1988). Creativity in manic-depressives, cyclothymes, and their normal relatives, and control subjects. *Journal of Abnormal Psychology, 97*(3), 281–288.

Sisson, D. P., & Fristad, M. A. (2001). A survey of stress and support for parents of children with early onset bipolar disorder. *Bipolar Disorders, 3*(Supp. 1), 58.

U.S. Department of Education. (1999). *21st annual report to congress on the implementation of the Individuals with Disabilities Education Act* [Online]. Available: http://www.ed.gov/offices/OSERS/OSEP/Research/OSEP99AnlRpt/DOC_Files/CH4.doc [2000, August 31]

Vuchinich, S., Vuchinich, R., & Wood, B. (1993). The interparental relationship and family problem solving with preadolescent males. *Child Development, 64*, 1389–1400.

15

Internet Support for Parents of Children with Early-Onset Bipolar Disorder

MARTHA HELLANDER, DORY P. SISSON, and MARY A. FRISTAD

One of the biggest stressors is the total isolation and lack of support. I *never* have a moment to myself, I have no friends, I have no life. I spend almost every day with a feeling of mortal terror that we will return to the horror before diagnosis and stabilization. No parent or child should ever have to experience what we and the many other parents I've met at CABF have had to go through. I am tired of this life. I grieve for the loss of what I thought motherhood would be. I grieve for my boys. The single greatest source of support, comfort, and education is CABF. No place else do I find the unconditional acceptance and support that I do there. It may be impossible to believe, but I feel a deeper bond to some of the pseudonymed, online friends than to my flesh-and-blood friends and family. If I did not have that lifeline, I don't know what I would do some nights. I can log on after a bad day and get the support and strength to start the new day with a smile so that I can be there for my boys.
—MOTHER OF A CHILD WITH BIPOLAR DISORDER

Early-onset bipolar disorder in one or more children impacts the entire family. The child or children struggle with the illness, siblings are affected, and parents must become specialized caregivers and case managers. The energy and patience required of these parents is daunting. Networking with other parents can reduce isolation, and peer support groups can provide much-needed information, resources, and education about parenting strategies that work. We anticipate that improved outcomes for children and adolescents can directly result from parents' access to online support.

In this chapter we review the literature on caregiver burden and how various forms of support can help families We then focus on the Internet as an emerging medium for delivering support services, and describe an example of the Internet's potential to create and sustain a supportive community for families raising children diagnosed with, or at risk for, bipolar disorder: the Child & Adolescent Bipolar Foundation, founded in 1999 by parents who met in early online support groups.

CAREGIVER BURDEN

Children with early-onset bipolar disorder are very challenging. Symptoms of the disorder and its frequently co-occurring conditions (e.g., anxiety disorders, attention-deficit/hyperactivity disorder, obsessive–compulsive disorder, substance use disorder, conduct disorder, and learning disabilities) can wreak havoc on family routines, exhaust family resources, and cause immense stress for the child's parents, in addition to producing the severe discomfort experienced by the child. Caregivers often suffer physical, emotional, and financial distress as a result. Siblings of the ill child are also affected, and parents struggle to balance the needs of all family members, including their own.

Behavior

A primary source of stress for caregivers, apart from the stress of watching their beloved child suffer from rejection by peers, school failure, severe anxiety, and even suicidality, is the unpredictability and volatility of the child's behavior when ill. Children experiencing mania or mixed states may be alternately demanding, hilariously funny, hostile, and in despair at various times during any given day. Intense and seemingly uncontrollable rages are common, and parents often must "walk on eggshells" to avoid triggering the child's fragile and hyperactive stress–response system. Families can become nearly homebound out of dread of yet another public episode. When rages occur in public (e.g., at the grocery store), parents suffer the dual challenge of calming their child and dealing with the misguided advice and stares of strangers. A raging child can be verbally dramatic and even abusive—it is common for a parent to hear "I hate you" and "You're so mean," and to endure a hail of obscenities, threats to call the police, and allegations of child abuse from one's young child or teenager while the parent is making extraordinary efforts to calm the child or restrain the child from leaping from a moving car, cutting him- or herself with a kitchen knife, destroying his or her own or his or her siblings' possessions, or frightening his or her younger siblings. The physical safety of the child and other family members may be at risk if a child becomes impulsively aggressive in the midst of a rage. Raging children may damage property, run away, or dash into the street with no thought of the consequences or of their safety. As a result, parents of symptomatic children with bipolar disorder often exist in a constant state of hypervigilance, wondering when the next episode of suicidality or raging will occur, and what the consequences will be. Parents are loathe to call authorities even when they are injured by their children, for fear of their fate in the foster care or juvenile justice system.

Finances

Financial strain is a given for families of children with bipolar disorder. Insurance coverage is rarely comprehensive enough to cover the child's extensive treatment needs. Inpatient hospitalizations and medications are expensive, and are not traditionally covered by insurance companies at a level equivalent to other medical conditions. It is estimated that 11% of children with special health care needs do not have any insurance (Newacheck et al., 1998). Additionally, many families find that it is necessary to have one parent or paid caregiver at home full time to manage their high-needs child or help with the younger siblings, at the expense of a second income, or, for single parents, their only income.

Medical Consequences

Caregivers of children with early-onset bipolar disorder may experience many medical problems as a result of the stress associated with their role. Exhaustion, headaches, and sleep disturbances are common physical consequences. There is evidence that providing care for a person with a chronic illness (e.g., Alzheimer's disease) is related to weakened immune functioning (Kiecolt-Glaser & Glaser, 1994). As childhood mood disorders are chronic and recurrent in nature, it is reasonable to expect that parents of children with early-onset bipolar disorder are also at risk for immunologic weakening. Psychiatric disorders are commonly reported. Parents may experience symptoms of depression or anxiety disorders as a result of the daily stress of caring for a child with early-onset bipolar disorder. After witnessing (or being in) a particularly intense rage or suicide attempt by the child, parents and siblings may exhibit symptoms (e.g., hypervigilance, reexperiencing) of posttraumatic stress disorder. Caregivers may also be dealing with their own preexisting mood or anxiety disorder in addition to that of their child, and instability in the parent or child may trigger onset of symptoms and exacerbate the other's condition.

Negotiating Uncharted Territory

Many children with early-onset bipolar disorder require special education services or become involved in the juvenile justice system. For parents and caregivers, this requires navigating a new system with its own language and interacting with a variety of authorities. Parents feel confused, misunderstood, and overwhelmed. Similarly, when dealing with mental health professionals, parents report that they often feel blamed for their child's problems, and perceive that their opinions and observations are not valued (Lefley, 1997).

Isolation

All of the above-mentioned sources of stress are exacerbated by the isolation experienced by children with bipolar disorder and their parents. Children with brain disorders and their parents are often stigmatized. They may feel too embarrassed to share their experiences with others. This leads to withdrawal from family gatherings, church and community events, and the support available from a diverse social network. Many parents report that their symptomatic children have no friends, or cannot handle the complex social interactions that occur on sports teams, church groups, or in other age-appropriate social groups.

SUPPORT GROUPS

Participation in a support group for families of individuals with brain disorders can alleviate caregiver burden. These self-help, or mutual help, groups can provide much-needed information, peer support, advocacy, coping skills, and respite from the strain of daily life with a chronically ill child. The recent growth of support groups for caregivers of children with brain disorders, including bipolar disorder, complements care provided by mental health professionals including basic information about the illness and its management.

In a time of reduced funding for mental health treatment within managed care systems, peer-led support groups may assume a greater role in helping families join together to form a consumer advocacy movement (Citron, Solomon, & Draine, 1999; Koroloff & Friesen, 1991). Additionally, it is estimated that more than 70% of Americans suffering from a diagnosable behavioral or mental disorder will never receive specialized mental health care, and instead will rely on self-help and mutual help options (Norcross, 2000).

Elements of Effective Support Groups

Members of mutual aid/self-help groups find themselves in a community of parents experiencing similar crises. Friendship often arises out of shared conditions, and social connections form that are crucial to improving the mental health of participants (Humphreys, 1997). Numerous interpersonal transactions occur within a support group. Specifically, two helping processes are particularly relevant to members: *giving* help and support, and *receiving* help and support (Roberts et al., 1999). Supportive comments and behaviors are often the most frequent interactions among support group members (Roberts et al., 1991; Wollert, Levy, & Knight, 1982), and serve an important function in forming social bonds within groups. Providing help can have a therapeutic effect by leading to increased feelings of competence and social usefulness, and by allowing members to perceive themselves as having strengths to offer others (Roberts et al., 1999).

Two primary types of support are prominent in mutual help groups: *informational support* and *emotional support*. One study by Roberts and colleagues (1999) found that members who provided informational support (e.g., guidance) showed improved social adjustment. Roberts and colleagues hypothesized that this improvement may be the result of the provider relying on his or her own experience with a similar problem, thereby reinforcing his or her own learning. Maton's (1998) research examining this *bidirectional support* (i.e., participating both in the giving and receiving of support) indicates that individuals who report experiencing bidirectional support also report better well-being and satisfaction with the group.

Benefits of Support Groups

Participation in support groups has been associated with lower reports of caregiver burden. In a study of members of a support group for parents of adult children with brain disorders, Cook, Heller, and Pickett-Schenk (1999) found that caregiver burden was significantly lower among support group participants than among nonparticipants.

An important goal of support groups is empowerment, so that families become more confident in their ability to evaluate the competency of professionals, seek better services, and have more positive interactions with service providers. Goldberg-Arnold, Fristad, and Gavazzi (1999) reported that over time, families participating in multifamily psychoeducation groups (MFPGs) showed an attitudinal shift toward more positive thinking about educational and mental health care systems (Goldberg-Arnold et al., 1999). Koroloff and Friesen (1991) found that members of parent support groups reported more utilization of information and services than did nonmembers.

Families who feel more empowered as a result of participation in a support group may also become active in advocacy efforts (Humphreys, 1997). Political activism such as lobbying for insurance parity and improved mental health services is one societal benefit of support groups. Singh and colleagues (1997) looked at empowerment in families of children with serious emotional disturbances, and found that membership in a parent support group was a strong predictor of family empowerment, particularly on the dimension of systems advocacy.

INTERNET SUPPORT

While it appears that many caregivers of children with early-onset bipolar disorder could benefit from membership in a "traditional" (i.e., in-person) support group, often this is not feasible. The format and limited time availability of face-to-face support groups (e.g., set meeting times a week or more apart, with only a brief hour or two for each meeting) is not conducive to the lifestyle and intense need of many families of children with brain disorders, especially when the children are symptomatic, first diagnosed, or experiencing a relapse. For these families, the Internet offers information and support in a more flexible, ever-available, and intimate environment.

Forms of Support

Support delivered via the Internet can occur in a variety of ways. A parent can visit a website from home via a personal computer. Educational content is immediately available, potentially very current (depending on the site), and may be accessed as long as one's time permits. One may read and respond to public postings on community message boards. Chat rooms offer the opportunity to participate in real-time discussions on designated topics at scheduled times, or participate in unstructured conversation during open times. Members in an e-mail support group may receive dozens of group-distributed comments each day from other members in a virtually never-ending group meeting, delivered to their personal e-mail account throughout the day or in a daily digest format. Some groups offer the option of reading e-mail on a website accessed with a password. There is increasing potential for these various forms of computer-mediated communication to serve as a means of program delivery. Many families use several or all of these forms of Internet support simultaneously.

Logistic Issues

Due to the fluctuating and unpredictable nature of early-onset bipolar disorder symptoms, many families find it difficult to attend scheduled appointments outside the home. Thus, a weekly support group meeting is not necessarily a practical option. The family may be unable to obtain childcare, or the meeting times and location may not be convenient. Other logistical challenges may include a lack of transportation, living in a remote area, or a long waiting list to join the group. The Internet removes all these barriers. It is accessible from any location at any time of day or night, and members can participate for as long or as short a time and as often as they like (Weinberg, Schmale, Uken, & Wessel, 1995).

Personal Issues

In addition to logistical barriers, there may be personal factors that draw individuals to the Internet as a more desirable form of support. Some people feel uncomfortable speaking in front of a group, or may be ashamed to discuss their issues with others face to face. Because of the stigma still attached to individuals with brain disorders, many caregivers are embarrassed to seek public help for their child's illness. The Internet provides anonymity, thereby allowing users to obtain educational information and to share personal information without revealing their identities.

Similar to in-person support groups, members of computer-mediated support groups seek advice, information, socialization, contact with others in similar situations, and emotional support (Bacon, Condon, & Fernsler, 2000). They communicate in ways characteristic of face-to-face groups, by offering support, acceptance, and positive feelings. Online groups in one study expressed high levels of emotional support and self-disclosure (Salem, Bogar, & Reid, 1997). Members may feel comfortable in self-disclosing because personal differences (e.g., race, gender, social status) are either minimized or not easily discernable. The shared problem becomes a common focus, and allows for an increased sense of similarity and unity (Salem et al., 1997).

THE CHILD & ADOLESCENT BIPOLAR FOUNDATION

The Child & Adolescent Bipolar Foundation (CABF) is an example of what can be accomplished when the Internet unites parents with a common goal. Parents of children with early-onset bipolar disorder started online support groups in the 1990s and began comparing information and experiences regarding their children (Hellander, 2000). In 1999, the leadership of these groups joined to form CABF. CABF is a national, not-for-profit organization of families raising children diagnosed with, or at risk for, bipolar disorder. Professionals may also become members. The CABF website, *www.bpkids.org*, receives over 100,000 unique visits per month. Over 6,000 families and a far greater number of visitors and subscribers receive regular support services and information.

CABF emphasizes that bipolar disorder can and does occur in childhood and adolescence. It advocates for early diagnosis and treatment of bipolar disorder in children to prevent a worsening course of illness, and to restore the child to wellness at the earliest opportunity so that the child may resume his or her normal tasks of child development. CABF informs its audience that medications known to be safe and effective in adults may be used to treat children, but more research on treatments for children and adolescents is needed. Controlled clinical trials have not been conducted to determine proven safety, efficacy, and optimal dosing strategy of most medications used to treat early-onset bipolar disorder, yet the consequences of not treating are significant (parents learn that the lifetime mortality rate is 18% for patients with this illness [Goodwin & Jamison, 1990]). Children and adolescents with bipolar disorders need and are entitled to flexible accommodations at school (e.g., individual education plans [IEPs]). CABF assists parents in learning the procedures and advocacy strategies required to make this happen. Children with early-onset bipolar disorder respond best to parenting and educational methods that take account of their neurobiological condition—parenting and educational strategies are provided on the website.

CABF also supports numerous public health initiatives, including

- increased funding for research on the causes, nature, treatment, and a cure for early-onset bipolar disorder
- access to appropriate evaluation and treatment for all children and adolescents with bipolar disorders
- education for schoolchildren about mood disorders
- screening for emerging mood disorders in children
- nondiscriminatory insurance coverage for individuals with mood disorders
- mandatory advice to parents by emergency and public safety personnel to remove or lock up guns kept in the home
- psychoeducational and support groups for children, parents, and families affected by early-onset bipolar disorder.

The CABF website (*www.bpkids.org*) is a "virtual community center" delivering information and support to parents of children with early-onset bipolar disorder. A key component to the website is science-based, current information regarding early-onset bipolar disorder. The *Learning Center* contains a selection of full-text medical journal articles, original educational content, and abstracts and citations to published scientific articles. The website describes the history of diagnosing bipolar disorder in children, and gives an overview of the psychiatric diagnostic and classification system for parents new to the diagnosis of early-onset bipolar disorder. Educational needs of children with bipolar disorder are also addressed, including a detailed chart of symptoms and their corresponding accommodation that might be included in an IEP. The *Learning Center* also includes tips for teachers, a discussion of home-schooling options, and a digest of laws governing school compliance.

The *Resources* page contains links to other advocacy organizations and information about insurance parity laws, legislative alerts, and nutritional supplements. It also contains a *drug database*, links to government sites on Social Security and Medicaid, and links to international resources. Families seeking to enroll in research studies of children with bipolar disorder can find a listing of current studies on the *Research Studies* page. The *Bookstore* consists of recommended books and articles for children, parents, and educators, selected and approved by the foundation's board of directors and professional advisory council. The *Gallery* of children's art and poetry displays creative works by the children themselves.

Among the most popular features of the site are *searchable databases* of doctors and mental health professionals, as well as local, in-person support groups. Support services available on the website include over 24 online *support groups* with over 2,000 families participating, *chat rooms* operating day and night, and numerous *message boards* that provide information on topics such as education, treatment, doctors, good news stories, news and announcements, support groups forming, and resources for children. Online support groups are available to parents and caregivers of children and adolescents diagnosed with, or at risk for, early-onset bipolar disorder. A team of two volunteer parent moderators leads each group

In a White Paper, commissioned by the National Institute of Mental Health, Martha Hellander, executive director and cofounder of CABF (2000), describes her observations of the impact of the CABF website:

> CABF is flooded with reports from families who have discovered the Web site and write to say how much better informed, and less stressed, they now feel. It appears that participation in on-line support groups and access to current science-based information and parenting strategies via the Internet lead to empowerment of families through understanding of bipolar disorder, reduced stress for parents, lower rates of depression, better coping skills for parents and children, better adjustment in school (and greater likelihood that families will obtain legally mandated services), better medication compliance for children, and better overall outcomes. (pp. 9–10)

THE PARENT STRESS AND SUPPORT SURVEY

To further document the stress experienced by caregivers of children with early-onset bipolar disorder, and the type of support received from the Internet and other sources, Sisson and Fristad (2001) administered a survey to users of the CABF website. Caregivers of children with early-onset bipolar disorder completed an online survey consisting of seven sections: Demographics, Stress Checklist, Illness History, Usage of the CABF website, Evaluation of the CABF website, Use and Evaluation of Face-to-Face Services, and Comparison of Internet versus Face-to-Face Services.

The survey was online for 9 weeks and received 723 responses. Demographic data reveal that users of CABF's website are primarily female (97%), Caucasian (97%), and married (75%). CABF survey respondents are a fairly well educated group, with 55% holding a college or graduate degree. Two-thirds (66%) of participants have an annual family income over $50,000, and many are professionals (e.g., doctors, teachers, social workers) who reported that even their training and expertise did not prepare them for dealing with this disorder in their own children. Consistent with previous research, a strong family history for brain disorders, specifically mood disorders, was reported by participants. A majority of the caregivers (79%) reported a family history of any brain disorder, with 59% reporting depression and 49% bipolar disorder. When asked about siblings of the identified child, 30% of participants reported a sibling with a diagnosis or symptoms of bipolar disorder, and 33% reported a sibling having a diagnosis other than bipolar disorder.

The stress checklist, the second subset of the Parent Stress and Support Survey, consists of 25 Likert-type items assessing caregiver stress due to a variety of factors related to raising a child with early-onset bipolar disorder (see Table 15.1). Question responses range from 0 (not at all stressful) to 4 (very stressful). The overall score can range from 0 (no stress) to 100 (high stress).

Results confirm that caregivers experience high levels of stress related to raising a child with early-onset bipolar disorder. Overall scores ranged from 9 to 93, with a mean of 58.2 (SD = 16.6). Mean ratings on individual items ranged from 0.7 to 3.3 (mean ratings for all 25 items appear in Table 15.1). While the Stress Checklist has not been normed on a population unaffected by early-onset bipolar disorder, an average score of 58 suggests that a caregiver might have endorsed every item with a score of 2 (somewhat stressful) or 3 (mostly stressful), or that approximately 15 items might have been endorsed as a 4 (very stressful). Given these high stress levels in this relatively affluent, educated, and resourceful group of parents, one might speculate that the stress experienced by other caregivers (e.g., single mothers, lower income families) would be significantly higher.

The primary limitation to this study was the inability to verify that respondents were really parents of children with early-onset bipolar disorder and that their children were accurately diagnosed with early-onset bipolar disorder. While directions for the survey indicated that the child should "be diagnosed with, or showing symptoms of early-onset bipolar disorder," it was the responsibility of the parent to determine if this description fit his or her child. No attempt was made to independently verify diagnoses—

TABLE 15.1. Stress Checklist

Item[a]	Mean rating
Walking on eggshells around your child to avoid rages	3.3
Trying to get your child to do chores or self-care	3.3
Having less time for taking care of yourself	3.2
Having less time to devote to your marriage or significant relationship	3.0
Having less time for your adult friendships	3.0
Trying to get your child to do homework	3.0
Witnessing self-harming or suicidal acts or hearing suicidal statements by your child	2.7
Not having enough time or energy to address your other children's needs	2.7
Feeling embarrassed by your child's public rages	2.7
Dealing with your own depression	2.5
Accusations from your child that you are a "mean" parent	2.5
Accusations or implications from your family that you are a bad parent or that you are at fault	2.3
Paying for costly medical bills not covered by your insurance company	2.2
Dealing with your insurance company or having no insurance coverage	2.2
Dealing with the stigma of having a child with a brain disorder	2.1
Finding a clinician who believed that there was something medically wrong with your child	2.1
Dealing with your own headaches	2.0
Accusations or implications from school personnel that you are a bad parent or that you are at fault	1.9
Not knowing how to disclose your child's disorder to family, school, etc.	1.9
Pressure from work because of absences due to your child's illness	1.8
Accusations or implications from your friends that you are a bad parent or that you are at fault	1.7
Dealing with your own multiple bouts of physical illness	1.7
Dealing with lost wages due to taking off work or quitting job	1.6
Accusations or implications from your child's treatment provider that you are a bad parent or that you are at fault	1.0
Divorce or separation as a result of raising a child with a brain disorder	0.7

Note. Potential range for the 25 items: 0 (not at all stressful) to 4 (very stressful).

[a] Listed from most to least stressful, based on survey results.

for example, through phone interviews using structured interviews with the respondents. However, due to the length of the survey, and the nature of the topic under investigation, it is not expected that "cheating" was a significant problem in data analyses. The most likely scenario is that some percentage of families who participated in the survey might receive diagnoses of "rule-out" bipolar disorder rather than a clear diagnosis of bipolar I or bipolar II disorder if they participated in a structured diagnostic interview with consensus conference review.

The Parents' Voices

Comments from parents who participated in the study provide poignant insight into the stress of raising a child with early-onset bipolar disorder, the benefits of Internet support in general, and the benefits of the CABF website specifically.

Parents consistently reported high levels of stress: "I grieve for the loss of what I thought motherhood would be"; "I have had no personal time in 9 years"; "That sickening feeling in the pit of my stomach when I hear the sound of his mania developing"; "Our home life revolves around my son. Everyone else is secondary"; "I feel that all I ever do is fight with various people or agencies to try to get them to help my children"; "Stress of daily rages directly caused depression"; "It's awful to see your child suffer so much"; "I frequently worry about my other children and how they will view their childhood in years to come."

Parents report that a primary advantage of the Internet is convenience: "When you are in the middle of a crisis you can get online and get support. You can't wait to get support on Tuesdays at 7:00 P.M. Your crisis will probably be over"; "Most of our free time is in the middle of the night"; "I can make a cup of tea when the kids are in bed and feel a part of a support group."

For some parents, the format of online interaction is more comfortable than face-to-face interaction: "I was able to type online without my tears getting in the way. In non-Internet settings I couldn't face people to get the help I needed"; "I am not as comfortable talking in a group because I am not as open in our community about my daughter's illness. I feel I can communicate more honestly via Internet communication."

Respondents overwhelmingly endorsed receiving support, despite the lack of face-to-face interactions: "I feel a real bond with these people. It has been a great source of support"; "We can be more supportive and more intimate with each other online. I have never met such accepting, loving, caring individuals"; "When something happens, good or bad, I turn to the online group because they are the only ones who understand."

Parents expressed gratitude for the role CABF played in fulfilling an unmet need: "This is the most comprehensive site on the net for early-onset bipolar disorder"; "Finding CABF saved my sanity and made me feel like a human being again"; "Gives me hope, information, and the knowledge I am not alone"; "The support lists [groups] literally have held me together over the years"; "Empowered me to demand better care"; "My only escape to validate my frustrations with bipolar"; "It has been my saving grace through this difficult time"; "This site saved my life . . . this site saved my child's life."

ADDITIONAL RESOURCES

In addition to the CABF website, other sources of Internet information and support appear in the Appendix. Many of these also appear as links in the CABF website. These websites vary in the amount of information and/or support they provide. Also in the Appendix is a list of recommended reading materials for families. These recommendations are routinely updated on the CABF website.

Due to the lack of regulation of content on the Internet, parents and clinicians should be cautious when evaluating information from online sources. Not all websites are strictly controlled, and some may provide inaccurate or misleading information regarding diagnosis and treatment of children with early-onset bipolar disorder. Parents should consult with physicians and therapists before acting on any suggestion regarding medication, treatment, or support groups.

CONCLUSION

Caregiving for children with early-onset bipolar disorder can be very challenging. The child's unpredictable behavior, financial pressures, mental and physical problems, and isolation all can exacerbate the stress felt by caregivers. Support networks are critical; for many families, the Internet is a convenient source of such support. The Child & Adolescent Bipolar Foundation (CABF) website is a virtual community for parents of children with early-onset bipolar disorder. The website contains informative resources, chat rooms, message boards, and e-mail support groups. Preliminary research suggests that while CABF website users experience high levels of stress due to raising a child with early-onset bipolar disorder, they also report finding support and guidance on the website. Further examination of the advantages and disadvantages of Internet versus face-to-face support is currently underway, as are the development of additional support materials (i.e., books on early-onset bipolar disorder written for parents and their children).

APPENDIX

Support/Advocacy Group Information

CABF (Child & Adolescent Bipolar Foundation)
1187 Wilmette Avenue, #PMB 331
Wilmette, IL 60091
(847) 256-8525
www.bpkids.org

DBSA (Depression and Bipolar Support Alliance)
730 North Franklin Street, Suite 501
Chicago, IL 60610-7204
(800) 826-3632, (312) 642-0049
www.ndmda.org

NAMI (National Alliance for the Mentally Ill)
Colonial Place Three, 2107 Wilson Boulevard, Suite 300
Arlington, VA 22201
(703) 524-7600, (800) 950-NAMI
www.nami.org

NIMH (National Institute of Mental Health)
6001 Executive Boulevard, Room 8184, MSC 9663
Bethesda, MD 20892-9663
(301) 443-4513
www.nimh.nih.gov

Further Reading

Most of these books are available in the online bookstore of the Child & Adolescent Bipolar Foundation at *www.bpkids.org/community/bookstore/*.

Anglada, T. (2001). *Brandon and the bipolar bear*. www.bipolar-children.bigstep.com
Cobain, B. (1994). *When nothing matters anymore: A survival guide for depressed teens*. Minneapolis, MN: Free Spirit.
Garland, E. J. (1997). *Depression is the pits, but I'm getting better: A guide for adolescents*. Washington, DC: Magination Press.
Greene, R. (1998). *The explosive child: A new approach for understanding and parenting easily frustrated, chronically inflexible children*. New York: HarperCollins.
Hallowell, E. (1996). *When you worry about the child you love: Emotional and learning problems in children*. New York: Simon & Schuster.
Irwin, C. (1999). *Conquering the beast within: How I fought depression and won . . . and how you can, too*. New York: Times Books/Random House.
Kutcher, S. (1997). *Child and adolescent psychopharmacology*. Philadelphia: Saunders.

Miklowitz, D. J. (2002). *The bipolar disorder survival guide: What you and your family need to know*. New York: Guilford Press.

Papalos, D., & Papalos, J. (1999). *The bipolar child*. New York: Broadway Books.

Simon, L. (2002). *Detour: My bipolar road trip in 4-D*. New York: Artria Books.

Sommers, M. A. (2000). *Everything you need to know about bipolar disorder and manic depressive illness*. New York: Rosen. (For teens age 13–19)

Steel, D. (1998). *His bright light: The story of Nick Traina*. New York: Delacorte Press.

Waltz, M. (2000). *Bipolar disorders: A guide to helping children and adolescents*. Sebastopol, CA: O'Reilly & Associates.

Wilens, T. E. (1999). *Straight talk about psychiatric medications for kids*. New York: Guilford Press.

REFERENCES

Bacon, E. S., Condon, E. H., & Fernsler, J. I. (2000). Young widows' experience with an Internet self-help group. *Journal of Psychosocial Nursing, 38*(7), 24–33.

Citron, M., Solomon, P., & Draine, J. (1999). Self-help groups for families of persons with mental illness: Perceived benefits of helpfulness. *Community Mental Health Journal, 35*(1), 15–30.

Cook, J. A., Heller, T., & Pickett-Schenk, S. A. (1999). The effect of support group participation on caregiver burden among parents of adult offspring with severe mental illness. *Family Relations: Interdisciplinary Journal of Applied Family Studies, 48*(4), 405–410.

Goldberg-Arnold, J. S., Fristad, M. A., & Gavazzi, S. M. (1999). Family psychoeducation: Giving caregivers what they want and need. *Family Relations, 48*, 411–417.

Goodwin, F. K., & Jamison, K. R. (1990). *Manic–depressive illness*. Oxford, UK: Oxford University Press.

Hellander, M. (2000). *Easing the burden: Childhood-onset bipolar disorder and the Internet*. Unpublished White Paper for the National Institute of Mental Health, Bethesda, MD.

Humphreys, K. (1997). Individual and social benefits of mutual aid self-help groups. *Social Policy, 27*(3), 12–19.

Kiecolt-Glaser, J. K., & Glaser, R. (1994). Caregivers, mental health, and immune function. In E. Light, G. Niederehe, & B. D. Lebowitz (Eds.), *Stress effects on family caregivers of Alzheimer's patients: Research and interventions* (pp. 64–75). New York: Springer.

Koroloff, N. M., & Friesen, B. J. (1991). Support groups for parents of children with emotional disorders: A comparison of members and non-members. *Community Mental Health Journal, 27*(4), 265–279

Lefley, H. P. (1997). The consumer recovery vision: Will it alleviate family burden? *American Journal of Orthopsychiatry, 67*(2), 210–219.

Maton, K. (1988). Social support, organizational characteristics, psychological well-being, and group appraisal in three self-help populations. *American Journal of Community Psychology, 16*, 53–77.

Newacheck, P. W., Strickland, B., Shonkoff, J. P., Perrin, J. M., McPherson, M.,

McManus, M., Lauver, C., Fox, H., & Arango, P. (1998). An epidemiologic profile of children with special health care needs. *Pediatrics, 102,* 117–123.

Norcross, J. C. (2000). Here comes the self-help revolution in mental health. *Psychotherapy, 37,* 370–377.

Roberts, L. J., Luke, D. A., Rappaport, J., Seidman, E., Toro, P. A., & Reischl, T. M. (1991). Charting uncharted terrain: A behavioral observation system for mutual help groups. *American Journal of Community Psychology, 19*(5), 715–737.

Roberts, L. J., Salem, D., Rappaport, J., Toro, P. A., Luke, D. A., & Seidman, F. (1999). Giving and receiving help: Interpersonal transactions in mutual-help meetings and psychosocial adjustment of members. *American Journal of Community Psychology, 27*(6), 841–868.

Salem, D. A., Bogar, G. A., & Reid, C. (1997). Mutual help goes on-line. *Journal of Community Psychology, 25*(2), 189–207.

Singh, N. N., Curtis, W. J., Ellis, C. R., Wechsler, H. A., Best, A. M., & Cohen, R. (1997). Empowerment status of families whose children have serious emotional disturbance and attention-deficit/hyperactivity disorder. *Journal of Emotional and Behavioral Disorders, 5*(4), 223–229.

Sisson, D. P., & Fristad, M. A. (2001). A survey of stress and support for parents of children with early-onset bipolar disorder. *Bipolar Disorders, 3*(Suppl. 2), 58.

Weinberg, N., Schmale, J. D., Uken, J., & Wessel, K. (1995). Computer-mediated support groups. *Social Work with Groups, 17*(4), 43–54.

Wollert, R. W., Levy, L. H., & Knight, B. G. (1982). Help-giving in behavioral control and stress coping groups. *Small Group Behavior, 13,* 204–213.

Index

Page numbers followed by f indicate figure, t indicate table

Academic functioning. *See* School functioning
Adolescent bipolar disorder
 course of, 13
 Oregon Adolescent Depression Project, 9
 prevalence rates, 54t
 symptoms, 8
 See also Pediatric bipolar disorder; Prepubertal and early adolescent bipolar disorder
Adoption studies, 251. *See also* Genetics
Adult-onset bipolar disorder, 46t
Affect-modulated startle, 183–189. *See also* Eyeblink response
Affective disorders
 comparison of clinical features, 207t
 EEG sleep variables, 226–228, 227t
 family studies, 247–250
 group A streptococcus, 202–203
Affective neuroscience
 applications of, 182–189, 183f
 description, 175, 189
 emotion and mood, 175–177
 emotion circuplex, 177–181, 178f–180f
Affective Posner paradigm, 187. *See also* Eyeblink response
Age of onset, NRHypo state, 148
Aggression
 attention-deficit/hyperactivity disorder, 84
 case example, 66–68, 95–99
 lithium, 257
 offspring studies, 118
 pervasive developmental disorders, 51
 risperidone, 65
 See also Symptoms
Agoraphobia, 91
Anger management, 278t, 281f–282f. *See also* Emotion
Antibody, 196t

Anticonvulsant
 carbomazepine, 259–260
 development, 262–263
 prepubertal and early adolescent bipolar disorder research, 44–45f
 prevention, 122
 valproate, 258–259
 See also Pharmacological treatment
Antidepressants
 affects of, 99–100
 description, 261
 development, 255
 effectiveness, 264
 PDD and bipolar disorder, 63–64
 prepubertal and early adolescent bipolar disorder research, 44–45f
 See also Pharmacological treatment; Selective serotonin reuptake inhibitors
Antimanic, prepubertal and early adolescent bipolar disorder research, 44–45f. *See also* Pharmacological treatment
Antimicrobial, 196t
Antineuronal antibodies, 196t
Antipsychotics
 immunosuppressive effects, 205
 PDD and bipolar disorder, 64–66
 See also Pharmacological treatment
Antiretroviral therapy, 206
Antisocial personality disorder
 attention-deficit/hyperactivity disorder, 84
 family history, 19t
Antiviral, 196t
Anxiety disorders
 case example, 95–99
 comorbidity rates, 11
 comparison of clinical features, 207t
 development, 90–91

Anxiety disorders (*continued*)
  family history, 19*t*
  genetic research, 93–94
  group A streptococcus, 202–203
  temperament, 91
Apoptosis, 196*t*
Approach, 175–176. *See also* Motivation
Arousal
  affective neuroscience, 189
  description, 176
  emotion circuplex, 177–181, 178*f*–180*f*
  physiological measures of, 182–183*f*,
    183–189
  See also Emotion
Arousal–cerebral fatigue theory, 222. *See
    also* Sleep–wake cycle
Asperger's disorder
  case example, 66–68, 69
  characteristics, 53*t*
  defining, 52, 53*t*
  genetics, 55–60, 56*t*
  neurobiology, 60–61
  prevalence rates, 54, 54*t*
  treatment of bipolar disorder and, 63–66
  See also Pervasive developmental disorder
Assessment
  development of anxiety disorders, 90–91
  General Behavior Inventory, 15–16
  Hypomanic Personality Scale, 16–17
  infectious illnesses and, 208
  offspring studies, 110–111
  pervasive developmental disorders, 61–62
  Psychosocial Schedule for School-age
    Children—Revised, 30
  Washington University in St. Louis
    Schedule for Affective Disorders
    and Schizophrenia, 29–32*t*
Attention, brain regions associated with,
    164
Attention-deficit/hyperactivity disorder
  carbomazepine, 260
  case example, 69
  comorbidity, 8, 11, 26, 80–82, 83–85,
    99–100
  compared to bipolar disorder, 2
  comparison of clinical features, 207*t*
  cytokine levels, 195
  diagnosis, 78
  DSM-IV criteria, 37*t*
  family history, 249
  genetic research, 94–95
  group A streptococcus, 202–203
  immune studies, 198*t*–199*t*
  infections illnesses and, 203–204
  offspring studies, 115–116
  prepubertal and early adolescent bipolar
    disorder, 47
  Sydenham's chorea, 202

treatment, 100
Atypical neuroleptics, 260. *See also*
    Neuroleptics; Pharmacological
    treatment
Autistic disorder
  case example, 68
  characteristics, 53*t*
  genetics, 55–60, 56*t*
  neurobiology, 60–61
  prevalence rates, 53–54*t*
  See also Pervasive developmental disorder
Autoantibodies
  assessment of, 197, 200
  definition, 196*t*
  immune studies, 198*t*–199*t*
  See also Immune system
Autoimmunity, 196*t*
Avoidance, 175–176. *See also* Motivation

Basal cortisol, 230, 231*t*, 232*t*
Basal ganglia
  comparison of clinical features, 207*t*
  neuroimaging studies, 204–205
Baseline exaggeration, 62. *See also* Func-
    tioning
Behavior
  affects on caregivers, 315–316
  baseline exaggeration, 62
  caregiver disagreement and, 298
  case example of problems related to,
    95–99
  emergency, 305–306
  managing, 275
  modification, 277
  neurobehavioral probes, 163–165, 166*t*–
    167*t*, 168
  offspring studies, 115
  parenting traps to avoid, 301–302
  separating from feelings, 282
  siblings, 297
Behavior disorders, 11, 99–100. *See also*
    Attention-deficit/hyperactivity dis-
    order; Conduct disorder
Behavior management, 275, 277
Behavioral inhibition
  case example, 95–99
  diagnosis, 94–95
  as a precursor to psychiatric illness,
    91
Biological markers, 119–121
Biological rhythms, 228–231*t*, 232*t*
Blood-oxygen-level-dependent techniques,
    163. *See also* Magnetic resonance
    imaging; Neuroimaging
Body language, 285–286
Borderline personality disorder, family his-
    tory, 19*t*
Brain imaging techniques, 159–163

Brain regions
attention and emotions, 164
pediatric bipolar disorder research, 169
recognition of facial affect, 165, 166*t*–167*t*, 168
Building the Tool Kit exercise
group therapy, 281*f*–282*f*
individual treatment, 289–290
treatment goals, 278*t*
See also Anger management; Emotion
Bulimia nervosa, 93–94

Carbomazepine, 259–260. *See also* Anticonvulsant; Pharmacological treatment
Central nervous system functioning
functional brain imaging techniques, 161–163
immune system, 194
NMDA receptors, 131–132
NRHypo state, 136, 141–142
PANDAS, 204
structural brain imaging techniques, 159–161
Sydenham's chorea, 201–202
Child & Adolescent Bipolar Foundation
description, 320–322
Parent Stress and Support Survey, 322–326, 324*t*
Childhood disintegrative disorder, 53*t*. *See also* Pervasive developmental disorder
Choices
group therapy, 283*f*
treatment goals, 278*t*, 282–284
Cholinergic activity
neurotransmitter regulation of sleep, 222–223
REM sleep regulation hypothesis, 226–228, 227*t*
Circadian rhythms
future research, 231–233
internal coincidence theory, 221
regulation of, 215–216
See also Sleep–wake cycle
Clomipramine, 63. *See also* Antidepressants; Pharmacological treatment
Clozapine, 138, 146–148. *See also* Pharmacological treatment
Cognition
deficits in, 62
disintegration, 62
NMDA receptors, 132–133
See also Functioning
Communication skills
family treatment, 303–304
intellectual distortions, 62

Naming the Enemy exercise, 288–292
treatment goals, 278*t*, 285–286*f*, 287, 288*f*
Comorbidity
affects on caregivers, 315
anxiety disorders, 87–90
attention-deficit/hyperactivity disorder, 26, 80–82, 115–116
behavior management, 275
case example, 95–99
caveats, 92
clinical view of, 99–100
comparison of clinical features, 207*t*
diagnosis, 61–62, 77–78, 100
genetics, 92–95
group A streptococcus, 202–203
offspring studies, 110
oppositional defiant disorder and conduct disorder, 83–85
Oregon Adolescent Depression Project, 10–11
pervasive developmental disorders, 51–52, 66–69, 69–70
prevalence rates, 8, 53–55, 54*t*
research, 78–80
school functioning, 307
substance use disorder, 85–87
suicidal behavior, 12*t*–13
Computed tomography, 159. *See also* Neuroimaging
Conduct disorder
comorbidity, 8, 83–85, 99–100
lithium, 257
offspring studies, 115
substance use, 87
Continuous cycling
prepubertal and early adolescent bipolar disorder, 39–40*f*
Washington University in St. Louis Schedule for Affective Disorders and Schizophrenia, 30, 32*t*
Coping skills
Building the Tool Kit exercise, 289–290
families, 301–305
group therapy goals, 276
Cortisol, 220–221
Creativity, 20–21
Cytokines
assessment of, 194–195, 197
definition, 196*t*
immune studies, 198*t*–199*t*
See also Immune system
Cytotoxicity, 196*t*

D2, 139–140
Dancing mania, 200–203. *See also* Sydenham's chorea

Delusions
  case example, 95–99
  NRHypo state, 132–133
  prepubertal and early adolescent bipolar
    disorder research, 39–40f
  psychosocial masking, 62
  See also Psychosis
Depression
  biological rhythms and, 228–231t, 232t
  childhood onset, 255–256
  EEG sleep variables, 217, 226–228, 227t
  emotion circuplex, 179–181, 180f
  family history, 19t
  family studies, 247–250
  immune studies, 198t–199t
  neurotransmitter regulation of sleep,
    222–223
  prepubertal and early adolescent bipolar
    disorder research, 39–40f
  process S theory, 218–219t
  sleep-associated depressogenic process,
    220–221
  sleep–wake cycle research, 223–226,
    225t
  suicidal behavior, 12t
  treatment, 100
  valence, 185–186
  See also Major depressive disorder;
    Mood disorders
Desynchrony, 218. See also Circadian
    rhythms; Sleep–wake cycle
Development
  anxiety disorders, 90–91
  case example, 95–99
  emotion circuplex, 181
  lithium and, 257
  NRHypo state, 137–139, 140–144, 148
  offspring studies, 111
  parenting, 303
  pharmacological treatment, 255–256,
    262–263, 264
  psychotherapy, 292
  sleep regulation, 226–228, 227t, 232–
    233
  temperament, 91
  in utero, 140–144
  See also Pervasive developmental disor-
    ders
Diagnosis
  case example, 95–99
  comorbidity, 78–80, 92–95, 99–100
  family history, 17–18, 19t
  infectious illnesses and, 208
  issues, 193
  NIMH Research Roundtable on
    Prepubertal Bipolar Disorder, 1–2
  overshadowing, 61–62
  pervasive developmental disorders, 61–62

prepubertal issues, 77–78
reconceptualization of, 94–95
stability of, 13
symptom overlap, 83–85
Diffusion imaging. See Magnetic resonance
    imaging
Disintegrative disorder. See Childhood
    disintegrative disorder
Distractibility
  case example, 66–68
  DSM-IV criteria, 39f
  pervasive developmental disorders, 62
Divalproex sodium
  description, 258–259
  PDD and bipolar disorder, 64
  vs. lithium, 261–262
  See also Mood stabilizers; Pharmacologi-
    cal treatment
Divide and Conquer technique, 291. See
    also Treatment
Dopamine
  NMDA glutamatergic systems, 139–140
  NRHypo hypothesis, 145
Dyskinesias, medication induced, 65

E-mail, 319–320. See also Internet support
EEG sleep variables
  carbomazepine, 260
  changes in mood disorders and, 226–
    228, 227t
  development, 233
  mood disorders and, 217–218
  research, 224–226, 225t
Ekman Facial Photographs. See Facial rec-
    ognition paradigms
Elation
  description, 33
  prepubertal and early adolescent bipolar
    disorder research, 39–40f
  See also Mania; Symptoms
Electroencephalagraphic sleep variables.
    See EEG sleep variables
Emotion circuplex, 189
Emotional regulation, 164
Emotional valence
  affective neuroscience, 189
  description, 175–176
  emotion circuplex, 177–181, 178f–180f
  physiological measures of, 182–183f
  startle eyeblink reflex, 183–189
Emotions
  affective neuroscience, 175–177, 189
  Building the Tool Kit exercise, 281f–
    282f
  emotion circuplex, 177–181, 178f–180f
  facial recognition paradigms, 164–165,
    166t–167t, 168
  physiological responses to, 182–189, 183f

sibling needs, 298
Thinking–Feeling–Doing exercise, 290–291
Thoughts/Feeling Charades exercise, 285–286
See also Anger management
Environment
circadian rhythms, 216
effects of, 117–118
emotions, 175–176
kindling theory, 108, 111
Epitope, 196*t*
Eyeblink response, 183–189. *See also* Emotions, physiological responses to

Facial recognition paradigms
description, 164–165, 166*t*–167*t*, 168
fMRI study, 171
See also Emotion; Functional imaging
Family history
case example, 66–69
Parent Stress and Support Survey, 323
prevention, 121–123
research, 17–18, 19*t*, 247–250
risk, 108
substance use, 86–87
See also Family studies; Genetics; Offspring studies
Family studies, 247–250. *See also* Family history; Genetics
Family treatment
caveats, 295–296
child's perspective, 296
coping strategies, 301–306
family's perspective, 300–301
parent's perspective, 298–300
sibling perspective, 296–298
support groups, 317–319
therapists' role, 311
See also Treatment
Fetal alcohol effects, 142–143. *See also* NRHypo state
Fetal alcohol syndrome, 142–143. *See also* NRHypo state
Film clip paradigm, 187. *See also* Eyeblink response
5-HT. *See* Serotonin (5-HT)
Fluoxetine, 63–64. *See also* Antidepressants
FMRI. *See* Functional magnetic resonance imaging
Functional imaging techniques
neurobehavioral probes, 163–165, 166*t*–167*t*, 168
results of research, 168–169, 170*t*, 171
techniques, 161–163
See also Functional magnetic resonance imaging; Magnetic resonance imaging; Neuroimaging

Functional magnetic resonance imaging
description, 162–163
neurobehavioral probes, 163–165, 166*t*–167*t*, 168
See also Magnetic resonance imaging; Neuroimaging
Functioning. *See also* School functioning
Divide and Conquer technique, 291
offspring studies, 118
Oregon Adolescent Depression Project, 10–11, 13–14*t*
pervasive developmental disorders, 61–62
psychotherapy, 272
sleep–wake cycle and, 233

Gating deficits, 188–189
Gender, comorbidity and, 93
General Behavior Inventory, 15–16. *See also* Assessment
Genetics
adoption studies, 251
comorbidity, 79–80, 82, 85, 90, 92–95
description, 55–60, 56*t*
development of anxiety disorders, 90–91
early-onset bipolar, 262–263
family studies, 247–250
kindling theory, 108, 111
NRHypo state, 141
segregation analysis, 251–252
substance use, 86–87
twin studies, 250
See also Family history
Glutatmate
description, 130–132, 131*f*
NRHypo state, 133–137*t*, 135*f*, 141
treatment, 146–148
See also NMDA receptor
Grandiosity
case example, 95–99
description, 33
DSM-IV criteria, 37*t*
prepubertal and early adolescent bipolar disorder, 35*t*
psychosocial masking, 62
See also Mania; Symptoms
Group A streptococcus
mania, 206–208, 207*t*
neuropsychiatric symptoms, 200–203
Group therapy
behavior management, 275
description, 274–275
developmental considerations, 292
goals of, 276
pilot study of, 273–274
support groups, 317–319

Group therapy (*continued*)
 treatment structure, 276–278*t*, 279*f*–
  283*f*, 284–285*f*, 286*f*, 287–288*f*
 See also Psychotherapy; Treatment
Hallucinations
 case example, 95–99
 NRHypo state, 132–133
 prepubertal and early adolescent bipolar
  disorder research, 39–40*f*
 See also Psychosis
Haloperidol
 compared to olanzapine, 66
 NRHypo state, 138–139
 PDD and bipolar disorder, 65
 See also Antipsychotics; Pharmacological
  treatment
Heart rate, shyness and, 91
Heritability. *See* Genetics
HPA activity, 229
Human Knot exercise
 group therapy, 286–287
 treatment goals, 278*t*
Huntington's disease, 188–189
Hyperactivity, 94–95. *See also* Attention-
 deficit/hyperactivity disorder
Hypersexual behaviors
 DSM-IV criteria, 38*f*
 prepubertal and early adolescent bipolar
  disorder, 36*t*, 38
 See also Symptoms
Hyperthymic temperament, 94–95. *See also*
 Temperament
Hyperthyroid state, 229–230
Hypomania scales
 General Behavior Inventory, 15–16
 Hypomanic Personality Scale, 16–17
 See also Assessment
Hypomanic Personality Scale, 16–17. *See
 also* Assessment
Hypothalamic–pituitary–adrenal activity,
 229
Hypothyroid state, 229–230

Immune system
 autoantibodies, 197, 200
 clinical presentations, 206–208, 207*t*
 cytokines, 194–195, 197
 infections illnesses, 203–204
 medication treatment and', 205–206
 neuroimaging studies, 204–205
 studies, 198*t*–199*t*
Immunoactivation, 196*t*
Immunogenetics, 196*t*
Immunomodulator, 196*t*
Immunoprotectant, 196*t*
Immunosuppressive, 196*t*
Impulsivity, 94–95. *See also* Attention-defi-
 cit/hyperactivity disorder

In utero development, 140–144. *See also*
 Development
Inattention, 94–95. *See also* Attention-defi-
 cit/hyperactivity disorder
Incidence rates, 9–10. *See also* Prevalence
Information processing
 cognitive disintegration, 62
 NMDA receptors, 132–133
Insurance
 Child & Adolescent Bipolar Foundation,
  321
 dealing with, 300, 316
Intellectual distortion, 62. *See also* Functioning
Interferon
 definition, 196*t*
 immune studies, 198*t*–199*t*
Interleukin, 196*t*
Internal coincidence theory, 219*t*, 221. *See
 also* Sleep–wake cycle
International Affective Picture System. *See
 also* Emotion
 description, 178, 179*f*
 physiological measures of, 182–
  183*f*
 startle eyeblink reflex, 183–189
Internet support
 Child & Adolescent Bipolar Foundation,
  320–322
 description, 319–320
 Parent Stress and Support Survey, 322–
  326, 324*t*
Intravenous immunoglobulin treatment,
 206
IQ, 119–120
Irritability
 case example, 66–68
 description, 26
 DSM-IV criteria, 39*f*
 prepubertal and early adolescent bipolar
  disorder research, 39, 39–40*f*
 See also Mood; Symptoms

Judgment
 DSM-IV criteria, 36, 38*f*
 pervasive developmental disorders, 62

Kindling theory
 anticonvulsants, 122
 description, 108, 111
 See also Offspring studies

Lamotrigine, 261. *See also* Pharmacological
 treatment
Left-handedness, 120. *See also* Offspring
 studies

Leukocytes
    immune studies, 198t–199t
    schizophrenics, 195
Lithium
    antiviral properties, 205
    description, 256–258
    development, 262–263
    offspring studies, 116
    PDD and bipolar disorder, 64
    prepubertal and early adolescent bipolar
        disorder research, 44–45f, 171
    prevention, 121
    relapse, 263–264
    vs divalproex sodium, 261–262
    See also Mood stabilizers; Pharmacologi-
        cal treatment
Longitudinal Interval Follow-up Evaluation,
    31
Lottery game, 187. See also Eyeblink
    response
Lymphocyte, 196t
Lymphocyte activation, 195, 197
Lymphocyte trafficking, 197t

Magnetic resonance imaging
    description, 160–161
    PANDAS, 204
    See also Functional magnetic resonance
        imaging; Neuroimaging
Magnetic resonance spectroscopy
    basal ganglia, 204–205
    description, 163
    results of research, 168–169, 170t, 171
    See also Magnetic resonance imaging;
        Neuroimaging
Major depressive disorder
    family history, 19t
    genetic research, 93–94
    immune studies, 198t–199t
    Sydenham's chorea, 202
    See also Depression; Mood disorders
Mania
    antiretroviral therapy, 206
    diagnosis, 81–82
    DSM-IV criteria, 36, 37f, 37t, 38
    emotion circuplex, 179–181, 180f
    identifying, 32–34t
    immune studies, 198t–199t
    parental management of, 305
    Putting on the Brakes technique, 292
    serotonin (5-ht), 228
    Sydenham's chorea, 200–203
Manic expansiveness, 62
Medication treatment
    antidepressants, 99–100
    case example, 66–69, 95–99
    Child & Adolescent Bipolar Foundation,
        321

description, 255–256
    group therapy, 280f
    immune system, 205–206
    NRHypo state, 136–137t, 138–139,
        146–148
    PDD and bipolar disorder, 63–66
    prepubertal and early adolescent bipolar
        disorder research, 44–45
    prevention, 121–122
    school functioning, 307
    treatment goals, 278t
Melatonin suppression, 120
Memory
    NMDA antagonists, 132
    NMDA receptors, 132–133
    NRHypo state, 139
Mesolimbic model, 60–61. See also Autis-
    tic disorder
Mitogen, 197t
Mixed mania
    mood stabilizers, 263
    prepubertal and early adolescent bipolar
        disorder research, 39–40f
    Washington University in St. Louis
        Schedule for Affective Disorders
        and Schizophrenia, 30, 32t
Mood
    affective neuroscience, 175–177, 189
    Divide and Conquer technique, 291
    DSM-IV criteria, 37t
    emotion circuplex, 179–181, 180f
    See also Irritability; Symptoms
Mood disorders
    comparison of clinical features, 207t
    EEG sleep variables, 226–228, 227t
    family studies, 247–250
    group A streptococcus, 202–203
Mood stabilizers, 64. See also Antidepres-
    sants; Pharmacological treatment
Motivation
    behavior management, 275
    emotional valence, 175–176
MRI. See Magnetic resonance imaging
MRS. See Magnetic resonance spectroscopy
Multifamily psychoeducation group
    pilot study of, 273–274
    structure, 276–278t, 279f–283f, 284–
        285f, 286f, 287–288f
    See also Psychotherapy; Treatment

N-acetyle aspartate, 120–121. See also Off-
    spring studies
N-Methyl-d-Aspartate receptors. See
    NMDA receptors
Naming the Enemy exercise
    group therapy, 279f–280
    individual treatment, 288–292
    treatment goals, 278t

National Institute of Mental Health,
    Research Roundtable on
    Prepubertal Bipolar Disorder, 1–2
Neuroanatomic structures, 158
Neurobehavioral probes, 163–165, 166*t*–
    167*t*, 168
Neurobiology, 57–58
Neuroimaging
    immune system, 204–205
    neurobehavioral probes, 163–165, 166*t*–
        167*t*, 168
    pediatric bipolar disorder research, 168–
        169, 170*t*, 171
    physiological paradigms, 188
    techniques, 159–163
    See also Magnetic resonance imaging;
        Positron emission tomography
Neuroleptics
    atypical, 260
    development, 262–263
    prepubertal and early adolescent bipolar
        disorder research, 44–45*f*
    See also Pharmacological treatment
Neuroplasticity, 197*t*
Neuropsychiatric symptoms, 200–203. *See
    also* Group A streptococcus; Symp-
    toms
Neurotransmitter regulation of sleep, 222–
    223. *See also* Sleep–wake cycle
Neurotrophic, 197*t*
NMDA receptors
    consequences of NRHypo state, 133–
        137*t*, 135*f*
    description, 3, 130–132, 131*f*
    symptoms, 132–133
    treatment, 146–148
    See also NRHypo state
Nocturnal enuresis, 188–189
Nonverbal learning disability, 59. *See also*
    Asperger's Disorder
NRHypo state
    age dependency, 137–139
    consequences of, 133–137*t*, 135*f*
    description, 149
    disinhibited, 139–140, 140–144
    implications, 144–148
    symptoms, 132–133
    See also NMDA receptor

OADP. *See* Oregon Adolescent Depression
    Project
Obsessive–compulsive disorder
    case example, 66–68, 69, 95–99
    comorbidity, 79, 87–90, 99–100
    comparison of clinical features, 207*t*
    cytokine levels, 195
    immune studies, 198*t*–199*t*
    neuroimaging studies, 204–205

PANDAS, 202–203
    prepulse inhibition, 188–189
    Sydenham's chorea, 200–202
    treatment, 100
Offspring studies
    challenges, 109–112
    description, 123–124
    markers for risk, 119–121
    phenomenology, 112, 113*t*–114*t*, 114–
        118
    psychosocial functioning, 118–119
    significance of, 107–109
    See also Family history
Olanzapine
    description, 260
    NRHypo state, 146–148
    PDD and bipolar disorder, 66
    See also Antipsychotics; Pharmacological
        treatment
Oligogenic model, 251. *See also* Genetics;
    Segregation analysis
Omega 3 fatty acids, 205–206
Oppositional defiant disorder
    comorbidity, 83–85
    offspring studies, 115
Oregon Adolescent Depression Project
    clinical implications, 18–21
    course of bipolar disorder, 13–14*t*
    demographics, 10–11
    description, 8–9
    hypomania scales, 15–17
    incidence and prevalence rates, 9–10
    suicidal behavior, 11–13, 12*t*

PANDAS
    description, 202–203
    neuroimaging studies, 204–205
    symptoms, 206–208, 207*t*
    See also Group A streptococcus; Obses-
        sive–compulsive disorder
Panic disorder
    comorbidity, 79, 87–90
    genetic research, 93–94
    temperament, 91
Paranoid ideation, 95–99
Parent Stress and Support Survey, 322–
    326, 324*t*
Parenting
    affects on, 315–317
    family treatment, 298–300
    Parent Stress and Support Survey, 322–
        326, 324*t*
    support groups, 317–319
Prepubertal and early adolescent bipolar
        disorder
    comparison to adult-onset bipolar disor-
        der, 46*t*
    DSM-IV criteria, 34, 36, 38

recovery, 41–44*f*, 42*t*, 43*f*
research methods, 27–32, 44–45
selection of a phenotype, 26–27
See also Adolescent bipolar disorder;
    Pediatric bipolar disorder
Pediatric autoimmune neuropsychiatric dis-
    orders associated with streptococ-
    cus. *See* PANDAS
Pediatric bipolar disorder
    genetics, 56*t*–60
    prevalence rates, 54*t*–55
    See also Adolescent bipolar disorder;
        Prepubertal and early adolescent
        bipolar disorder
Peer relationships
    description, 310–311
    social functioning, 118–119
    See also Relationships
PENN Facial Photographs. *See* Facial rec-
    ognition paradigms
Pervasive developmental disorders
    assessment and diagnosis, 61–62
    case examples, 66–69
    comorbidity, 51–52, 69–70, 99–100
    defining, 52–53*t*
    genetics, 55–60, 56*t*
    prevalence rates, 53–55, 54*t*
    treatment of bipolar disorder and, 63–66
PET. *See* Positron emission tomography
Pharmacological treatment
    antidepressants, 99–100, 261
    atypical neuroleptics, 260
    carbamazepine, 259–260
    case example, 66–69, 95–99
    Child & Adolescent Bipolar Foundation,
        321
    description, 255–256, 263–264
    development, 262–263
    group therapy, 280*f*
    immune system, 205–206
    lithium, 256–258
    NRHypo state, 136–137*t*, 138–139,
        146–148
    PDD and bipolar disorder, 63–66
    prepubertal and early adolescent bipolar
        disorder research, 44–45
    prevention, 121–122
    research, 261–262
    school functioning, 307
    treatment goals, 278*t*
    valproate, 258–259
Phenomenology, 112, 113*t*–114*t*, 114–118
Plasma exchange, 206
Plasma melatonin levels, 230
Polygenic model, 251. *See also* Genetics;
    Segregation analysis
Positron emission tomography
    description, 162

mania, 204–205
neurobehavioral probes, 163–165, 166*t*–
    167*t*, 168
results of research, 169, 170*t*, 171
See also Neuroimaging
Prepubertal bipolar disorder
    family history, 249–250
    mania, 33–34*t*
    Oregon Adolescent Depression Project, 9
    pharmacological treatment, 262–263
    recognition of, 76–77
    symptoms, 8
    See also Prepubertal and early adoles-
        cent bipolar disorder
Prepulse inhibition, 188–189. *See also*
    Eyeblink response
Prevalence
    comorbidity with substance use disor-
        ders, 85–86
    lifetime, 7
    Oregon Adolescent Depression Project,
        9–10
    prepubertal bipolar disorder, 76–77
Prevention
    future research and, 231–232
    goal of, 18
    offspring studies, 121–123
    research, 107–109
Problem solving
    family treatment, 304–305
    treatment goals, 278*t*, 284, 285*f*
Process S theory, 218–219*t*. *See also* Sleep–
    wake cycle
Prostaglandin, 197*t*
Psychoeducation, 311. *See also* Treatment
Psychological markers, 119–121
Psychosis
    case example, 66–68, 95–99
    comparison of clinical features, 207*t*
    NMDA antagonists, 132
    NRHypo state, 132–133
    prepubertal and early adolescent bipolar
        disorder research, 39–40*f*
    prepulse inhibition, 188–189
Psychosocial factors, 118
Psychosocial masking, 62. *See also* Func-
    tioning
Psychosocial Schedule for School-age
    Children—Revised
    prepubertal and early adolescent bipolar
        disorder research, 30
    recovery rates, 42, 43*f*, 44*f*
    See also Assessment
Psychotherapy
    description, 274–275
    development, 292
    individual, 288–292
    pilot study of, 273–274

Psychotherapy (*continued*)
  structure, 276–278*t*, 279*f*–283*f*, 284–
    285*f*, 286*f*, 287–288*f*
  See also Treatment
Pupillary dilation, 91
Putting on the Brakes technique, 292. *See
  also* Treatment

Racing thoughts
  case example, 66–68
  DSM-IV criteria, 37*t*
  prepubertal and early adolescent bipolar
    disorder, 37*t*
  See also Symptoms
Rapid cycling
  immune studies, 198*t*–199*t*
  lithium and, 205
  lymphocyte activation, 195, 197
  mood stabilizers, 263
  prepubertal and early adolescent bipolar
    disorder research, 39–40*f*
  prepubertal bipolar disorder, 52
  sleep–wake cycle, 216–217
  Washington University in St. Louis
    Schedule for Affective Disorders
    and Schizophrenia, 30, 32*t*
Rapid eye movement sleep. *See* REM
  sleep
Recovery, 41–44*f*, 42*t*, 43*f*, 46–47
Relapse, 41–44*f*, 42*t*, 43*f*, 46–47
Relationships
  group therapy, 276, 276–277
  peer, 118–119, 310–311
  social functioning, 118–119
  See also Peer relationships
REM sleep
  depression and, 217–218
  EEG sleep variables, 226–228, 227*t*
  internal coincidence theory, 221
  process S theory, 218–219*t*
  research, 224–226, 225*t*
  sleep-associated depressogenic process,
    220–221
  temperature regulation, 229
  See also Sleep–wake cycle
REM sleep regulation hypothesis, 221–222.
    See also REM sleep; Sleep–wake
    cycle
Research
  family history, 17–18, 19*t*
  Oregon Adolescent Depression Project,
    8–9
Responsibility
  group therapy, 283*f*
  treatment goals, 278*t*, 282–284
Retroviruses, 197*t*
Rett's disorder, 53*t*. *See also* Pervasive
  developmental disorder

Rheumatic fever
  immune studies, 207*t*–208
  seasonal affective disorder, 206
  Sydenham's chorea, 201–202
Risk factors
  identifying, 232
  markers of, 119–121
  offspring studies, 107–109, 123–124
Risperidone
  description, 260
  PDD and bipolar disorder, 65
  See also Antipsychotics; Pharmacological
    treatment
Role functioning, 10–11. *See also* Func-
    tioning

Schizoaffective disorder, *in utero* develop-
    ment, 143–144
Schizophrenia
  autoantibodies, 197, 200
  cytokines, 194–195, 197
  immune studies, 198*t*–199*t*
  prepulse inhibition, 188–189
  treatment, 146–148
  in utero development, 143–144
School functioning
  Child & Adolescent Bipolar Foundation,
    321
  description, 306–310, 308*t*
  offspring studies, 119
  Oregon Adolescent Depression Project,
    10–11
  See also Functioning
Seasonal affective disorder
  diagnosis, 206–207
  plasma melatonin levels, 230
Segregation analysis, 251–252. *See also*
    Genetics
Selective serotonin reuptake inhibitors
  description, 261
  development, 255
  effectiveness, 264
  See also Antidepressants; Pharmacologi-
    cal treatment
Self epitopes, 197*t*
Self-injury, 51. *See also* Symptoms
Sensorimotor gating, 188–189
Sensory information processing, 132–133
Sensory integration disorder, 95–99
Separation anxiety disorder
  case example, 95–99
  immune studies, 198*t*–199*t*
  as a precursor to psychiatric illness, 91
Serotonin (5-HT)
  neurotransmitter regulation of sleep, 223
  REM sleep regulation hypothesis, 227–
    228
Sexual abuse, 38

Shyness
case example, 95–99
diagnosis, 94–95
as a precursor to psychiatric illness, 91
Siblings, perspective of, 296–298
Side effects
carbomazepine, 260
lithium, 256–257
valproate, 258–259
Single-photon emissions computed tomography
description, 161
results of research, 169, 170t, 171
See also Neuroimaging
Sleep-associated depressogenic process, 219t, 220–221. See also Sleep–wake cycle
Sleep–wake cycle
DSM-IV criteria, 37t
future research, 231–233
mechanisms of, 218–223
mood disorders and, 216–218
prepubertal and early adolescent bipolar disorder, 35t
as a precursor to psychiatric illness, 91
research, 223–226, 225t
See also Circadian rhythms; Symptoms
Slow-wave sleep suppression, 222. See also Sleep–wake cycle
Social functioning
group therapy, 276–277
offspring studies, 118–119
Oregon Adolescent Depression Project, 10–11
See also Functioning
Social intelligence, 60–61
Social learning disability, 66–68
Social phobia, 87–90
Social skills, 62
SPECT. See Single-photon emissions computed tomography
Speech, 39f
SSRIs. See Selective serotonin reuptake inhibitors
St. Vitus dance, 200–203. See also Sydenham's chorea
Startle response, 183–189. See also Eyeblink response
Stimulants, 44–45f. See also Pharmacological treatment
Stop–Think–Plan–Check exercise, 278t, 284, 285f. See also Treatment
Stress
cognitive disintegration, 62
Parent Stress and Support Survey, 322–326, 324t
parental management of, 306
shyness, 91

Structural brain imaging, 159–161. See also Neuroimaging
Structural MRI. See Magnetic resonance imaging
Substance use
comorbidity, 11, 79
family history, 19t, 249
genetic research, 93–94
Substance use disorder, 85–87
Subsyndromal bipolar disorder
clinical implications, 18–21
course of, 13
family history, 19t
prevalence rates, 9–10
suicidal behavior, 12t
symptoms, 10–11
Suicidality
adoption studies, 251
medication treatment and, 99–100
Oregon Adolescent Depression Project research, 11–13, 12t
parental management of, 305
prepubertal and early adolescent bipolar disorder research, 39–40f
research, 18, 20
Support groups
description, 317–319
Internet, 319–320
Parent Stress and Support Survey, 322–326, 324t
Suprachiasmatic nucleus, 216. See also Circadian rhythms
Sydenham's chorea
description, 200–203
neuroimaging studies, 204–205
symptoms, 206–208, 207t
Symptoms
affects on caregivers, 315–317
case example, 95–99
Divide and Conquer technique, 291
DSM-IV criteria, 34, 35t–37t, 38f–41f
emotion circuplex, 180f–181
genetic influence, 92–93
group A streptococcus, 200–203
group therapy goals, 276
individual treatment, 288–292
managing, 274–275
NRHypo state, 132–133, 144–145
Oregon Adolescent Depression Project, 10–11
overlap, 83–85, 92, 99. See also Comorbidity
school functioning, 307
Sydenham's chorea, 200–202
treatment goals, 278t, 279f–280f
variability of, 8, 295
Synaptogenesis stage, 141–142, 142–143. See also Development; NRHypo state

Temperament
  diagnosis, 94–95
  as a precursor to psychiatric illness, 91
Temperature rhythm, 228–229
Temporal lobe epilepsy, 188–189
Testosterone levels, 259
Thinking–Feeling–Doing exercise
  group therapy, 282–284, 283*f*
  individual treatment, 290–291
  treatment goals, 278*t*
  See also Treatment
Thoughts/Feeling Charades exercise
  group therapy, 285–286
  treatment goals, 278*t*
  See also Treatment
Thyroid-stimulating hormone
  association with bipolar disorder, 229–
    230
  sleep–wake cycle, 219
Thyroid studies, 230, 231*t*, 232*t*
Tic disorders
  comparison of clinical features, 207*t*
  infections illnesses and, 203–204
  neuroimaging studies, 204–205
  Sydenham's chorea, 202
Topiramate, 261. *See also* Pharmacological
    treatment
Tourette's syndrome
  autoantibodies, 197
  comorbidity, 99–100
  prepulse inhibition, 188–189
Treatment
  affect on substance use, 86
  case example, 95–99
  comorbidity, 69–70, 99–100
  description, 274–275
  developmental considerations, 292
  future research and, 231–232
  individual, 288–292
  NRHypo state, 146–148
  offspring studies, 123–124
  PANDAS, 205–206
  PDD and bipolar disorder, 63–66
  prepubertal and early adolescent bipolar
    disorder research, 44–45
  prevention, 121–123
  sleep–wake cycle research, 233
  structure, 276–278*t*, 279*f*–283*f*, 284–
    285*f*, 286*f*, 287–288*f*
  See also Family treatment; Psychotherapy

Tricyclic antidepressants, 255. *See also*
    Antidepressants; Pharmacological
    treatment
TSH. *See* Thyroid-stimulating hormone
Twin studies, 250. *See also* Genetics

Ultradian (continuous) rapid cycling
  prepubertal and early adolescent bipolar
    disorder, 39–40*f*
  prepubertal bipolar disorder, 52
  Washington University in St. Louis
    Schedule for Affective Disorders
    and Schizophrenia, 30, 32*t*
Ultrarapid cycling
  prepubertal and early adolescent bipolar
    disorder, 39–40*f*
  Washington University in St. Louis
    Schedule for Affective Disorders
    and Schizophrenia, 30, 32*t*

Valence, emotional
  affective neuroscience, 189
  description, 175–176
  emotion circuplex, 177–181, 178*f*–
    180*f*
  physiological measures of, 182–
    183*f*
  startle eyeblink reflex, 183–189
Valproate
  cytoprotective protein, 205
  description, 258–259
  PDD and bipolar disorder, 64
  See also Mood stabilizers; Pharmacologi-
    cal treatment
Vulnerability markers, 232

Washington University in St. Louis Sched-
    ule for Affective Disorders and
    Schizophrenia
  description, 2
  offspring studies, 111
  prepubertal and early adolescent bipolar
    disorder, 29–32*t*

Zeitgebers, 215–216. *See also* Circadian
    rhythms